Vascular Disease Nursing and Management

Edited by

SHELAGH MURRAY RN, BSc(Hons)
Senior Clinical Nurse, Vascular Surgery, St George's Hospital, London

W

WHURR PUBLISHERS
LONDON AND PHILADELPHIA

First published 2001
by Whurr Publishers Ltd
19b Compton Terrace
London N1 2UN England and
325 Chestnut Street, Philadelphia PA 19106 USA

British Library Cataloguing in Publication Data

A catalogue record for this book
is available from the British Library.

ISBN 1 86156 219 5

Printed and bound in the UK by Athenaeum Press Ltd,
Gateshead, Tyne & Wear.

Contents

Contributors

Jill Arthur RGN
Vascular Nurse Specialist, Torbay Hospital, Torbay

Janet Chesworth RGN, BSc(Hons)
Night Coordinator, Staffordshire General Hospitals Trusts, Stafford

Frances Collins RN, BSc(Hons)
Formerly Vascular Nurse Specialist, St Mary's Hospital, London

Samantha Donohue RGN, BSc(Hons), PGCE
Ward Sister, John Radcliffe Hospital, Oxford

Krzysztof S. Gebhardt RGN, PhD
Clinical Nurse Specialist in Pressure Sore Prevention, St George's Hospital, London

Jane Holden RGN, BA(Hons), RNT, PGDip
Clinical Nurse Specialist Plastic and Reconstructive Surgery, St George's Hospital, London

Soraya Jones RN, RNT, BSc(Hons), MSc
Senior Lecturer, Faculty of Health and Social Care Sciences, St George's Hospital Medical School, London

Belinda Litchfield RGN, PGCEA, BSc(Hons), MSc
Senior Lecturer, Kingston University, and Faculty of Health and Social Care Sciences, St George's Hospital Medical School, London

Christine Moffatt RGN, DN, MA
Director, Centre for Research and Implementation of Clinical Practice (CRICP), Wolfson Institute of Health Sciences, Thames Valley University, London

Shelagh Murray RN, BSc(Hons)
Senior Clinical Nurse, Vascular Surgery Department, St George's Hospital, London

Carolyn Nocton RN
Vascular Nurse Specialist, Princess Margaret Hospital, Swindon

Lindsey J. Ockenden DipN, RN, BSc(Hons), MSc
Formerly Senior Lecturer, Faculty of Health and Social Care Sciences, St George's Hospital Medical School, London

Nicola Stubbing RGN, RVT
Clinical Nurse Specialist/Vascular Technologist, Staffordshire General Hospitals Trusts, Stafford

Penny Sutton-Woods BSc(Hons), MCSP, SRP
Senior Physiotherapist, Physiotherapy Department, St George's Hospital, London

Kathryn Vowden RGN, FETC, DPSN(TV)
Clinical Nurse Specialist (Vascular and Wound Healing), Department of Vascular Surgery, Bradford Royal Infirmary, Bradford

Peter Vowden MD FRCS
Consultant Vascular Surgeon, Department of Vascular Surgery, Bradford Royal Infirmary, Bradford

Lyn Ward RGN
Acute Pain Team Leader, Department of Anaesthetics, St George's Hospital, London

Louise M. Wilson RGN, BSc(Hons)
Vascular Nurse Specialist, Eastbourne District General Hospital, Eastbourne, Sussex

Preface

Caring for patients with vascular disease has always been a challenging and complex area of care for both nurses and other healthcare professionals. The last decade has seen major changes in healthcare provision and the development of knowledge and skills as well as technological advances have all enhanced practice, particularly within the field of vascular surgery. One of the key effects of these changes has been the development of specialist areas of practice. In the past, patients with vascular disease were cared for under the umbrella of 'general surgery'. There is now a clearer understanding of the need to provide specialist nursing to meet the needs of vascular patients.

An ageing population has meant an increase in patients developing vascular disease. The nature of vascular disease and its impact on lifestyle, employment and relationships require expert nursing input, advice and support through all phases of this chronic condition. Earlier hospital discharge has emphasised the importance of a multidisciplinary approach which allows the provision of effective, 'seamless' and holistic care within acute and community settings.

This book aims to help nurses and other healthcare professionals involved in caring for vascular patients to update and expand their knowledge of developments in conservative, radiological and surgical aspects of care. All contributors are experts within their fields of practice, providing an individual approach to different aspects of vascular nursing. Each chapter may be read individually for reference, or as part of a whole.

Despite these differences in approach, all the contributors share an enthusiasm and commitment to a patient-centred philosophy of care. Although the authors concentrate on the principles of care and allow the readers to apply them using their own nursing model of choice, the approach also acknowledges that knowledge previously seen as 'medical' plays a legitimate role in nursing vascular patients.

The book addresses all aspects of care and management of different vascular conditions and stages of the disease process which nurses encounter. Guidance is given in dealing with some of the very challenging aspects of vascular nursing such as pressure sore prevention, pain and wound management, as well as palliative care for patients with end-stage vascular disease.

Care plans and case studies have been included in some chapters to outline nursing management, and to illustrate how patients' lives have been affected by this chronic disease.

Health promotion is paramount in helping to empower patients to take responsibility for their health and reduce the incidence of vascular disease. The very complex issues which surround adult learning are discussed, to assist practitioners to develop an understanding and acquire the skills to help promote health.

It is expected, that the book will be suitable for a wide range of nurses studying for pre-registration diploma or degree courses, and post-registration courses. The book also provides a ready reference for nurses and other health professionals caring for vascular patients in a variety of settings, including dedicated vascular surgery units, general surgery wards or the community.

Shelagh Murray

Acknowledgements

I would like to thank all the contributors for their commitment during the last couple of years to this valuable project. Gratitude is also extended to all my nursing colleagues at St George's Hospital, London, for their support and encouragement, and also to my surgical colleagues (Professor John Dormandy, Mr Robert Taylor, Mr Tom Loosemore, and Ms Stella Vig) for their advice and guidance.

I should also like to thank my friends and family, especially my partner, Neville, for supporting me through the book's development.

Acknowledgement is also given to all the companies who provided photographs for the book.

Finally, a special word of thanks is extended to the patients with vascular disease as, without them, this book would never have been written.

Shelagh Murray

CHAPTER 1

Anatomy and Physiology of the Vascular System

SORAYA JONES

The circulatory system consists of three components: the heart, the blood vessels and the blood. The heart is the pump and the driving force of this system while the blood vessels provide the route by which blood reaches all parts of the body. The whole purpose of this system is to deliver nutrients to the cells and collect their waste. In addition to this role the circulatory system performs other functions. The heart and blood vessels respond to haemodynamic changes and adjust the volume and the pressure of blood within the circulation. Some of the vasoactive substances produced by the heart and the blood vessels, as well as producing circulatory effects, influence the body's metabolism.

This chapter aims to explore the structure and function of blood vessels and the factors that affect these, and therefore tissue perfusion, with particular emphasis on the role of the endothelium as the major contributor to vascular disease. The circulation is described and an outline of the role of the lymphatic system in fluid exchange is provided. Finally, the structure of the skin is described in association with inflammation and healing, which is discussed in Chapter 14.

Blood vessels

The blood vessels undergo segmental changes to perform their specific functions. They are made up of a number of tissues (see Figure 1.1):

- epithelium
- muscle

- connective tissue
- neural and vascular supply

General features of endothelial tissue

The epithelium that lines the blood vessels is termed *endothelium*. This tissue has a number of important functions and has become the subject of increasing interest in recent years. For this reason a further section, later in this chapter, is devoted to its role in the development of vascular disease.

The endothelium consists of squamous epithelial cells on a basement membrane. The cells are connected together in two ways:

1. *Tight junctions* in which the walls of neighbouring endothelial cells are tightly attached to allow substances to pass from the blood into the intercellular space. The presence of slits in the tight junctions allows some fluid and small solutes to get through to the intercellular space. For this reason the tissue fluid contains only a small amount of protein. Tight junctions allow cell-to-cell communication between endothelial cells.

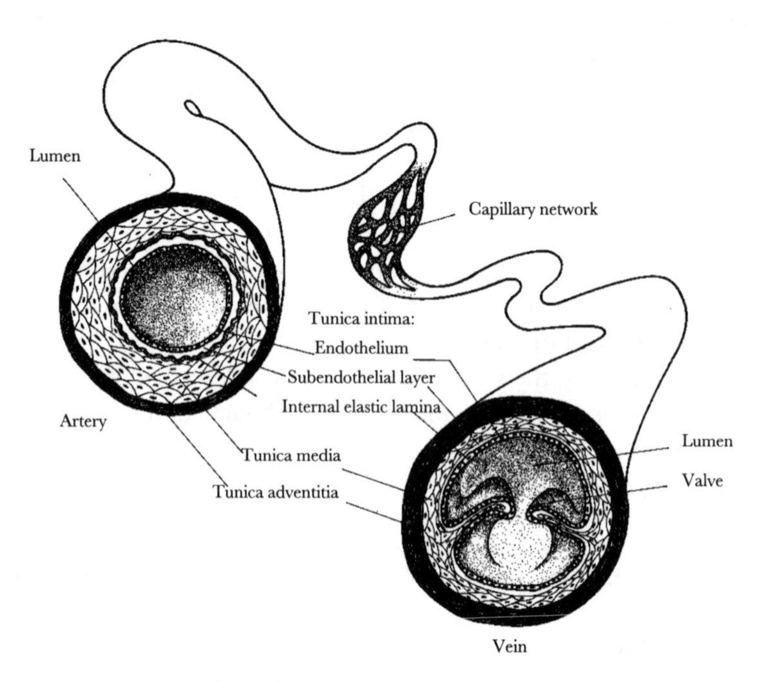

Figure 1.1 The structure of blood vessels.

2. *Gap junctions* in which there are gaps or holes in the wall-to-wall attachment of endothelial cells to allow exchange of solutes between the plasma and intercellular space as well communication between adjacent endothelial cells. The total number and ratio of tight to gap junctions vary in different segments of blood vessels and according to the nature of exchange that occurs in that segment. For example, tight junctions are more frequent in the endothelium of the arteries.

At capillary level the endothelium functions as a semi-selectively permeable membrane interposed between the blood and the tissue fluid. The structure of the endothelium is designed to facilitate bi-directional flow of solutes of small size and to restrict the passage of larger size substances.

Plasmalemmal vesicles are infoldings of the endothelial cells, and their function is to transport water-soluble substances to and from the blood. The endothelial cells have prominent and elongated nuclei. The presence of certain metabolic enzymes suggests that these vesicles may be involved in hormonal transport and synthesis of some of the vasoactive substances produced by the endothelial cells.

The endothelial surface and the blood are both negatively charged and therefore repel each other. The intact surface of the vessel wall is not attracted to and does not interact with the blood. This renders the endothelium non-thrombogenic (non-thrombus forming). The subendothelial layer, by contrast, is attracted to and interacts with the blood and is therefore thrombogenic. Factors such as deposition of low-density lipoproteins, histamine, toxins and microorganisms can damage the endothelium and promote aggregation of platelets at the site of injury. Aggregation of platelets leads to clot formation.

The endothelial cells rarely divide and have a lifespan of 100 to 180 days. Damaged endothelial cells are replaced by blood cells, underlying smooth muscle cells, subendothelial layer and adjacent endothelial cells.

The basement membrane of the endothelium consists of collagen, which is attached to the endothelial cells by a glycoprotein layer called *laminin*. The collagen gives the endothelium adequate strength to withstand the pressure of flowing blood, although the pressure is small due to the reduced radius of the capillary. The collagen fibres do not act as a barrier to the passage of protein out of the capillary, except in kidneys where they hold back large molecules such as ferritin.

Vascular smooth muscle

The vascular smooth muscle is composed of small, spindle-shaped cells (myocytes) with a single nucleus. The cells or muscle fibres are arranged in a helical or circular pattern in the blood vessels. The endothelial cells lining the blood vessels project between the myocytes, and this arrangement is thought to represent a close functional relationship between the two structures. The vascular myocytes are anchored to the elastic fibres, which facilitates the transmission of contractile force to the elastic fibres. The degree of contraction of myocytes determines the vessel radius or 'tone' and therefore the quantity of blood going through the blood vessel. The vascular smooth muscle is innervated by the *sympathetic nervous system.*

Neural stimulation leads to contraction, which is dependent on calcium. Extracellular calcium enters the smooth muscle fibre and causes release of intracellular calcium from the endoplasmic reticulum–'calcium-induced calcium release'. The rise in the intracellular calcium causes the actin and myosin filaments to 'slide' over each other. As a result the fibres shorten and develop tension, which is the mechanism by which the vascular smooth muscle contracts. The smooth muscle fibres contract slowly, but develop high force, which can last for a long period of time. Any agent that blocks the entry of calcium into the vascular smooth muscle fibre would prevent its contraction and cause vasodilatation. The muscle fibres are linked by 'gap junctions' which facilitate conduction of impulses from one fibre to another. The wave of electrical activity then spreads to several cells at the same time (functional syncytium) leading to simultaneous contraction of adjacent fibres. The smooth muscle of blood vessels has receptors through which the neural stimulation reaches the muscle. Generally α-receptors are excitatory and increase contraction and β-receptors are inhibitory and cause vasodilatation. Many substances act directly on the smooth muscle of blood vessels and cause vasoconstriction, e.g. prostaglandin, angiotensin, dopamine and serotonin. Others cause vasodilatation, such as nitric oxide, atrial natriuretic peptide, histamine and local metabolites.

Vascular connective tissue

The connective tissue supports and connects various structures that form the blood vessels. It consists of cells surrounded by an intercellular matrix. The matrix is composed of a ground substance and extracellular fibres. These fibres are: elastic, reticular and collagen. The elastic fibres are made of protein and elastin, which provide strength as well as allowing the fibre to be stretched. The reticular and collagen fibres are made of collagen, which provide strength for the vessel wall. The collagen fibres are tough and resistant to stretch.

The cells of the connective tissue have many functions: they secrete the proteins elastin and collagen; they also produce, store and secrete many vasoactive substances such as histamine and serotonin; they have phagocytic action through macrophages; and they provide some of the immunological reactions which involve plasma cells and eosinophils.

Vascular blood and nerve supply

The blood vessels receive their own blood supply from a network of vessels called *vasa vasorum*. The blood vessels also have a rich lymphatic supply. With the exception of capillaries, the nerve supply to the blood vessels is generous. The nerve supply consists of sympathetic motor neurons, which reach the outer connective tissue that covers the blood vessels and the muscular layer, and stimulates muscle contraction. Sympathetic sensory nerve endings supply the outer connective covering and form a variety of receptors. These receptors convey information about blood pressure, pH, oxygen and carbon dioxide levels from the blood vessels to the higher centres in the brain.

Types of blood vessels

There are three types of blood vessels:

- arteries
- veins
- capillaries

Arteries and veins have a similar wall structure which consists of three layers:

- an outer layer (*tunica adventitia* or *externa*)
- a middle layer (*tunica media*)
- an inner layer (*tunica intima*)

Tunica adventitia is mainly composed of connective tissue and some collagen fibres. The tunica media is composed of smooth muscle and the tunica intima consists of endothelium on a basement membrane.

Arteries

Arteries (Figure 1.2) convey blood from the heart to different parts of the body. There are three types of arteries: *elastic* arteries, *muscular* arteries and *arterioles*.

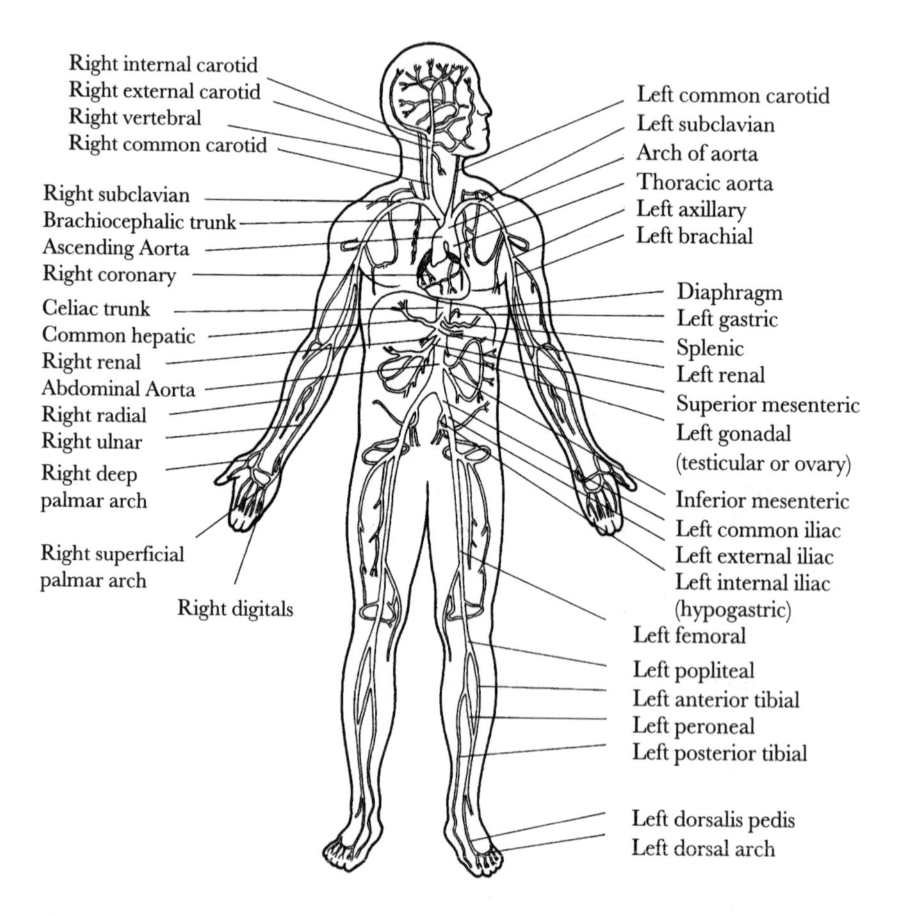

Figure 1.2 The arterial component of the vascular system.

Elastic arteries

Elastic arteries are large arteries into which the ventricles eject blood with each contraction of the heart. These arteries are also known as the *conducting arteries*. The tunica media of elastic arteries consists chiefly of elastic fibres, which stretch to accommodate the volume and the pressure of the blood they receive from the ventricles during systole. In diastole, when the ventricles are not contracting and no blood is pushed into the arteries, the elastic fibres recoil to maintain pressure within the arteries. The aorta, pulmonary artery, common carotid, subclavian and common iliac are examples of elastic arteries. The elastic arteries house the baroreceptors and the chemoreceptors which are located in the carotid artery and the aorta.

Muscular arteries

The muscular arteries are also known as the *distributing arteries*. The tunica media of muscular arteries is composed mainly of smooth muscle fibres which have a circular arrangement. These fibres contract in response to sympathetic stimulation. The diameter of the muscular arteries is therefore determined by the degree of sympathetic activity reaching the circular fibres in their tunica media. For example, during exercise, when the skeletal muscle requires more oxygen, the blood vessels in this area dilate while the arteries supplying the gastrointestinal tract constrict so that blood is diverted to the skeletal muscle where it is most needed. The axillary, brachial, radial, intercostal, splenic, mesenteric, femoral, popliteal and tibial are examples of muscular arteries.

Arterioles

Arterioles are the very small arteries in which the smooth muscle in the tunica media is reduced to one or two layers only. The diameter of these vessels becomes progressively smaller as they approach the capillaries. In some arterioles, the smooth muscle becomes thicker to form a sphincter (the precapillary sphincter) just before a capillary. The role of the sphincter is to determine the quantity of blood going through the capillary, although these sphincters are not present in all arterioles. The last section of the arterioles, the terminal part which joins the capillary, is called the *metarteriole*. Metarterioles can constrict to shut off blood to certain capillaries. In this way metarterioles regulate the number of functioning capillaries. As the arterioles become gradually smaller, they can offer a huge resistance to blood flow which is known as the *peripheral resistance.* The size of these blood vessels has a major effect on the blood pressure: when they constrict, the blood pressure is elevated and when they dilate, the blood pressure is reduced.

Veins

The main function of veins (Figure 1.3) is to carry blood back to the heart. There are also other functions attributed to veins: they form a

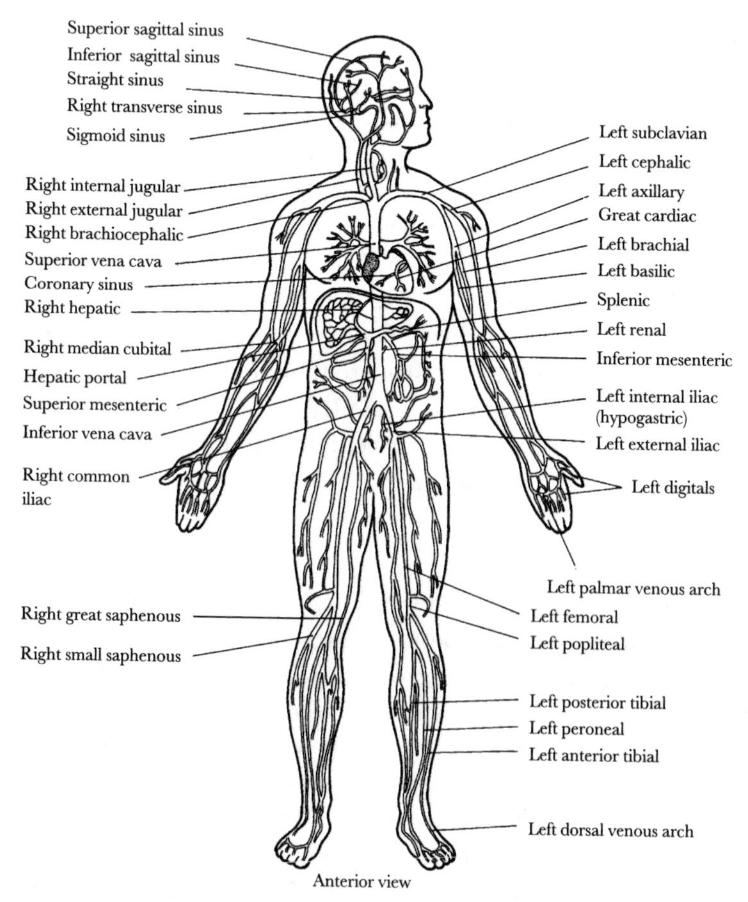

Figure 1.3 The venous component.

selective barrier for reabsorption of fluids; redistribute blood volume to dampen pressure; maintain the filling pressure of the heart by providing adequate venous return and increasing the orthostatic (relating to upright position) tolerance of the body. They also produce vasoactive substances in the same way that arteries do and they can stimulate angiogenesis, although in these two latter functions they may not be as effective as arteries.

The general structure of the veins is similar to the arteries in that there are three layers: tunica externa, tunica media and tunica intima. However, the walls of veins are much thinner than the arteries and the distinction between the different layers is not as clear. Furthermore, the structure is modified in different veins. For example, in large veins such as the vena cava, external jugular, pulmonary, external iliac, renal, splenic and portal, the walls are very thin. In some parts of the vena cava, the tunica media is absent. In parts of the vena cava and in the pulmonary arteries, cardiac muscle is found over a short section of the veins that lie closer to the heart. Some veins are rich in smooth muscle, which may be arranged longitudinally in all three layers as well as circularly in the middle layer. Examples of such veins are the popliteal, femoral, saphenous, uterine and mesenteric. The reinforced muscular layer adds extra strength to the superficial veins which do not have the support of the skeletal muscles. In other veins, such as the veins of the abdominal cavity, longitudinal smooth muscle fibres are in the adventitia. The veins of the retina, meninges, the nail beds and placenta have no smooth muscle fibres.

The veins that empty into the heart are called *draining* veins and those that carry blood away from various tissues and towards the heart are *propelling* veins. The walls of the draining veins are very thin compared to the walls of arteries and consist mainly of elastic fibres with some collagen fibres. These veins are highly distensible. The smooth muscle fibres are arranged circularly and some longitudinally. The longitudinal muscle fibres change the length of the vein when necessary.

Superficial veins lie beneath the skin. They are large and have muscular walls. Examples of superficial veins are the external jugular, the cephalic and the saphenous (Figure 1.3). *Deep veins* are less muscular and lie deep within the body, close to an artery of the same name. The *perforator veins* connect the superficial and deep veins.

Examples of these are the six medial calf perforators. These join the posterior tibial veins to the greater saphenous veins through a network of superficial veins called the *posterior arch veins*.

Veins have *valves* which help to propel blood towards the heart. The valves are more numerous in the veins closer to the surface of the body. The valves are made of tunica intima of the veins, reinforced in the centre with connective tissue. Elastic fibres are arranged on the borders of the valves. Endothelial folds form the leaflets of the valves. There are usually two leaflets but some veins have only one. The section of the vein close to the attachment of the valve dilates to form a *pouch* or a *sinus*. These sinuses can be seen as swelling on the distended superficial veins, as a guide to the location of the valves. The role of the valves is to help overcome the force of gravity. The leaflets of the valves move upwards and in the direction of the heart. This movement allows the blood to flow forwards. When the leaflets return to their original position, in which they are in apposition, the vein is closed. This prevents back-flow of blood within the veins (Figure 1.4). Muscle contraction, during exercise, acts as a pump (*the muscle or foot pump*) to squeeze blood through the valves. The valves also help to prevent a rise in pressure in the venous end of the capillary during contraction of the muscles surrounding the vein.

The veins have a much richer vascular supply than the arteries, as the vasa vasorum of the veins reaches the intima more closely than in arteries.

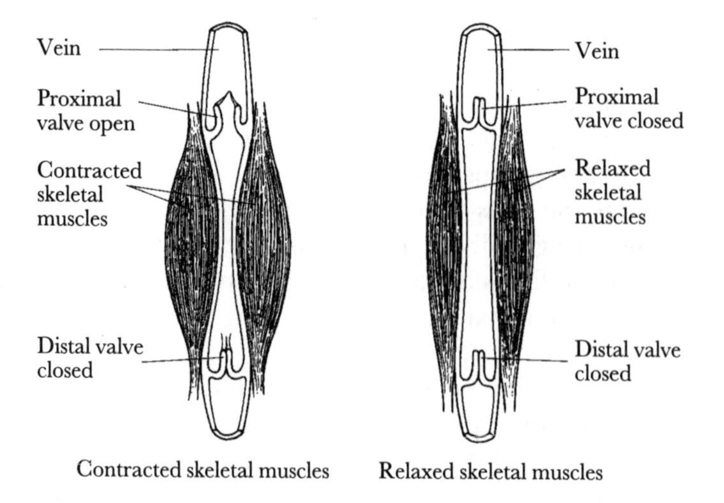

Figure 1.4 The muscle pump and the venous valves.

Venules

The structure of the venules is of particular interest as they have an important role in the process of inflammation. The part of the venule closest to the capillary (the postcapillary venule) consists of cells known as *pericytes.*

The intima of these venules is an endothelium in which there are relatively large spaces between some cells through which the white cells can migrate to the tissue. To enhance this function of the endothelium in the venules, pericytes contain actin filaments which are thought to enable pericytes to change size and shape. This change in the shape of the pericytes can increase the space between the endothelial cells. The opening between the endothelial cells can increase in response to histamine, bradykinin, serotonin and other agents active in the inflammatory process, and facilitates leakage of fluid into the tissue in inflammation. A distinct tunica media is absent in postcapillary venules. Instead, the actin filaments in pericytes give these cells the appearance of smooth muscle cells. The adventitia of the postcapillary venules contains fibroblasts and a variety of blood cells such as mast cells, macrophages and plasma cells. These empty into larger venules called the collecting venules, which have a slightly thicker media consisting of a very thin layer of collagen and elastic fibres. In turn, the collecting venules form the muscular venules, which have one or two layers of smooth muscle fibres in their tunica media. The number of venules far exceeds that of arterioles.

The venules lead to capillaries which separate the arterial and venous system (Figure 1.5). However, not all arterioles are separated from the venules by capillaries. Some arterioles join the venules directly. These are called *arteriovenous anastomoses* or *shunts.* In this arrangement the arterioles have a rich muscular tunica media generously supplied with sympathetic nerves. The arteriovenous shunts are sensitive to thermal and chemical stimulation, and their presence in places such as the skin (where they are numerous) helps to conserve heat as the blood bypasses the capillary bed.

Capillaries

The function of the circulation is to deliver nutrients to the cells of the organism and remove waste. This exchange takes place in the

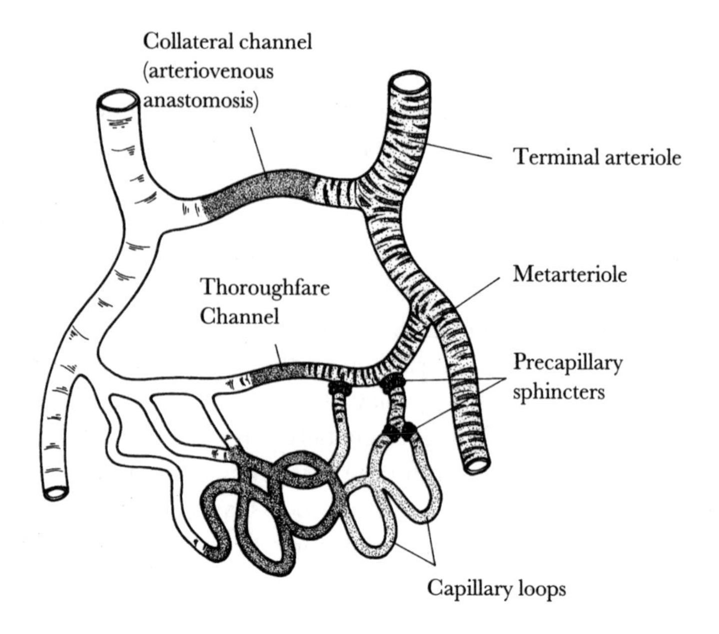

Figure 1.5 The capillary and arteriovenous anastomosis.

capillary (*microcirculation*). The thin wall of capillaries consists of endothelium, basal lamina and a few pericytes. The diameter of a capillary is large enough to allow a red cell to pass through to the venous side. There are three types of capillaries: continuous, fenestrated and discontinuous (Figure 1.6).

Continuous capillaries

The wall of continuous capillaries consists of one or two layers of endothelial cells resting on a basement membrane. A pericyte surrounds the endothelial cell. This cell contains contractile elements which are thought to influence the permeability of the endothelial cell. The endothelial cell or cells of the continuous capillary form tight junctions through which exchange of some solutes takes place. Many of the capillaries in the brain are of this type. These capillaries restrict exchange of solutes of certain molecular weight, and have a protective function in which passage of agents that may be harmful to the sensitive brain cells are barred. This capillary network is known as the *blood–brain barrier*.

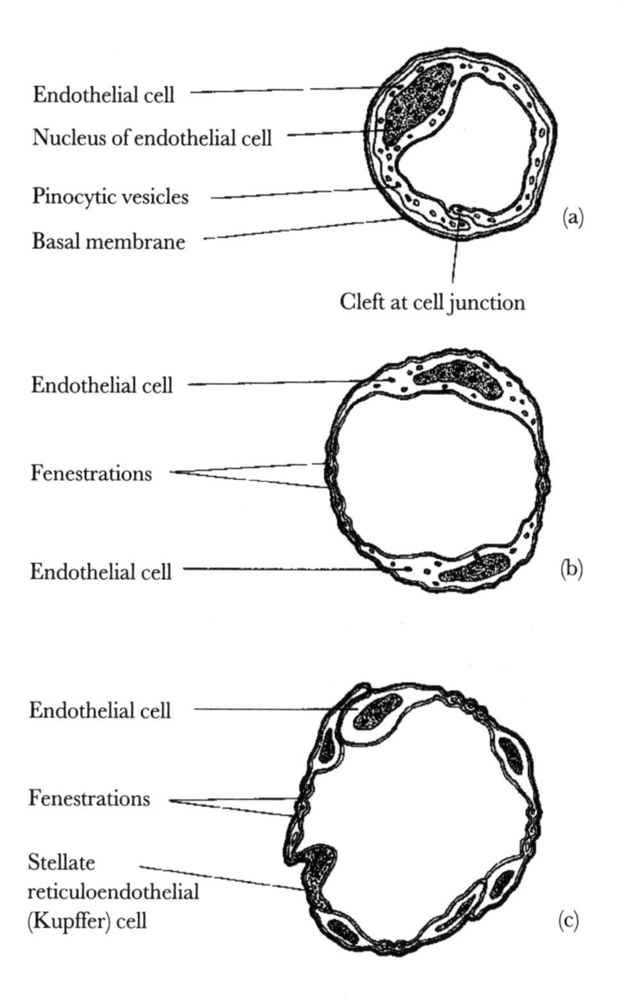

Figure 1.6 Three types of capillary: (a) continuous; (b) fenestrated; (c) discontinuous.

Fenestrated capillaries

The fenestrated capillaries have holes or fenestrae and are therefore more permeable to water and solutes than are continuous capillaries. They are located in parts of the body concerned with fluid exchange such as the kidneys, gastrointestinal mucosa and exocrine glands.

Discontinuous capillaries

These capillaries have larger pores that allow the passage of solutes of larger size such as plasma proteins and blood cells. The discontinuous capillaries are often called *sinusoids* and they are sited in the liver, spleen and bone marrow where red cells need to move freely in and out of the capillaries.

Exchange of fluid and solutes across the capillary

The fluid and solutes are exchanged across the capillary in a number of ways.

Diffusion

Oxygen and nutrients diffuse across the capillary membrane and metabolic waste enters the capillary by the same process (moving from an area of high concentration to an area of low concentration). The exchange of nutrients and waste at capillary level depends on blood flow (flow-limited exchange) and how easily solutes can cross the capillary membrane (diffusion-limited exchange). When the blood flow is increased to an area, the quantity of solutes crossing the capillary in either direction is increased. In addition, fast running circulation reduces the capillary crossing time of those solutes that are a little too large to get through the pores with ease (diffusion-limited exchange). However, increased flow recruits capillaries that are not normally perfused, facilitating exchange by increasing the surface area of diffusion.

Osmosis

Fluid movement across the capillary is dependent on two factors: blood pressure and the colloid osmotic pressure (oncotic pressure) exerted by the plasma proteins, mainly albumin. At the arteriole end of the capillary, the blood hydrostatic pressure exerts a force which tends to push fluid out of the capillary and into the intercellular space (filtration). The force opposing this movement is the colloid osmotic pressure of the albumin in the plasma, which tends to attract movement of fluid towards the capillary and back into circulation (absorption). At the arterial end, the hydrostatic pressure of blood is greater than the osmotic pressure of plasma albumin. This causes a net movement of fluid out of the capillary and towards the intercellular space. As the blood courses through a capillary which has no tone, its pressure drops and by the time it reaches the venous end of the capillary the blood pressure is below the colloid osmotic pressure of the plasma albumin. This leads to a net movement of fluids back into the capillary to join the circulation. This is the sequence of events in the idealised capillary. In some capillaries, filtration occurs throughout with some absorption. In others, where blood pressure is relatively low, absorption is predominant. Two factors are therefore of utmost importance in fluid dynamics across the capillary: (1) the hydrostatic pressure of blood, and (2) the osmotic force exerted by the albumin fraction of plasma proteins. In conditions where the blood pressure is low, the net movement of fluid tends to be towards the intravascular compartment. This influences the venous pressure of the blood which, measured at the vena cava (*central venous pressure*), becomes elevated. When the plasma proteins are depleted (starvation, malnutrition, renal failure) the volume of fluid moving into the tissue exceeds that entering the circulation, leading to oedema which may be regional (ascites) or general.

Fat solubility

If a solute is fat-soluble, it will readily cross the membrane of the endothelial cell which forms the capillary. Oxygen and carbon dioxide are fat-soluble and cross the capillary wall many times faster than glucose, which is fat-insoluble.

Some fat-insoluble substances cross the capillary in places where the capillary wall has water-filled channels. In the brain, fat-insoluble glucose needs a carrier in order to diffuse out of the capillary.

The distance between the cells and capillaries is important. The shorter the distance, the better the exchange between the cells and the blood. Where a great number of capillaries are packed into a relatively small space, the distance between the blood and the cells is reduced. In skeletal muscle, for example, the capillary density is high to enable the muscle to get adequate oxygen for contraction and physical work. In the brain and the heart muscle the capillary density is even greater, so much so that each myocyte in the myocardium has its own capillary. In addition to reducing the blood-to-cell distance, capillary density provides a larger surface area for exchange of nutrients and waste.

The role of endothelium in development of vascular disease

There has been a surge of interest in the function of endothelium and its potential role in the genesis of vascular disease. Vasoactive substances such as *nitric oxide* and angiotensin II are important determinants of vascular disease (Gibbon, 1997).

The endothelium is the interface between the blood and the vascular wall. It is therefore the primary recipient of all haemodynamic fluctuations imposed upon the blood vessels by the circulating blood. The endothelium can stimulate changes in the vascular muscle tone and growth, haemodynamic and inflammatory responses and anti-thrombotic activity.

There is overwhelming evidence that the vascular endothelium is an important regulatory tissue in maintaining cardiovascular homeostasis. The anti-platelet, anti-thrombotic and anti-fibrinolytic properties of endothelium maintain the fluidity of the blood. Damage to the endothelium disrupts its function and leads to vasospasm, thrombosis and atherosclerosis. It is suggested that the therapeutic effects of angiotensin-converting enzyme (ACE) inhibitors may be due to their overcoming the endothelial dysfunction associated with the cardiovascular disease process.

Muscle tone

Arterial tone is a major factor in determining blood pressure. It is the result of a balance between *vasodilatation* and *vasoconstriction* of the arterial wall. The arterial endothelium produces relaxing and constricting factors which act on the smooth muscle of the arteries. It has been established that the relaxing factor is *nitric oxide* (NO) (Palmer et al., 1987), although there is increasing evidence to suggest that in addition to NO, there are other agents that bring about relaxation of the arterial wall (Quilley et al., 1997). Important endothelial vasodilators are prostacyclin, bradykinin, NO, and endothelium-derived hyperpolarising factor (Ruschitzka et al., 1997). The constricting factors released by the endothelial cells are identified as *endothelins*, which occur in three distinct types, and activators of cyclooxygenase such as thromboxane (TXA^2) and prostaglandin H^2 (PGH^2).

Nitric oxide is produced in the endothelium and the smooth muscle cells of the arteries. It is also produced in other sites in the body such as the brain, kidneys, macrophages and the peripheral nerves. In the endothelium, NO is produced in response to shear stress caused by the flow of blood (flow-induced vasodilatation). Other agents that cause release of NO are bradykinin, serotonin, adenosine triphosphate (ATP), adenosine diphosphate (ADP), thrombin, cytokines, tumour necrosis factor (TNF), substance P (Schiffrin, 1994) and possibly oestrogen (Griendling and Alexander, 1996). Bradykinin also causes release of prostaglandins and endothelium-derived hyperpolarising factor, both of which are vasodilators (Horing and Drexler, 1997). Nitric oxide diffuses from the endothelium to the underlying smooth muscle of the arterial wall. It inhibits the influx of calcium into the muscle cells and thus prevents the release of intracellular calcium and, thereby, contraction of the vascular smooth muscle. Nitric oxide is released, apparently unstimulated in certain regions, but it can only work locally as it has a short half-life (Paulus, 1994). Endothelium-mediated responses vary in the same arteries of different species and in different vessels in the same species (Shepard and Zovonimir, 1991). The endothelium of the veins also produces similar substances, although the level of these vasoactive agents seems to be lower than that produced by arteries (el Khatib et al., 1991).

In recent years there has been a vast interest in the potential role of NO in the pathogenesis of cardiovascular disease. Experimental work has revealed that changes in production of NO may in fact trigger the onset of some of these conditions or contribute to their progression. Evidence suggests that either the production of NO is reduced, or that once produced, it is degraded more rapidly in hypertensive patients (Schini et al., 1994). In atherosclerosis there is also evidence of reduced NO production, which has many effects. Hypercholesterolaemia and atherosclerosis impair the release of endothelium-dependent relaxation of arterial smooth muscle. This mechanism is also impaired in coronary arteries where there is no overt atherosclerosis (Ludmer et al., 1986; Zeirher et al., 1991).

Nitric oxide also has anti-aggregatory and anti-adhesive properties. Reduced NO not only causes increased tone in arteries (including coronary arteries), but also thickens the underlying muscle layer and increases aggregation of platelets on the inner surface of the arteries (Vane and Botting, 1992). It is thought that one cause of reduced NO production is damaged endothelium. In atherosclerosis this is conducive to platelet deposition and thrombosis, and eventually formation of plaque. Various constrictor and dilator stimuli work simultaneously to maintain the balance between the arterial blood supply and tissue perfusion in the intact endothelium. Damaged endothelium seems to alter the influence of agents that normally induce release of NO and relaxation of arterial smooth muscle. For example, in the presence of damaged endothelium, serotonin and thrombin cause contraction by acting directly on the vascular smooth muscle. Furthermore, damaged endothelium is thought to release endothelin, which is a potent vasoconstrictor. Chronic hypoxia causes reduced NO release and release of endothelin (Cohen, 1995). Abnormalities in endothelial function can increase the arterial tone in other ways. Damaged endothelium reduces the activity of baroreceptors and decreases inhibition of vasomotor activity, with consequential increases in sympathetic outflow and vasoconstriction. Endothelial damage also causes decreased inhibition of the renin–angiotensin system.

There is profound endothelial dysfunction in diabetes which is thought to be due to reduced NO (Tesfamariam et al., 1990) and increased endothelin (Weisbrod et al., 1991). The endothelial damage in diabetes may be due to glycosylation products and deposition of unmetabolised glucose in the basement membrane of blood vessels. Deficiency of NO may also be involved in impotence in diabetes, as NO is the mediator of vasodilatation in the corpus cavernosum (Rajfer et al., 1992).

In addition to substances that induce dilatation, blood vessels produce vasoconstrictor agents. The best known and most potent vasoconstrictor substance released by the endothelium is *endothelin.* Endothelin 1 is found in humans and production may be modulated by sex hormones. The levels of endothelin are found to be lower in women and higher in men (Schiffrin, 1994).

In atherosclerosis, endothelin release may be directly involved in pathogenesis or may be the trigger for the disease process. The pattern of smooth muscle growth and migration into the intima of the arterial wall in atherosclerosis suggests involvement of endothelin (Ruschitzka et al., 1997).

Endothelin also stimulates protein synthesis and tissue growth. There is some evidence that endothelin levels may be elevated in patients with hypertension (Chua et al., 1992). Over-production of endothelin can lead to thickening of the arterial wall and hypertension, while deficiency of endothelin may cause postural hypotension and syncope (Kurihara et al., 1994). Endothelin is increased in Raynaud's disease (Smits et al., 1991) and renal failure (Tomita et al., 1989).

Haemodynamic response

At the interface between the blood and the vascular wall, the endothelium is exposed to changes in the pressure and flow of circulating blood. These changes act as mechanical stresses which evoke structural and functional responses in endothelial cells. Mechanical stress appears to determine the arrangement of the endothelial cells in the vascular wall, in that they become elongated and aligned with the direction of blood flow. Physical forces imposed on the endothelium trigger biochemical signals which lead to changes in vascular muscle tone, vascular wall growth and white cell migration adhesion. It has been demonstrated that shear stress is a potent regulator of NO (Nishida et al., 1992) and it is likely that the biochemical signals influence the production of NO by the endothelial cells.

The interaction between blood and the venous endothelium plays an important role in the pathology of varicose veins and more serious complications of venous disease such as thrombosis (Dormandy, 1996). Endothelial dysfunction involves an imbalance between vasoactive substances, and disturbances in the regulation of tone, homeostasis and vessel structure, resulting in the development of cardiovascular diseases such as hypertension, atherosclerosis and heart failure.

Inflammatory response

Cytokine (TNF) inhibits release of NO from the endothelial cells (Nishida et al., 1992), and inhibits the source of NO in the smooth muscle cells (Schini et al., 1994). This latter effect of cytokines may be related to the function of NO in the inflammatory response and promotion of healing in the injured tissue. In atherosclerosis, high cholesterol levels in the plasma contribute to increased oxygen free radicals which in turn inhibit release of NO, causing vasoconstriction. In addition, the likelihood of local inflammation in the affected blood vessels is increased because NO normally inhibits white cell adhesion.

Anti-thrombotic activity

Intact endothelium repels platelets and therefore inhibits clotting. When thrombin is present it becomes bound to the anti-thrombin III found on the endothelial cells and in this way it is deactivated. If the integrity of the endothelium is lost, as in atherosclerosis, the endothelial cells synthesise and release coagulants which triggers thrombin formation. Production of thrombin stimulates the endothelial cells to release platelet-aggregating factors such as fibrinolytic, growth and endothelium-relaxing factors and increase capillary permeability. In addition, thrombin activates leukocytes and promotes their adhesion and migration to the vessel wall.

Tissue growth

The endothelial cells regulate the growth of smooth muscle in the vascular wall. They also play a major role in growth and proliferation of blood vessels (angiogenesis). Endothelium produces both growth-promoting and growth-inhibiting factors which regulate both mitogenesis and angiogenesis of the vascular wall.

Peripheral vascular disease

One of the substances produced by and stored in the endothelial cells is von Willebrand factor. This factor, when released, mediates platelet aggregation and adhesion. Many studies suggest that the levels of von Willebrand factor (vWf) are markers of endothelial damage (Lip and Blann, 1997). Close association between vWf and thrombus formation also suggests that this factor may be a useful indirect indicator of atherosclerosis. It has been suggested that levels of vWf may have diagnostic value in patients with ischaemic heart disease, peripheral vascular disease and inflammatory vascular disease. Leukocyte adhesion to the endothelial cells appears to be another process that leads to atherosclerosis of the peripheral vessels. Many cell adhesion molecules coordinate this process. It has been suggested that, in peripheral vascular disease, an insulin-like growth factor may be the cause of adhesion of leukocytes to the endothelial cells by upregulating some of the cell adhesion molecules (Schiffrin, 1994). There is evidence that antibodies against endothelial cells are present in some patients with severe atherosclerotic peripheral vascular disease (Schiffrin, 1994).

Circulation

Composition of blood

The volume of circulating blood is about 5 litres in an adult. This volume varies with age, gender, weight and other factors such as level of physical activity. The blood volume or *intravascular* volume consists of the fluid contained in the plasma (3 litres) and that within the red cells (2 litres). Blood consists of two main components: plasma and the formed elements. Plasma consists of 91.5% water and 8.5% solutes. Plasma proteins constitute about 7% of the formed elements. Gases such as *nitrogen*, *oxygen* and *carbon dioxide* are carried in the blood. Oxygen is carried combined with haemoglobin in the red cells, whereas the other two gases are dissolved in the plasma. Blood has a pH (power of hydrogen) of 7.4 at rest. The plasma bicarbonate acts as a buffer to maintain this pH, which has a very narrow normal range.

At rest, close to 60% of the blood volume is held in the venous system compared to 15% in the arteries and 5% in the capillaries. For this reason, the venous system acts as the *blood reservoir* for the body. The major reservoirs in the venous system are the blood vessels of the gut, liver, spleen and skin. The function of these reservoirs is to divert blood to where it is needed in times of stress, for example in exercise when the skeletal muscle requires a greater blood flow, and in cases of severe fluid loss such as haemorrhage.

Haemostasis

Tissue injury evokes haemostasis. There are three components to haemostasis: *vasoconstriction*, *platelet formation* and *coagulation*. Simultaneously, fibrinolysis is initiated in order to dissolve the clot. It is the balance of these two mechanisms, clot formation and dissolution, that stops bleeding and promotes healing.

Coagulation

Tissue injury to a blood vessel stimulates the release of *thrombokinase*. This substance (in the presence of calcium) converts *prothrombin* to *thrombin*. Thrombin converts another plasma protein, *fibrinogen*, to *fibrin*, which traps red cells to form a clot. Sometimes clotting occurs spontaneously and without the stimulus of external injury. In such cases the surface of the endothelium is roughened or damaged and the collagen of the vascular wall is exposed. This attracts platelets which aggregate and adhere to the surface of the endothelium and the mechanism of clotting is initiated. Clotting caused by trauma and external injury is termed *extrinsic*. Clotting in the absence of external injury is termed *intrinsic*. Clotting time is about 5 to 8 minutes. *Prothrombin time* (PT) is an indication of the amount of prothrombin in the blood. This is measured by adding tissue extracts to a sample of blood which converts prothrombin to thrombin. This reaction requires calcium and takes about 12 seconds. Because formation of thrombin requires thrombokinase, the speed with which this substance is activated is an important factor in clotting (APTT; *activated prothrombin time*). *Heparin* prevents formation of thrombin and therefore delays clotting whereas *warfarin* prevents production of prothrombin by impairing synthesis of vitamin K. *Aspirin* combines with the enzyme *cyclooxygenase* in the platelets and inhibits synthesis of *thromboxane* A_2 (TXA^2), which is a potent platelet aggregator. Low-dose aspirin therapy may also reduce viscosity of the blood via an anti-fibrin activity, an effect that is enhanced when aspirin is combined with *ticlopidine* (Rupprecht et al., 1998).

Velocity and flow

Velocity refers to the volume of the blood passing through a tissue at a given time. The greater the velocity the shorter the transit time, or the time during which the nutrients and waste are exchanged between the tissue and the blood. Velocity is inversely proportional to the diameter of the blood vessel; the smaller the diameter the greater the velocity. Each time a major blood vessel divides to form smaller vessels, the velocity is decreased because the total cross-sectional area of the smaller vessels is larger than the cross-sectional area of the dividing vessel. The velocity is lower in the branches of the aorta compared to the aorta itself. Velocity is therefore lowest in the capillary. Similarly, as the capillaries join to form a venule, velocity increases.

Blood enters the right atrium via the inferior and superior vena cavae, and the left atrium via the pulmonary veins. From the atria it enters the ventricles through the atrio-ventricular valves. Contraction of the ventricles pushes blood into the systemic and pulmonary circulation, following which the ventricles relax. The time course of blood through the heart is known as the *cardiac cycle*, each lasting about 0.8 seconds. This means that in adults there are approximately 75 cardiac cycles in one minute. The time taken for the blood to travel from the right ventricle to the lungs, then to the left ventricle, through the rest of the body and back to the right ventricle is called the *circulation time*, which is approximately one minute.

The vascular system contains about 5 litres of blood. More correctly, the volume of blood ejected from the heart in one minute is about 5 litres in adults. This is known as the *cardiac output*. The cardiac output is the product of stroke volume and heart rate as follows:

Cardiac output (ml/min) = stroke volume (ml/beat) × heart rate (beats/min)

The amount of blood ejected from each ventricle in one contraction, or beat, is about 70 ml; as the heart rate is about 70 beats per minute the quantity of blood ejected from the heart in one minute is 4900 ml, or nearly 5 litres. This is one of the fundamental equations of circulatory physiology.

Pulse

The ejection of blood into the aorta creates a wave of expansion and pressure which travels through the arterial system; this is the *pulse*. The pressure wave is strongest in the arteries closest to the heart and although it becomes weaker the further it gets from the heart, it can easily be felt in the arteries passing over a bone and close to the surface of the body. The pulse is commonly felt in the radial artery but can also be palpated in the temporal, facial, common carotid, brachial, femoral, popliteal, posterior tibial and dorsalis pedis arteries (Figure 1.2).

Blood pressure

Blood pressure is the pressure exerted on the arterial wall by the circulating blood. It is the pressure of blood that makes the exchange of fluid between capillary and tissue possible. Without blood pressure, little would reach the tissues in the form of nutrients and fluid. Blood pressure is dependent on the following factors:

- contraction of the heart
- volume of circulating blood
- elasticity of the arteries

The contraction of the heart muscle must generate a force capable of producing an adequate stroke volume. A good stroke volume, however, is dependent on the amount of blood that reaches the heart (*venous return* or *preload*). The size of the preload determines the extent of cardiac muscle fibre stretch. The more the ventricular muscle fibres stretch, the greater the force of contraction of the heart (Starling law of the heart). The arteries respond to the pressure of blood by expanding. When the pressure falls, the arteries contract to compensate for the drop in pressure. However, as the arteries divide and form smaller blood vessels their diameter becomes narrower. This has two effects: (1) flow is difficult and *resisted*; (2) pressure is increased.

The arterioles, being the narrowest of arteries, offer the most resistance to blood flow (*peripheral resistance*). The two factors that determine blood pressure are, therefore, the cardiac output and peripheral resistance:

Blood pressure = cardiac output × peripheral resistance

Cardiac output is determined by the quantity of blood that reaches the heart (*venous return*), and stretches the ventricles (*preload*).

Viscosity increases the pressure of circulating blood. Many factors influence the blood pressure: age, weight, diet, drugs, level of hormones and physical activity. While there is no convincing evidence that there is a reduction in cardiac output with age, there is evidence that the elasticity of the arteries is reduced as a result of the ageing process.

Local blood circulation

We tend to think of the circulation as a system that delivers nutrients to the tissues. However, an equally important function of the circulation is to remove waste from the tissues. Often it is the accumulation of waste that causes equal if not more harm than shortage of nutrients, and these two factors are important regulators of local circulation.

It is thought that the regulation of local circulation falls into two categories: *short term* and *long term*. Blood flow to a tissue may fluctuate depending on the metabolic activity of that tissue. For example, in the resting muscle blood flow is very low. During exercise metabolism increases, leading to an increase in flow. The increase in blood flow is achieved by vasodilatation. Two possible mechanisms have been put forward for local vasodilatation:

1. Increased metabolic activity leads to release of vasodilator substances such as adenosine, carbon dioxide, histamine, potassium ions, lactic acid and hydrogen ions, and any of these or their combination may act as a vasodilator. Increase in temperature as a result of increased metabolism is also thought to be a vasodilator.
2. Shortage of oxygen and nutrients acts as a vasodilator. It is thought that in the absence of oxygen and nutrients, muscle is not able to contract and the arteriolar tone is therefore lost. These two are known as the *metabolic mechanisms* of local blood flow control. These mechanisms can be observed in *active* and *reactive hyperaemia*. Active hyperaemia is the increased flow to a tissue whose metabolic activity is increased, as in exercising muscle. If the blood supply to a tissue is temporarily cut off, for example when a tourniquet is applied to the arm, then re-established, the tissue becomes red and feels warm due to increase in flow. This is known as reactive hyperaemia because lack of oxygen and nutrients leads to release of vasodilator substances which increase the flow above its previous levels.

While the short-term regulation of local blood flow is fast, it is always below the nutritional requirement of the tissue and therefore inadequate. To meet increased requirement in times of increased metabolic activity lasting over a long period of time (weeks and months), a long-term response is produced. In this case there is a gradual increase in the vasculature of the tissue (*angiogenesis*). It is thought that shortage of oxygen causes release of substances such as endothelial cell growth factor, fibroblast growth factor and angiogenin which promote growth of blood vessels. In athletes, the tissue extraction of oxygen is also increased during exercise. These mechanisms provide a blood flow that matches the nutritional needs of the tissue. However, the extent of the long-term response varies in different individuals. An important factor is the age of the person. The increase in vascularity is greater the younger the individual. In neonates the increase in vascularity provides a blood flow that exactly matches the tissue's need, whereas in the older person the growth of new vessels may fall well short of tissue requirement. Furthermore, the increase in vascularity in the neonate commences within days, whereas in the elderly the response may take weeks, months and even years to develop. Certain agents such as cortisone impair growth of new vessels. The growth of new blood vessels is also promoted when an artery or a vein is blocked. In this case the new growth develops around the blockage in order to readjust the blood supply (*collateral circulation*), which can result from both, short- and long-term response of the tissue to changes in blood flow.

In addition to local factors, substances released by other tissues in the body can lead to changes in the arteriolar tone. Adrenaline and noradrenaline cause vasoconstriction particularly in the skin, but also mild vasodilatation of the coronary arteries. Pain and stress are associated with the release of neuroendocrine factors such as adrenaline and cortisone. Angiotensin and vasopressin (ADH, antidiuretic hormone) are two of the most potent vasoconstrictors. However, under normal conditions the quantity of ADH is too small to cause a significant vasoconstriction, and it is only in cases of severe hypovolaemia that marked increases in ADH levels have been observed.

Most tissues in the body release vasodilator substances such as *histamine, bradykinin*, *serotonin* and *prostaglandin*. These agents are mostly vasodilators, although the role of serotonin in regulation of the circulation is in doubt. Prostaglandins are several chemically-related substances, some of which have vasoconstrictor activity but the majority are vasodilators.

Whereas tissue blood flow is regulated by local agents, the most powerful regulator of the circulation as a whole is the central nervous system. The heart and blood vessels are innervated by the autonomic nervous system. The heart is supplied with both *sympathetic* and *parasympathetic* nervous systems, whereas the blood vessels receive only the sympathetic nervous supply. Sympathetic activity elevates the blood pressure in two ways:

1. An increase in the rate and force of contraction of the heart.
2. A simultaneous increase in peripheral resistance.

Parasympathetic activity reduces the rate and force of contraction of the heart, but as the blood vessels do not have a parasympathetic supply it does not have an effect on peripheral resistance. The pressure exerted on the arteries at certain locations (e.g. the carotid artery and the arch of the aorta) is sensed by nerve endings which are normally present in these areas (*baroreceptors*). When the pressure is increased, the baroreceptors are stretched and fire impulses to the vasomotor centre; this reduces the sympathetic tone to the blood vessels and consequently the blood pressure falls. When the pressure is low and the baroreceptors are not stretched, their rate of firing is reduced and the vasomotor centre is free to increase the sympathetic activity, which results in vasoconstriction and a rise in blood pressure.

Lymphatic circulation

The lymphatic circulation is another route by which fluid can leave the tissue space and enter the circulation (Figure 1.7). In addition, the lymphatic system removes from the interstitial space, proteins and particles that are too large to be absorbed into the capillaries. The removal of these proteins maintains the colloid osmotic pressure gradient across the capillary and facilitates the return of fluid into the capillary. This is an extremely important function without which life could not be sustained beyond 24 hours. The lymphatic circulation also absorbs fat from the gastrointestinal tract. The lymphatic system has a major protective function. The white cells of the lymph, i.e. the lymphocytes and macrophages, provide both specific and non-specific immunity against microorganisms. The macrophages are monocytes which, when mature, leave the bloodstream and enter the lymph or become resident in various tissues such as the skin, where they are called *histocytes*, or the liver, where they are called *Kupffer cells*.

The lymphatic fluid is essentially the tissue fluid that courses through the lymphatic vessels. The lymphatic system begins as close-ended capillaries located in between the cells. The lymphatic capillaries converge to form lymphatic vessels which are similar in structure to veins except that they have thinner walls and more valves. In the skin, respiratory, gastrointestinal and genitourinary tract, the lymph capillaries are numerous, whereas in the brain they are absent. The permeability of lymph capillaries increases in certain conditions such as application of pressure sufficient to block the lymph vessel, rise in temperature, and presence of histamine.

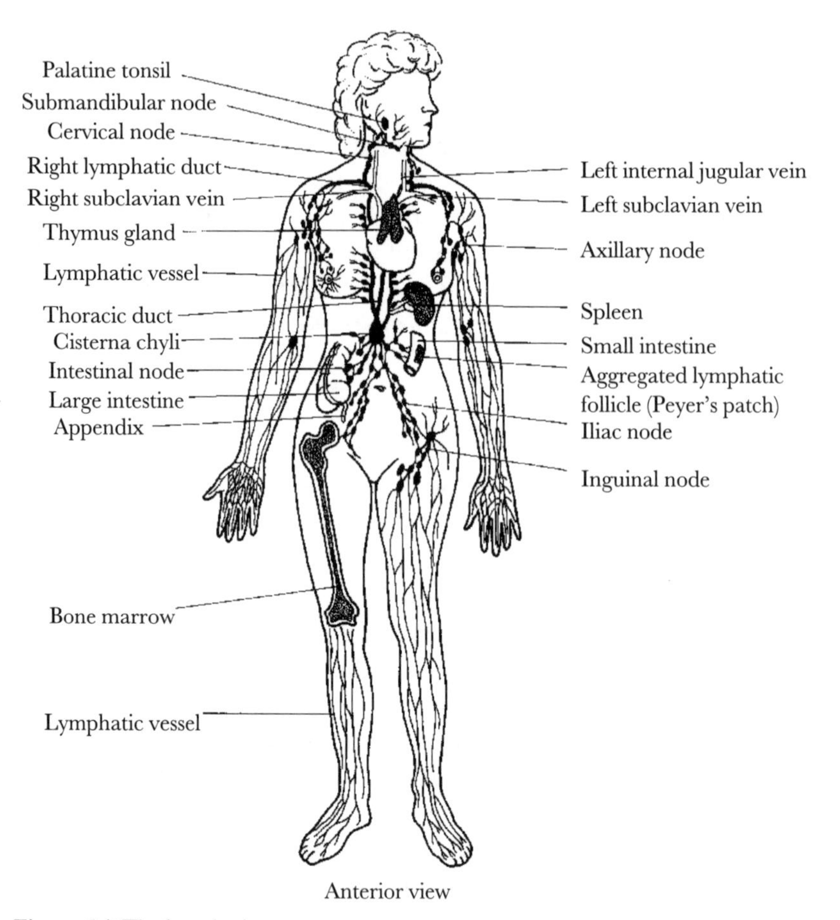

Figure 1.7 The lymphatic system.

The lymph vessels pass through lymph nodes. A lymph node consists of a meshwork of reticulum in which lymphocytes, macrophages and other free cells are arranged. The node is encapsulated and ovoid in shape and it is supplied with nerve, lymphatic and blood vessels. Each node is divided into compartments by connective tissue. Lymphocytes line the outer aspect of these compartments in dense clusters called *nodules*. The *germinal layer* is the centre of the nodule where the lymphocytes are produced. There are numerous nodes within the lymphatic system. Some are placed strategically, e.g. cervically, abdominally, thoracically, to engulf microorganisms before they reach the circulation. The tonsils, thymus gland and the spleen are lymphoid organs which consist of lymphoid tissue similar to the lymph nodes.

The skin

The skin provides a waterproof layer which prevents fluid entering and leaving the body. It helps to regulate body temperature, is a major organ of sensation, synthesises vitamin D from sunlight, has an excretory role and an important protective function (Figure 1.8). The cells found in the skin are: *keratinocytes* (produce keratin), *macrophages* and melanin-producing cells, *melanocytes*.

The thickness of the skin varies in different parts of the body. Two layers form the skin: *epidermis* (upon the dermis) and *dermis*. The epidermis consists of stratified epithelium, forming two layers: an outer *horny zone*, which is further divided into horny cells, clear cells and granular cells, and an inner *germinal zone*, which is divided into prickle cells and basal cells. The epidermis is devoid of blood vessels and nerves. Under the influence of the *protein epidermal growth factor*, the horny cells are shed and replaced by the basal cells. The rate of this replacement is greatest in early life and declines in old age.

Dermal papillae connect the epidermis to the dermis. The dermis is the major component of the skin. It consists of collagen, reticular elastic fibres and connective tissue arranged in a strong and flexible meshwork. The dermis is rich in blood, nerve and lymph

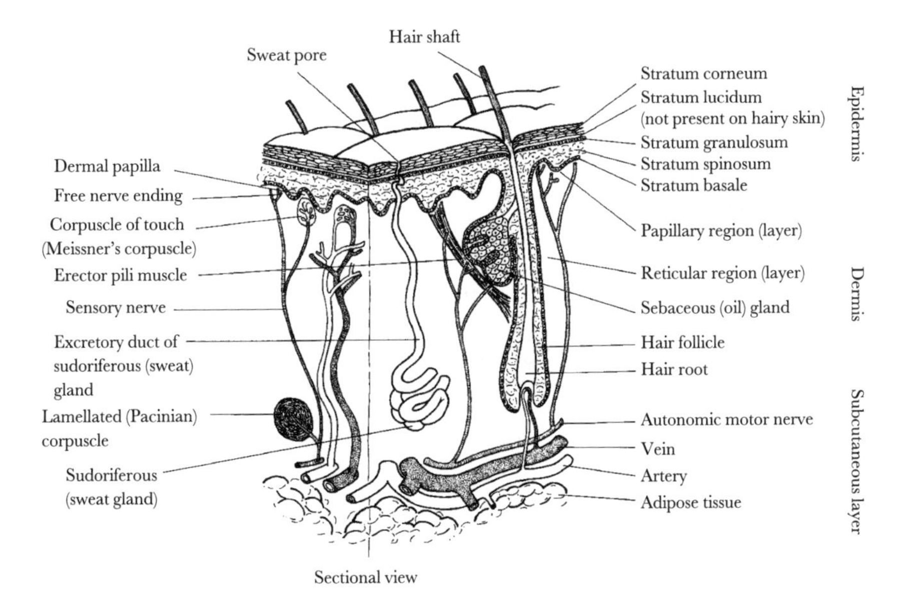

Figure 1.8 The structure of the skin.

supplies. When exposed to severe irritation the blood vessels of the dermis dilate and leak fluid, which accumulates between the dermis and epidermis, forming *blisters*. The layers of the dermis are the *papillary* and the *reticular*. The collagen fibres of the dermis are arranged in a particular pattern in different parts of the body (*cleavage lines*). Surgical incisions made along the cleavage lines heal faster and with minimum scarring. *Hypodermis* is the layer below the dermis. It is also called the *subcutaneous* layer. The hypodermis is much thicker than the dermis and has richer blood, nerve and lymphatic supplies. The sweat glands and hair follicles are contained within the hypodermis, whereas the sebaceous glands are found in the dermis. The physiology and stages of wound healing are discussed in Chapter 14.

References

Chua BHL, Krebs CJ, Chua CC, Diglio CA (1992) Endothelium stimulates protein synthesis in smooth muscle cells. American Journal of Physiology 262: E412–E416.

Cohen RA (1995) The role of nitric oxide and other endothelium-derived vasoactive substances in vascular disease. Progress in Cardiovascular Disease 38(2): 105–128.

Dormandy JA (1996) The influence of blood cells and blood flow on venous endothelium. International Angiology 15(2): 119–123.

el Khatib H, Lupinetti FM, Sanofsky SJ, Behrendt DM (1991) Production of endothelium-dependent relaxation responses by saphenous vein grafts in the canine arterial circulation. Surgery 110(3): 523–528.

Gibbon GH (1997) Vasculoprotective and cardioprotective mechanisms of angiotensin-converting enzyme inhibition: the homeostatic balance between angiotensin II and nitric oxide. Clinical Cardiology 20(11 Suppl 2): II-18–25.

Griendling KK, Alexander RW (1996) Endothelial control of the cardiovascular system: recent advances. FASEB Journal 10(2): 283–292.

Horing B, Drexler H (1997) Endothelial function and bradykinin in humans. Drugs 54(Suppl 5): 42–47.

Kurihara Y, Kurihara H, Suzuka H, Kodama T, Maemura K, Nagai R, Oda H, Kuwaki T, Cao WH, Kadama N, Jishagi K, Ouchi Y, Azuma S, Toyoda Y, Ishikawa T, Kudoma M, Yazaki Y (1994) Elevated blood pressure and craniofacial abnormalities in mice deficient in endothelin-1. Nature 368: 703–710.

Lip GY, Blann A (1997) von Willebrand factor: a marker of endothelium dysfunction in vascular disorder. Cardiovascular Research 34(2): 255–265.

Ludmer PL, Selwyn AP, Shook TL, Wayne RR, Mudge GH, Alexander RW, Ganz P (1986) Paradoxical vasoconstriction induced by acetylcholine in atherosclerotic coronary arteries. New England Journal of Medicine 315: 1046–1051.

Nishida K, Harrison DJ, Nava JP, Fisher AA, Dockery SP, Uematsu M, Nerem RW, Murphy TJ (1992) Molecular cloning and characterization of constitutive bovine aortic endothelial nitric oxide synthase. Journal of Clinical Investigation 90: 2092–2096.

Palmer RMJ, Ferrige AC, Moncada S (1987) Nitric oxide release accounts for biological activity of endothelial-derived relaxing factor. Nature 327: 524–526.

Paulus WJ (1994) Endothelial control of vascular and myocardial function in heart failure. Cardiovascular Drugs and Therapy 8: 437–446.

Quilley J, Fulton D, McGiff JC (1997) Hyperpolarization factors. Biochemical Pharmacology 54(10): 1059–1070.

Rajfer J, Aronson WJ, Bush PA, Doey FJ (1992) Nitric oxide as a mediator of relaxation of corpus cavernosum in response to noradrenergic, noncholinergic neurotransmitters. New England Journal of Medicine 36: 90–94.

Rupprecht HJ, Darius H, Borkowski U, Voigtlander T, Nowak B, Genth S, Meyer J (1998) Comparison of antiplatelet effects of aspirin, ticlopidine, or their combination after stent implantation. Circulation 97(11): 1046–1052.

Ruschitzka FT, Noll G, Luscher TF (1997) The endothelium in coronary artery disease. Cardiology 88 (Suppl 3): 3–19.

Schiffrin EL (1994) The endothelial control of blood vessels function in health and disease. Clinical and Investigative Medicine 17(6): 602–620.

Schini VB, Busse R, Vanhoute PM (1994) Inducible nitric oxide in vascular smooth muscle. Arzneimittel-Forschung 44: 432–435.

Shepard JT, Zovonimir KS (1991) Endothelium-derived vasoactive factors: I. Endothelium-dependent relaxation. Hypertension 18 (Suppl III): 76–85.

Smits P, Hofman H, Rosmalen F, Wollersheim H, Thein T (1991) Endothelin-1 in patients with Raynaud's phenomenon. Lancet 337: 236.

Tesfamariam B, Brown ML, Deykin D (1990) Elevated glucose promotes generation of endothelium-derived vasoconstrictor prostanoids in rabbit aorta. Journal of Clinical Investigation 85: 929–932.

Tomita K, Nakanishi T, Tomura S, Matsuda O, Ando K, Hirata Y, Marumo F (1989) Plasma endothelin levels in patients with acute renal failure. New England Journal of Medicine 321: 1127.

Vane JR, Botting RM (1992) The role of chemical mediators released by the endothelium in the control of the cardiovascular system. International Journal of Tissue Reactions 14(2): 55–64.

Weisbrod RM, Brown ML, Cohen RA (1991) Elevated glucose alters endothelial cell nitric oxide and prostanoid production. Circulation 84(Suppl II): 11–43.

Zeirher AM, Drexler H, Wollschlager H, Just H (1991) Modulation of coronary vasomotor tone in humans – progressive endothelial dysfunction with different early stages of coronary atherosclerosis. Circulation 83: 391–401.

CHAPTER 2

Aetiology and Pathology of Vascular Disease

LINDSEY J. OCKENDEN

This chapter explores the causes and incidence of vascular disease in the adult population. Vascular disease includes pathological processes affecting both the arterial and venous circulations.

Atherosclerosis

Atherosclerosis is the commonest cause of arterial disease, and is responsible for nearly 90% of all Western world arterial disease (Robertson, 1967); it will therefore be discussed first.

Atherosclerosis is a common disease process that affects the muscular arteries throughout the body, although its distribution is not uniform. Atherosclerosis is responsible for the following clinical conditions:

- Brain:
  Cerebral vascular disease
  Transient ischaemic attacks
  Cerebral thrombosis (stroke)
- Heart:
  Coronary artery disease
  Stable angina
  Unstable angina
  Myocardial infarction
- Thorax and abdomen:
  Aortic artery disease
  Aortic dissection
  Aortic aneurysm

- Renal:
  Renal arteries
  Renal failure
  Hypertension
- Gut:
  Mesenteric artery disease
  Intestinal angina
- Lower limbs:
  Peripheral arterial disease
  Intermittent claudication
  Critical limb ischaemia
  Acute limb ischaemia

The term atherosclerosis is derived from the Greek word for 'porridge' or 'gruel' (*athere*), whilst sclerosis infers 'scar formation', hence the term 'hardening' of the arteries. This is exemplified by the term atherosclerotic plaque, a lesion within the intima of the arterial wall that consists of a lipid pool (atheroma) surrounded by a fibrous or (sclerotic) cap.

Atherosclerotic disease is caused by the development of atherosclerotic plaques within the intima of the artery wall. This was previously thought to be a slow, progressive process but greater understanding of the pathological processes involved has shown that atheroma formation is a dynamic and not a static process, resulting in both acute and chronic vascular disease progression (Libby, 1996).

Atherosclerosis is described as occurring in a number of stages (Figure 2.1). The first stage involves the development of fatty streaks within the intima of the vessel. These fatty streaks do not reduce the lumen of the vessel and are not associated with symptoms of diminished blood flow (Stary et al., 1995). Although present in the intima of the artery in the majority of individuals under the age of 30 years (Davies, 1994; Fuster et al., 1996), it is only after the age of 30 years that the atheromatous plaques become more pronounced and only cause symptoms when the arterial lumen becomes stenosed by more than three-quarters (Shah, 1997).

Additionally, the presence of atheroma within the intima of the artery also interferes with endothelial function. Vessel endothelium affects vascular tone by releasing relaxing factors such as prostacyclin and nitric oxide that induce vasodilatation, whilst endothelin-1

Type I lesion

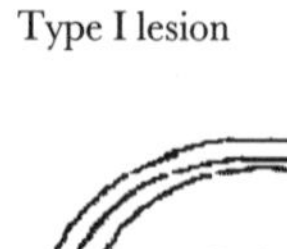

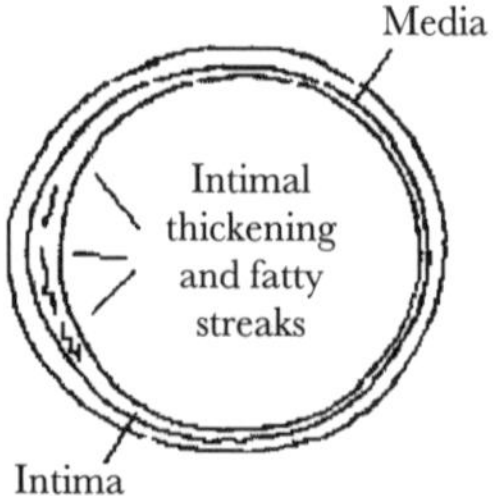

Type II lesion

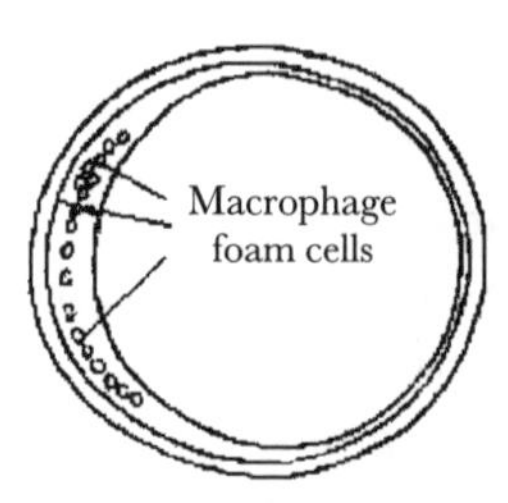

Type I and II lesions are sometimes referred to as early lesions appearing in the coronary arteries of infants and children and also adults.

Type III lesion

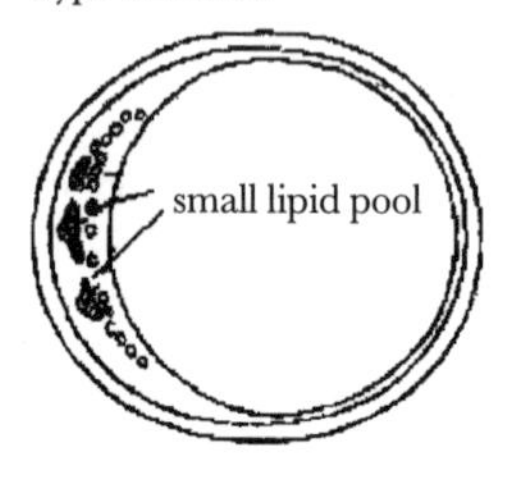

A pre-atheromatous lesion, the stage between early and advanced lesions.

Type IV lesion

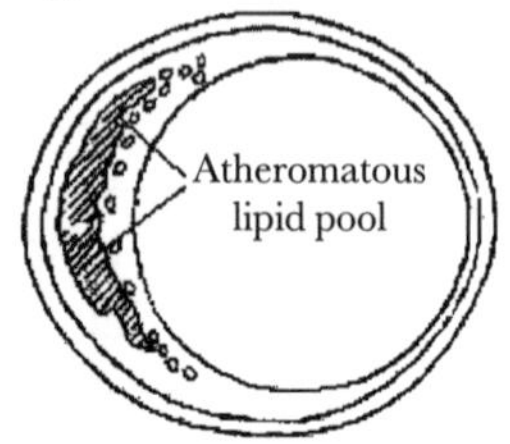

Advanced atheroma from the 3rd decade of life.

Type V lesion

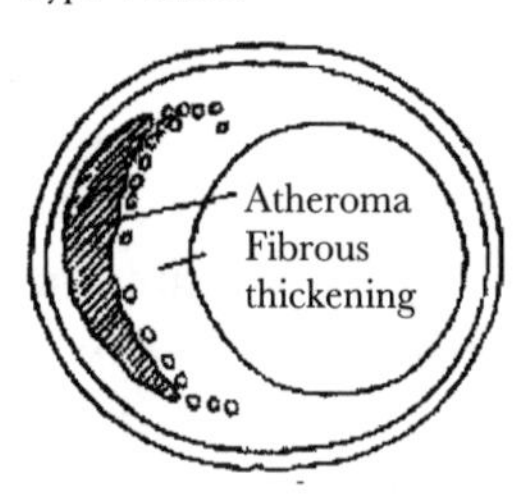

Fibrous thickening (fibroatheroma) of the intima surrounding the atheroma leading to a narrowed lumen.

Type VI lesion

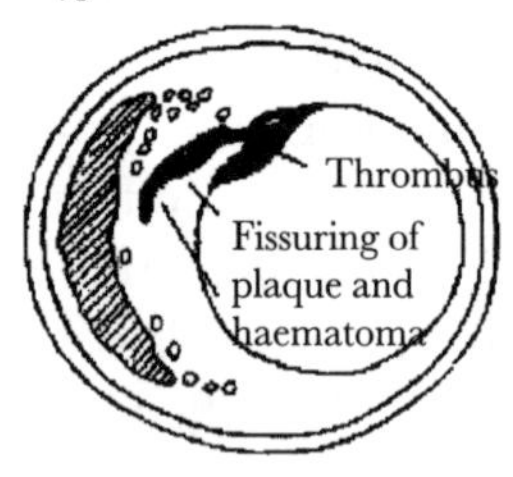

Complex lesion showing plaque rupture, bleeding and thrombus formation, further narrowing the lumen resulting in unstable coronary syndromes.

Figure 2.1 Developmental stages of atherosclerosis. (Adapted from Stary et al., 1995.)

opposes vasodilatation by causing vasoconstriction (see Chapter 1). It is thought that the vasodilatory effects of nitric oxide release predominate in the healthy vessel, but this is reversed in vessels with atheroma, resulting in greater release of constricting factors which further diminish blood flow and worsen ischaemia (Fuster et al., 1996; Toutouzas et al., 1998).

The atheromatous plaques can be stable or unstable. Stable atherosclerotic plaques consist of a hard crystalline cholesterol interior with a thick fibrous cap (Shah, 1997). This protects and separates the lipid thrombogenic core from the blood in the lumen and thus thrombus formation and occlusion do not occur.

Once the atherosclerotic plaque has reduced the vessel lumen by more than 75%, blood flow and oxygen supply to the tissues are reduced. A narrowed artery may supply sufficient blood at rest, but during exercise blood flow may be inadequate to meet tissue oxygen requirements. This situation causes *ischaemic pain.*

The strength of the fibrous cap influences the probability of plaque rupture (Davies, 1997); if rupture occurs the plaque becomes unstable.

An unstable atherosclerotic plaque is characterised by a soft lipid-rich core, deficient in supporting collagen covered by a thin fibrous cap that is vulnerable to rupture or fissuring (Doering, 1999).

It is not entirely clear why the plaque should rupture but evidence suggests that both internal and external triggers are involved (Doering, 1999). Internal triggers may be induced by immune cells such as macrophages and other inflammatory cells that infiltrate the plaque pool. These cells release a cocktail of destructive chemicals that weaken the shoulders of the fibrous cap (Cooke, 1997; Shah, 1997). It is possible that an immune reaction causes fissuring or cracking of the fibrous cap with resultant thrombus formation. There is growing evidence that infection by *Chlamydia pneumoniae*, a respiratory pathogen, is another internal trigger; the stimulus of inflammation may be responsible for further atheroma development and plaque rupture (Knight, 1999). Further studies are required to establish this hypothesis, but post-mortem studies have found the presence of *C. pneumoniae* in 85% of atherosclerotic coronary lesions compared to none in normal arteries (Kuo et al., 1995). In a recent study (Gurfinkel et al., 1997), patients with acute unstable coronary syndromes due to plaque rupture who were treated with an antichlamydial drug were found to have fewer adverse cardiac events such as myocardial infarction than a similar untreated group of patients. These studies need to be repeated, but provide further evidence of an infective/immune influence in atherosclerosis and its sequelae.

Plaque rupture may be caused by external triggers such as sudden increases in pulse and blood pressure; and in the heart increased contractility and coronary blood flow (Doering, 1999). These physiological events are triggered by an increase in stress hormone levels including adrenaline. Such raised levels occur in the first hour after awakening, cold environments, emotional stress and vigorous exercise (Gronholdt et al., 1998).

Plaque rupture is sometimes silent, and therefore asymptomatic, if the plaque rupture causes a small non-occlusive thrombus that is spontaneously lysed by the thrombolytic system (Knight, 1999). If, however, the plaque rupture results in the formation of a large or complete thrombus, this will be accompanied by acute tissue ischaemia if the vessel occlusion is partial, or tissue necrosis if the vessel is totally occluded (Davies, 1997). Thus an acute picture is seen when the plaque ruptures, compared with a chronic one when the stable plaque slowly enlarges.

The location of the artery affected by these pathological events will result in a number of acute clinical conditions such as myocardial infarction in the heart, or limb ischaemia if lower limb arteries are involved, or a stroke when cerebral arteries are affected.

Aetiology

There are a number of risk factors associated with the formation of atheromatous plaques (Furberg et al., 1996). These are considered to be modifiable when lifestyle changes or medical interventions can reduce them or slow the progress of atheroma (Gensini et al., 1998); non-modifiable risk factors cannot be reduced (risk factors are further discussed in the next chapter in relation to health promotion). These risk factors have been identified and can be seen in Table 2.1.

Table 2.1 Modifiable and non-modifiable risk factors for the development of atherosclerosis

Modifiable risk factors	Non-modifiable risk factors
Cigarette smoking	Age
Low density lipoprotein cholesterol	Gender
Physical inactivity	Family history
Obesity	
Diabetes mellitus	
Hypertension	
Homocysteine (raised levels)	
Thrombogenic factors	

Source: Pasternak et al. (1996).

Modifiable risk factors

Smoking

The evidence that cigarette smoking is responsible for atheroma formation is overwhelming and is considered proven (Anon, 1964; Doll and Peto, 1976; McBride, 1992). Smoking increases cardiovascular mortality by 50% by accelerating atherosclerosis and enhancing the effects of other risk factors such as diet, hyperlipidaemia and hypertension (Pasternak et al., 1996). The duration of smoking and the quantity of cigarettes smoked have a strong influence on the development of atheroma. Additionally, the risk of cardiovascular disease is particularly high in those smoking before the age of 15 years (Wood et al., 1998). The exact mechanisms by which smoking induces atherosclerosis are not yet fully understood; however, it appears that smoking causes endothelial dysfunction, elevates blood fibrinogen levels, (Gensini et al., 1998; Wood et al., 1998), enhances platelet activity and increases blood viscosity due to secondary polycythaemia. All these factors facilitate thrombus formation (Fuster et al., 1996). Smoking causes vasoconstriction by increasing vascular tone and reduces the protective effects of high density lipoproteins (HDL) (Fuster et al., 1996). Stopping smoking reduces the risk of further atherosclerosis in those with established disease to levels seen in those who have never smoked within 2–3 years (Wood et al., 1998).

Blood lipids

Diets rich in saturated fats are an important risk factor for the development of atherosclerosis. Cholesterol is manufactured in the liver and is absorbed from the gut and is essential for cell membrane function. Cholesterol is found in a variety of forms in the body, and when bound to plasma proteins it forms lipoproteins. Collectively, cholesterol and triglycerides found in the blood plasma are referred to as blood lipids.

The size of lipoproteins plays a role in their ability to cause atherosclerosis. High density lipoproteins (HDL) are the smallest lipoproteins that can enter and leave the arterial wall easily without causing atherosclerosis. Low density lipoproteins (LDL), intermediate density lipoproteins (IDL) and very low density lipoproteins (VLDL) are also able to enter the artery wall; however, if these lipoproteins are oxidised by macrophages, they are detained within the artery wall to cause the lipid pools of atherosclerotic plaques (Wood et al.,

1998). Dietary saturated fats increase LDL cholesterol and the risk of developing atherosclerosis. HDL cholesterol on the other hand is thought to have protective effects by removing cholesterol from the arterial wall and transporting it to the liver. HDL is lowered by smoking, obesity and physical inactivity, and low plasma HDL levels are associated with increased risk of developing atherosclerosis (Wood et al., 1998; Anon, 1998).

Obesity

Obesity is associated with a number of adverse influences on the development of atherosclerosis. Obesity is defined as an increased body mass index (BMI) above 30.0 kg/m^2 (Wood et al., 1998). Obesity increases the risk of developing hypertension, raises plasma LDL cholesterol and triglycerides, and causes glucose intolerance. Central obesity (an increase in intra-abdominal fat), assessed by waist to hip circumference ratio, is strongly associated with the development of insulin resistance leading to type 2 diabetes mellitus and cardiovascular disease (Wood et al., 1998).

Diabetes

Diabetes mellitus type 1 (insulin-dependent) and type 2 (non-insulin-dependent) are associated with a markedly increased risk of developing atherosclerosis. Although the reasons for this are not fully understood, it is thought that hyperglycaemia plays a direct role in the acceleration of atheroma formation (Wood et al., 1998). Diabetes appears to increase endothelial permeability for calcium and LDL cholesterol, which are deposited within the media of the artery wall. Additionally, poor glucose control causes abnormalities of lipoprotein metabolism, resulting in an elevation of plasma triglycerides and an enhanced susceptibility to oxidation of LDL cholesterol, which are associated with an increased risk of thrombus formation (O'Brien et al., 1998).

Hypertension

Hypertension is a modifiable risk factor for the development of atherosclerosis (Wood et al., 1998). The mechanisms by which hypertension contributes to vascular disease are not currently understood. However, it is thought that hypertension may cause functional damage to the vascular endothelium, allowing the influx of proteins, lipoproteins and cells into the arterial intima and thereby promoting formation of lipid pools and the development of atherosclerosis (O'Brien et al., 1998). Additionally, hypertension alters shear stress on the endothelium, leading to damage and subsequent platelet deposition (O'Brien et al., 1998) which may reduce the vessel lumen size by altering its morphology or shape.

Homocysteine

Homocysteine is a by-product of protein metabolism, and raised plasma homocysteine levels are associated with an accelerated development of atherosclerosis and an increased thrombotic tendency (Cooke, 1997; Gensini et al., 1998; Kassianos, 1999). Homocysteine appears to have a graded, linear relationship with vascular risk just as cholesterol does, and there is an increased risk with each 5 μmol/l rise in homocysteine (Hankey and Eikelboom, 1999). Elevated homocysteine is also associated with the development of premature vascular disease. Elevated levels appear to enhance the effects of other risk factors such as smoking, hypertension and hyperlipidaemia. Deficiencies of vitamin B_6, B_{12} and folate are associated with raised plasma homocysteine; however, it is unclear whether vitamin replacement reduces the risks of developing atherosclerosis when homocysteine is elevated (Wood et al., 1998; Gensini et al., 1998; Hankey and Eikelboom, 1999).

Thrombogenic factors

Fibrinogen is a plasma protein involved in platelet aggregation and clot formation. It also influences blood viscosity and serves as a non-specific marker of inflammation (Campbell, 1998a). Recent evidence suggests that an elevated plasma fibrinogen level is an independent risk factor for a vascular event such as tissue ischaemia or infarction in those with atherosclerosis. Smoking and physical inactivity are associated with raised fibrinogen levels (Wood et al., 1998; Gensini et al., 1998).

Physical inactivity

A sedentary lifestyle is linked to the development of many of the risk factors previously discussed. Regular physical activity has the following favourable effects: it decreases LDL cholesterol and increases the protective effects of HDL cholesterol by raising levels, it reduces blood pressure and improves glucose tolerance. These, along with improved cardiovascular and pulmonary functional capacity, have a protective effect against the development of atherosclerosis (Fuster et al., 1996).

Non-modifiable risk factors

The contribution of non-modifiable risk factors to the atherosclerotic process will be discussed briefly.

Age

The risk of developing symptomatic atherosclerosis increases with age (Rivard et al., 1999), which is also influenced by the number of modifiable and non-modifiable risk factors affecting the individual. The incidence of vascular disease in relation to age and sex can be illustrated by results from a study by Kannel et al. (1970) which investigated the risk of atherosclerosis causing intermittent claudication in men and women of different ages. They found that 6 per 10 000 men between the ages of 30 and 44 years were affected, increasing ten times to 61 per 10 000 in men aged 65–74 years. The incidence in women was 3 per 10 000 between the ages of 30 and 44 years, rising to 54 per 10 000 in the 65–74 year age group.

Gender

Advanced lesions of atherosclerosis develop about 20 years earlier in men than in women (Fuster et al., 1996), although the incidence of atherosclerotic vascular disease is similar in men and women following the menopause. Age-specific mortality from atherosclerotic vascular disease is lower in premenopausal women than in men of the same age range (Sans et al., 1997).

Family history

The best way to avoid atherosclerosis is to 'choose one's parents wisely' (Fuster et al., 1996). A history of atherosclerosis is more important in a first-degree relative (parent, sibling) than in a second-degree relative (grandparent, uncle) (Wood et al., 1998).

Clinical conditions caused by atherosclerosis

It is clear from the discussion of the pathology and aetiology of atherosclerosis that it is a complex disease. It causes a number of clinical conditions, which will now be discussed.

Peripheral arterial occlusive disease

The major cause of peripheral arterial occlusive disease (PAOD) is atherosclerosis affecting the large arteries of the lower limbs; as the disease advances, the smaller arteries also become affected (Cooke, 1997).

Progressive atherosclerotic plaque formation causes increasing arterial stenosis and reduction in blood flow to the lower limb. At rest, blood flow is adequate and patients are asymptomatic. However, during exercise, when oxygen and blood flow demands are increased and not met, tissue metabolism is compromised leading to ischaemic pain.

The first symptom of PAOD is *intermittent claudication*, leg pain that occurs during physical activity. The location of pain provides an indication of the artery affected by atherosclerosis. Buttock, hip or thigh pain indicates aortoiliac disease whilst calf pain indicates femoropopliteal artery involvement (McGrae-McDermott and McCarthy, 1995) (see Chapters 1 and 9).

The reduced blood supply to the leg causes various physical changes. There may be dusky erythema of the foot where the blood vessels dilate in an attempt to increase blood supply to the oxygen-deprived tissues, hair loss from the limbs, and absent or diminished foot pulses with decreased capillary refill times due to arterial insufficiency to the skin (see Chapter 4). The reduced blood supply to the skin also promotes the formation of ischaemic arterial foot or leg ulcers (O'Brien et al., 1998). Fortunately, only a minority of patients, about 7.5%, go on to develop ischaemic rest pain or gangrene (McGrae-McDermott and McCarthy, 1995). Patients with PAOD also have a high risk for cardiovascular disease, resulting in significant morbidity and mortality (Criqui et al, 1997).

Diabetes mellitus

Diabetics not only have an increased risk of PAOD which is associated with heavily calcified large vessels, they also develop microangiopathy (microvascular disease) with thickening of arterial and basement membranes. Diabetics also develop peripheral neuropathies (decreased sensation in periphery). This may lead to foot ulceration because of injury (Ierardi and Shuman, 1998). Diabetics are also prone to infected ulcers, pulp spaces and osteomyelitis because of reduced immune defences. They are therefore more likely to develop critical and chronic limb ischaemia leading to amputations (Ierardi and Shuman, 1998).

Critical limb ischaemia

Critical limb ischaemia is a continuum of PAOD where blood flow to the limb is so reduced that pain occurs at rest rather than during exercise (*rest pain*). Worsening of the existing ischaemia, an acute event, is caused by further partial occlusion of the artery either due to increasing arterial stenosis induced by the atheroma or from thrombus developing over a ruptured atherosclerotic plaque. The partially occluded artery by either means results in markedly reduced blood flow to the tissue beyond the affected artery, causing a very high risk of ischaemic ulceration, tissue necrosis, and the affected limb developing gangrene for which surgical amputation is the only treatment option (Dormandy et al., 1999a). The catastrophic effects of critical leg ischaemia may be reversed if blood flow can be rapidly increased by pharmacological, surgical or radiological interventions (see Chapter 10). Critical limb ischaemia is a continuum of intermittent claudication and therefore shares the same risk factors responsible for the development of atherosclerosis and intermittent claudication.

Acute limb ischaemia

Acute limb ischaemia (ALI) is not dissimilar to critical limb ischaemia, the affected limb becoming acutely ischaemic due to sudden cessation of blood flow, in contrast to the partial occlusion seen with critical leg ischaemia. This causes acute ischaemic pain at rest, and if blood flow is not rapidly restored, the tissues of the limb quickly become necrotic leaving amputation as the only treatment option. Unlike chronic ischaemia, the suddenness of the acute occlusion does not allow time for the formation of collateral blood vessels which can otherwise reduce ischaemia and limit tissue damage.

The affected artery becomes totally occluded by *thrombus* or an *embolism* which prevents blood flow to the tissues beyond the obstruction.

- Thrombus may have originated from a segment of the already diseased artery, e.g. the abdominal aorta or iliac artery due to fissuring or rupture of an atherosclerotic plaque. A number of cardiac conditions cause thrombus formation which may embolise, one of the commonest being the cardiac arrhythmia atrial fibrillation (AF) (Campbell, 1998b). Thrombus can form within the fibrillating atria due to loss of coordinated contraction and reduced blood flow, which becomes entirely passive in AF. If the thrombus breaks away from the atrium wall it becomes an embolism that can then occlude an artery elsewhere in the body.
- Embolisms originate elsewhere in the body and are of various types. An embolism can be made up of air that may have been inadvertently injected into the circulation; fat embolisms are released following bone fracture; amniotic fluid embolism is a complication of pregnancy; or an embolism may be a thrombus that has been dislodged from elsewhere in the cardiovascular system. The embolism, whatever its cause, has the potential to occlude any vessel in which it becomes trapped. These can occur at any age, as can be deduced from the causes previously discussed, but embolisms consisting of thrombus are more common in those in their 50s and 60s. Embolisms may also occur following invasive investigations, vascular surgery, trauma, diabetes, compression syndromes and injection of illegal drugs (Dormandy et al., 1999b).

Coronary artery disease

Atherosclerosis can affect any artery of the body; 40–60% of patients with PAOD will also have coronary artery disease (Dormandy et al., 1999c). Coronary artery disease (CAD) affects large numbers of the adult population, and is the leading cause of mortality in men over 45 years and women over 65 years (Wood et al., 1998). In comparison to PAOD, the clinical presentation of CAD is dependent on an atheromatous plaque affecting blood flow within the coronary circulation. Patients with stable angina experience chest pain during physical activity, whereas patients with intermittent claudication get limb pain during physical activity. When coronary artery disease becomes unstable the patient is at risk of developing unstable angina, pain at rest, which can be compared with the patient with critical limb ischaemia who also gets pain at rest. Myocardial infarction is associated with complete occlusion of a coronary artery that left untreated rapidly causes necrosis of part of the myocardium, which may lead to ventricular failure (Grubb and Fox, 1999). Again these coronary vascular events can be contrasted with those of acute limb ischaemia; these vascular events require immediate medical intervention to prevent or limit the extent of tissue damage due to insufficient or occluded blood flow.

The symptoms resulting from atherosclerosed arteries will vary depending on the tissues and organs affected. All of the symptoms and signs caused by atherosclerosis are due to the effects of reduced or occluded blood flow to that tissue which results in pain, dysfunction and at the worst end of the spectrum, tissue death.

Upper arm claudication

Arterial disease of the upper limbs is far less common than disease of the lower limbs, because of a more extensive collateral blood supply that is able to compensate for altered blood flow in the major arteries (Fahey, 1994). Branches off the subclavian artery supply the arm and hand with blood. This major upper extremity vessel can be affected by atherosclerosis causing a rare condition, *subclavian steal syndrome*. This syndrome occurs when there is stenosis of the subclavian artery proximal to the origin of the left vertebral artery causing retrograde blood flow via a 'siphoning' effect. Blood is siphoned from the vertebrobasilar artery to the arm resulting in a wide variety of neurological symptoms such as syncope, dizziness, confusion and headache (Cosgrove, 1995). These symptoms may be incorrectly attributed to cerebrovascular disease.

Renal artery stenosis

Atherosclerosis and subsequent stenosis of one or both renal arteries reduces blood flow through the kidney, causing activation of the renin–angiotensin–aldosterone system. These potent hormones cause arteriolar constriction, salt and water retention which in turn elevates blood pressure leading to hypertension (Kumar and Clark, 1998). Hypertension is an important risk factor for the development of coronary artery disease, cerebrovascular disease and renal failure (Wood et al., 1998).

Arterial impotence

Sexual dysfunction can occur because of atherosclerotic disease of the helicine arteries of the penis and in association with aortoiliac disease leading to *Leriche syndrome.* This syndrome causes effort-produced ischaemic discomfort in the low back, buttocks and thighs and the reduced blood flow may cause impotence (Schlant and Alexander, 1994).

Coeliac and mesenteric vessel stenosis

Atherosclerosis reducing arterial blood flow to the vessels of the gut may lead to severe abdominal pain after meals (*intestinal angina*). In severe cases the gut can become severely ischaemic, leading to gut necrosis.

Cerebrovascular disease

The arterial circulation of the brain is also vulnerable to atherosclerosis, embolism and aneurysms. These pathologies are responsible for stroke caused by cerebral infarction, and transient ischaemic attacks (TIA) leading to reversible neurological dysfunction. TIA is an important prognostic indicator of stroke, since 40% of patients will have a stroke within 5 years of developing TIA (Kumar and Clark, 1998). Stroke is the third leading cause of death in the developed world (Wolf et al., 1999), and it is estimated that one person will suffer a stroke every 5 minutes in the UK (Maitland, 1999).

Pathophysiology of cerebrovascular disease

Reduced blood flow to the brain causes cerebral ischaemia and subsequent symptoms of TIA. A number of pathologies are responsible for the disturbance of cerebral blood flow. Thromboembolism is responsible for 80% of TIAs and 70% of strokes (Kumar and Clark, 1998). Major embolic sources of thrombus arise from the left side of the heart due to the following: atrial fibrillation, prosthetic heart valves, mitral valve disease and left ventricular aneurysms (Overell, 1999). These microemboli only partially interfere with blood flow, causing transient symptoms such as loss of vision in one eye because of retinal artery involvement (*amaurosis fugax*), whilst disruption of the posterior circulation causes episodes of amnesia and confusion. These symptoms are transient, lasting for minutes or hours, but resolve in less than 24 hours (Kumar and Clarke, 1998). A disrupted atherosclerotic plaque that reduces blood flow within the carotid or cerebral circulation will have the same effects as microemboli. Reduced blood flow can also be caused by cardiac failure.

A stroke causes cerebral infarction because of acute obstruction to blood flow through carotid or cerebral arteries (see Chapter 13), whilst complete occlusion of the retinal artery may lead to permanent loss of vision.

Aneurysmal disease

Aortic aneurysms

An aneurysm is a segment of an artery that has become dilated to twice its normal width (Sternbergh et al., 1998). Aneurysms are classified as *true aneurysms* or *false aneurysms* (Figure 2.2). *True aneurysms* are the commonest and involve dilatation of all three layers of the artery wall (Lilly, 1992). False aneurysms do not involve dilatation of all three layers; the dilated area is restricted to the adventitia and is caused by a hole that allows blood to track along and form a bulge within the adventitia (Lilly, 1992). False aneurysms are generally caused by infection or trauma due to arterial puncture during surgery or from arterial catheterisation during radiological angiograms (Davis et al., 1997).

True aneurysms are further classified according to their shape and can be fusiform, where the entire circumference of the affected aorta is dilated, or saccular, where only a portion of the aorta is dilated (Lilly, 1992).

Although the emphasis here is on abdominal aortic aneurysms, they can occur throughout the peripheral arterial tree; for example, iliac, popliteal, femoral, carotid subclavian and renal arteries, and others can be affected. Aneurysms affecting the aorta are described according to their location within the aorta. Thoracic aneurysms

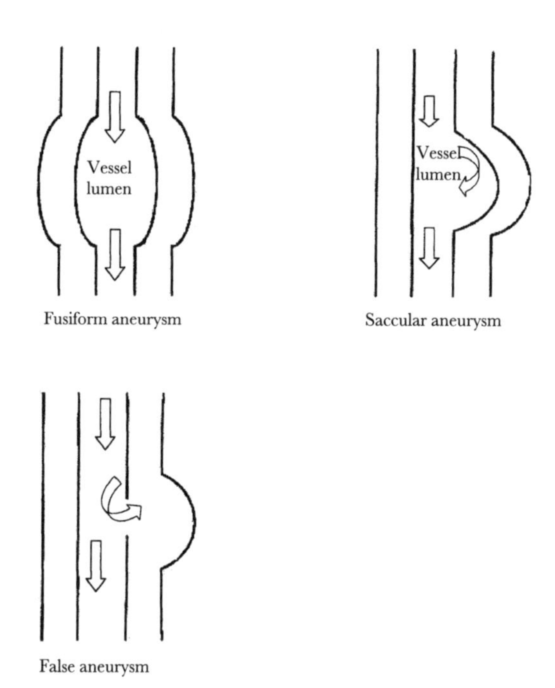

Figure 2.2 Types of aortic aneurysm. Arrows show direction of lumen blood flow and blood accumulating within the adventitia via a tear in the intima and media. (Adapted from Lilly, 1992.)

may be located at the aortic annulus, ascending aorta, aortic arch and descending aorta. Abdominal aortic aneurysms (AAAs) are located within the abdominal cavity but may extend to the thoracic region, hence the term thoraco-abdominal aneurysm.

Aetiology and pathogenesis of true aneurysms

Aneurysms are a disease of the elderly. Abdominal aortic aneurysms are the most frequent site of aneurysm formation and affect 2–5% of the male population over the age of 60 years, with a male:female ratio of 4:1 (Sternbergh et al., 1998). The exact mechanism responsible for aneurysm formation is unclear, although a variety of factors would appear to play a role. Defects in the proteins elastin and collagen responsible for recoil and strength of the vessel walls cause aortic pathology and are responsible for the collagen problems of *Ehlers–Danlos syndrome* (Izzat et al., 1994; Greenberg and Risher,

1998). Other possible mechanisms responsible for aneurysm formation may be due to increased activity of collagenase, elastase and other proteolytic enzymes that cause degeneration of the aortic wall (Sternbergh et al., 1998). Atherosclerosis may contribute to aneurysm formation, although this has been recently questioned as a direct cause, and untreated hypertension is also implicated (Sternbergh et al., 1998). There may be a genetic predisposition to aneurysms since there is a family history of AAA in 15% of patients (Sternbergh et al., 1998). Syphilis is attributable to 5% of thoracic aneurysms and classically produces saccular aneurysms (Greenberg and Risher, 1998). Aneurysms can also be caused by infections such as *Staphylococcus* and *Salmonella* (mycotic aneurysm). Bacteria gain access to the artery wall, and in combination with an inflammatory reaction, cause structural damage to the artery, inducing dilatation of the affected segment (Sunthareswaran and Horton-Szar, 1998).

Another important cause of aneurysms is *Marfan's syndrome.* This is an autosomal dominant inherited disorder linked to a genetic mutation in the fibrillin-1 gene (Greenberg and Risher, 1998). The syndrome is classically characterised by elongation of the skeletal system, e.g. long 'spider-like' fingers and asymmetry of the face. This complex disorder results in progressive aortic dilatation and aneurysm formation. The ascending portion of the aorta is particularly affected and may involve the annulus of the aortic valve. Dilatation of the valve annulus causes aortic valve regurgitation and eventually left ventricular hypertrophy and failure. Aneurysms can also occur in the peripheral vessels such as the popliteal arteries.

Other less common causes of aneurysm are trauma, particularly from deceleration injury resulting in blunt thoracic trauma (Greenberg and Risher, 1998).

Whatever the cause of the true aneurysm, the strength of the aortic wall is affected resulting in loss of elastin, which normally gives the aorta its recoil abilities, and the structural strength provided by collagen is reduced. Together with the reduction of collagen and elastin there is progressive dilatation of the aortic walls. As the diameter of the affected segment dilates, the tension within the weakened aortic wall increases (LaPlace's law), dilating it further (Greenberg and Risher, 1998). The bulging aneurysm is also responsible for turbulent blood flow in the area of dilatation which may lead to thrombus formation and become a potential source of emboli (Greenberg and Risher, 1998).

Aneurysms are frequently asymptomatic, unless the bulging wall of the aorta compresses other structures. A large abdominal aneurysm may cause erosion of the vertebrae resulting in back pain (see Chapter 12), whilst a thoracic aneurysm exerting pressure on the oesophagus can cause dysphagia, or respiratory symptoms (Lilly, 1992). Thrombus may form within the aneurysm and embolise, causing peripheral arterial symptoms such as *blue toe syndrome*.

Popliteal aneurysm

The popliteal artery is the second commonest site, with an incidence of 70% of all peripheral aneurysms; 5% are associated with abdominal aortic aneurysms (McCollum et al., 1983). The aneurysm can cause neurovascular compression leading to paresis, paraesthesia and venous compression with subsequent calf swelling (Kester and Leveson, 1981).

Splenic artery aneurysm

These are the second commonest intra-abdominal aneurysm, affecting women four times as commonly as men, especially during childbearing years. The aneurysm may be asymptomatic but may rupture in the last trimester of pregnancy (Macfarlane and Thorbjarnarson, 1966).

A major problem associated with aneurysms is the risk of rupture, which carries a high mortality. A leaking or ruptured abdominal aneurysm results in mortality rates of 50–70% (Bell, 1996). As a rule, the enlargement of an aneurysm increases the risk of rupture (see Chapter 12).

Aortic dissection

Aortic dissection is a sudden catastrophic event where blood penetrates the intima of the artery through a tear and gains access to the artery media, causing dissection of these layers (Figure 2.2). This creates an additional but false lumen which limits blood flow and obstructs arterial side branches.

Aetiology and pathogenesis

Aortic dissection commonly occurs in men in their 50s and 60s. It is strongly associated with hypertension. Marfan's syndrome is another cause due to its association with cystic medial necrosis causing fragmentation and weakening of the elastic tissue of the aorta.

The dissection can occur in the ascending aorta just above the aortic valve, and can extend up to the aortic arch and down the descending aorta (DeBakey type I dissection). This type of dissection can affect aortic valve function. If the dissection involves the adventitia of the artery, blood creates a false lumen in this layer that is continuous with the pericardium and left pleura, which can cause cardiac tamponade or haemo-pneumothorax (Izzat et al., 1994).

Type II dissections are confined to the ascending aorta, and type III dissections begin distally to the left subclavian artery and involve the descending aorta. Dissections can occlude blood flow into the arterial branches of the aorta, depriving limbs and organs of blood. The dissected aorta can also rupture into the mediastinum and retroperitoneally resulting in massive haemorrhage and sudden death (Izzat et al., 1994).

Inflammatory vascular disease

Although atherosclerosis is the commonest cause of peripheral vascular disease, other disease processes can mimic the symptoms of atherosclerosis. These diseases are caused by an immune mediated inflammatory process affecting arteries and sometimes veins. Inflammation of the artery, or arteritis or vasculitis, can reduce the size of the lumen and subsequent blood flow through the narrowed segment. The following presents an overview of inflammatory vascular disease.

Systemic vasculitides is a term that refers to a collection of vascular diseases characterised by an inflammatory process that damages the vessel walls, resulting in a vasculitis. The trigger of the inflammatory process may be infective, immune-mediated or idiopathic (Senthareswaran and Horton-Szar, 1998).

The vasculitides are classified as a medical emergency, since a delay in diagnosis and treatment may result in organ damage and failure (Savage, 1998a).

The following provides an overview of the vasculitides according to the vessels affected.

Large vessel vasculitis

Large arteries are classified as the aorta and the largest branches that supply major body organs, the extremities, head and neck (Jennette et al., 1994). Two idiopathic disease processes affecting these vessels are giant cell (temporal) arteritis and Takayasu's arteritis.

Giant cell (temporal) arteritis

This was first described in 1889. Giant cell arteritis affects about 20/100 000 of the worldwide population, and is four times more common in women than in men after the age of 50 years. It typically affects large and medium size arteries such as the temporal, vertebral, ophthalmic and posterior ciliary vessels, and in about 15% of patients the aorta is also affected (Gordon, 1998).

The inflammatory process involves infiltration of the vessel adventitia, media and internal elastic lamina by the following immune cells: lymphocytes, macrophages and multinucleated giant cells (Gordon, 1998). These immune cells can initiate or release a cocktail of destructive chemicals that damage the vessel wall (Lilly, 1992). This cellular infiltration also results in granuloma formation. The subsequent healing process causes the replacement of elastic tissue with fibrotic scar tissue and destruction of the vasa vasorum, the small blood vessels that supply the walls of larger vessels (Gordon, 1998). The damaging effects of inflammation and subsequent healing process cause irregular intimal thickening of the affected vessels. In some cases this will result in narrowing or stenosis of the vessel, and may also cause aneurysm formation.

The combination of inflammation and stenosis causes ischaemia of the tissue downstream to the affected vessels, which may give rise to the following symptoms: *temporal artery arteritis* causes a unilateral, temporal, throbbing headache. The diseased artery may also cause facial pain and claudication of the jaw muscles when speaking or chewing, both of which will increase blood supply demands that may not be met due to the narrowed vessel lumen. Occipital headaches, vertigo, hearing loss and ataxia may occur with *vertebrobasilar arteritis* (Gordon, 1998).

Complete or partial visual loss may occur with ocular artery involvement, and blindness may occur if treatment is not started promptly (Gordon, 1998).

Takayasu's arteritis

Also called 'pulseless' disease, this was first described in 1908. This form of arteritis shares a similar pathological process to giant cell arteritis but affects a much younger age group (<40 years). It affects ten times more women than men, and is more common in Asia and the Far East (Gordon, 1998)

Takayasu's arteritis affects the large arteries such as the aorta and its main branches. Aortic arch syndrome occurs when the disease affects arteries of the upper extremities, heart and neck. This may result in arm claudication, and absence of brachial and radial pulses. Aortic valve regurgitation may occur because of aortic root dilation and there is also a risk of aortic aneurysm and dissection (Gordon, 1998). Inflammation and subsequent narrowing of the brachiocephalic or carotid artery can cause cerebrovascular ischaemia, whilst affected coronary arteries cause myocardial ischaemia (Lilly, 1992).

Both giant cell arteritis and Takayasu's arteritis cause non-specific symptoms associated with inflammatory disease such as: fever, night sweats, malaise and weight loss (Gordon, 1998).

Polyarteritis nodosa (PAN)

PAN is another form of vasculitis which affects medium and small arteries and occasionally arterioles. It is sometimes associated with hepatitis B virus infection which would appear to lead to the formation of immune complexes that may have a role in the causation of arteritis. PAN may also follow acute respiratory infection and acute haemolytic streptococcus infection. PAN may occur as a side effect of drugs such as sulphonamides, penicillin and immunisations. It is uncommon in the UK and affects both men and women over the age of 50 years (Savage, 1998b).

Cells of the immune system (neutrophils and mononuclear cells) infiltrate all three vessel layers, causing fibrinoid necrosis and occlusion of the lumen. The elasticity of the vessel wall is disrupted, which weakens the wall and leads to dilatation and aneurysm formation.

Occlusion of the vessel lumen results in tissue ischaemia downstream to the affected vessel. The resultant ischaemia and/or occlusion of medium size arteries are responsible for renal infarction leading to renal failure, angina, myocardial infarction, gastrointestinal tract haemorrhage, infarction or perforation (Savage, 1998b).

Kawasaki disease

This form of arteritis affects medium size arteries, and in particular the coronary arteries. It affects children between 6 months and 8 years of age, and is commonest in Japanese children (Savage, 1998b).

There is a seasonal variation in the disease, which suggests an infective cause. Various microorganisms and their toxins are implicated, such as staphylococcal enterotoxins, toxic shock syndrome toxin and streptococcal erythrogenic toxin (Gordon, 1998). The toxins of these microorganisms would appear to trigger a T-cell immune mediated response that causes a number of immune cells to infiltrate all three layers of the artery wall (Gordon, 1998). The damaging effects of the activated immune response affect the ostia (opening) and entire length of the coronary artery, resulting in the formation of aneurysms causing weakening of the arterial wall. Thrombus can form within the aneurysm; if this occludes the vessel, myocardial infarction will occur and is the main cause of death. Healing of the coronary lesions causes thickening of the artery wall and narrowing of the lumen, which may result in angina and late deaths due to myocardial infarction (Gordon, 1998). The disease can affect other medium size arteries with similar outcomes to the tissues of the affected arteries.

Thromboangiitis obliterans (Buerger's disease)

Thromboangiitis obliterans (TAO) is also known as Buerger's disease after Leo Buerger first described it in 1908 (cited by Aqel and Olin, 1997). TAO produces the same symptoms and complications as intermittent claudication but has a different epidemiological and pathological profile.

TAO has a worldwide distribution but is more prevalent in Middle, Near and Far Eastern countries than in Western Europe and North America. Age at presentation of the disease tends to be in the 15–40 year age group, which is a much younger age range in comparison to those affected by PAOD due to atherosclerosis (Mishima, 1996).

TAO was at first thought to be exclusively a disease of men who are heavy smokers and rare in women (Mills and Porter, 1993). There is an increasing incidence of TAO in women, probably because an increasing number of women are smoking. Although smoking clearly influences the progression of TAO, and stopping smoking prevents its progression (Terry et al., 1998), it is not clear how smoking influences the disease process.

TAO is a hypercellular, occlusive thrombotic process due to inflammation that affects small and medium arteries, and veins, predominantly of the lower limbs, although it can affect vessels of the upper limbs (Mishima, 1996; Aqel and Olin, 1997). It has been hypothesised that some patients may be allergic to some of the chemicals inhaled from cigarette smoke, which provokes an inflammatory immune response (Aqel and Olin, 1997) affecting all layers of the vessel. The vessel wall inflammation is associated with an occlusive thrombus which is surrounded by various cells of the non-specific immune system such as neutrophils, basophils and eosinophils, although the vessel wall above and below the thrombus remains unaffected (Mishima, 1996; Aqel and Olin, 1997).

The presence of the thrombus impedes forward blood flow, depriving tissues beyond the thrombus of oxygen and nutrients. This results in ischaemic limb pain. Typically, patients present with symptoms of intermittent claudication of their feet, calf and sometimes the hands. A proportion of patients go on to develop ischaemic cutaneous ulcers and gangrene of the toes and fingers (Aqel and Olin, 1997). Severe ischaemia also causes paraesthesia of the affected limb. Venous involvement results in thrombophlebitis of the superficial veins.

Raynaud's phenomenon

First described by Maurice Raynaud in 1862, Raynaud's phenomenon (RP) is a blanket term describing cold-related vasospasm of the microvascular circulation (Ho and Belch, 1998). The patient experiences episodic spasm of cutaneous digital arteries of the hands, feet, nose, ears, and sometimes the nipples; subsequently the skin becomes dry, the nails brittle and ulceration and gangrene can occur (Turton et al., 1998). The arterial spasm causes arterial insufficiency resulting in digital ischaemia. The sufferer experiences cyanosis and pallor of the affected tissues, which may also be associated with numbness and tingling (Turton et al., 1998). When blood flow returns, there is reactive hyperaemia causing rubor or red flushing of the affected tissues (Khan, 1999). The vasospasm can be induced by cold environmental temperature, emotional stress, smoking and hormonal changes, as well as trauma caused by local vibration from vibrating tools (Khan, 1999).

The prevalence of Raynaud's is 16% in men and 21% in women (Turton et al., 1998). Studies reported by Chetter et al. (1998) have found this to rise to 50% in those involved in using vibrating tools such as electrical drills and food processors.

The pathophysiological mechanisms of this disease are not clearly defined although it would appear that patients have microvascular hyperreactivity to sympathetic nervous stimulation. This, along with increased sensitivity and/or density of peripheral alpha-adrenergic receptors, causes episodic vasoconstriction (Khan, 1999). Other pathological factors thought to have an influence on vasospasm induction are endothelial damage resulting in inactivity of the potent vasodilator nitric oxide (NO), along with possible haematological factors causing coagulation, fibrinolysis and reperfusion injury (Turton et al., 1998; Khan, 1999).

Thoracic outlet compression syndrome

Thoracic outlet compression syndrome (TOCS) causes a variety of symptoms and signs because of compression of the nerves of the brachial plexus, subclavian artery and vein (Atasoy, 1996). According to Atasoy (1996), the brachial plexus is most commonly affected by compression followed by the subclavian vein and lastly the artery.

Compression of the brachial plexus causes pain, paraesthesia, motor weakness, and in rare cases atrophy of the upper limbs (Atasoy, 1996).

Compression of the subclavian vein increases intravenous pressure within the vessels of the arm and hand, causing pain, oedema, venous distension, cyanosis, and thrombus formation because of venous stasis and collateral vein formation (Atasoy, 1996).

Compression of the subclavian artery may cause loss of brachial and radial pulses, motor weakness, claudication, thrombosis with peripheral emboli and necrosis. Symptoms may be very similar to those associated with Raynaud's phenomenon (Atasoy, 1996).

Brachial plexus compression is more common than vascular compression, and is also more difficult to diagnose because of insufficient measurable signs and symptoms at examination (Atasoy, 1996; Novak and Mackinnon, 1996).

The causes of TOCS are osseous or soft tissue related, both of which can cause narrowing of the thoracic inlet which can compress the nerves and vessels running through this channel. Osseous causes of TOCS affect 30% of patients and include a prominent cervical rib affecting 0.4% of the population; this is a bony process from the C7 vertebra. Other causes are prominent callus formation from fractures of the first rib or clavicle and congenital rib abnormalities (Atasoy, 1996).

Soft tissue causes of TOCS may result from the formation of congenital bands and ligaments which restrict the thoracic inlet. Trauma to the scalene muscle causes inflammatory changes that result in spasm, scarring, contractures and increases in muscle fibre mass, causing narrowing of the thoracic inlet and symptoms of compression (Atasoy, 1996). Scalene hypertrophy leading to TOCS also occurs in gymnasts, swimmers and body builders.

Popliteal artery entrapment syndrome

First described by a medical student in 1879, this condition was thought to be rare; although the true incidence of this condition is unknown, it is now thought that there is a higher prevalence of bilateral disease than previously indicated (Levien and Veller, 1999). The condition can occur when the origin of the medial gastrocnemius muscle head is abnormal and can be caused by other muscles compressing the popliteal artery during contraction; it also involves the popliteal vein in up to one-third of cases (Levien and Veller, 1999). It is seen in young patients who are athletes or those in military service (Levien and Veller, 1999).

Patients usually present with intermittent claudication, often in the absence of risk factors for atheroma. Acute ischaemic symptoms of critical limb ischaemia may occur if the vessel becomes thrombosed or aneurysmal (Levien and Veller, 1999).

Vascular tumours

Vascular tumours are very uncommon and may be either benign or malignant.

Benign vascular tumours

Angiomas are a collection of dilated capillaries and are better described as malformations than tumours.

A *glomus* tumour is an angioma that has developed within specialised skin thermoregulatory organs. The majority of these are found on the arm, with 50% located on the fingers and a third under the fingernails. Women are more likely to develop these lesions on their fingers whilst men develop them on their trunks. These lesions affect adults in their 20s. Glomus tumours are very painful, causing a severe burning sensation.

Malignant tumours

Angiosarcoma

These rapidly growing tumours develop in young men and women, forming a fragile vascular tumour which manifests in the lung. Angiosarcomas may arise from longstanding angiomas. If an existing angioma starts to enlarge, this should be suspected.

Kaposi's haemangiosarcoma

The incidence of these malignant skin lesions has increased with the advent of AIDS. Prior to AIDS these lesions were associated with old age. They start to form in the lower limbs as a bluish-red spot, which is followed by the formation of multiple spots that coalesce into one. These then metastasise to the lungs and liver and have a poor prognosis.

Carotid body tumour

These are rare tumours found equally in men and women with a peak incidence in the 5th decade of life. There may be a genetic component to their cause, and a possible link with chronic hypoxia. They may have the potential to become malignant, and as they enlarge the risk of metastases to lymph nodes, liver and lungs increases.

Hyperhidrosis

Hyperhidrosis, although not a vascular disease, is traditionally treated by vascular surgeons. The condition causes excessive sweating from the eccrine glands located over the entire body surface. They are particularly abundant on the palms, soles, face and axillae (Leung et al., 1999). Hyperhidrosis affects between 0.6 and 1% of the general population, with more women than men seeking treatment (Leung et al., 1999). The cause of this condition is unknown but the sweat glands and their sympathetic nerve supply are normal. However, there are numerous factors, such as emotion, environmental temperature, exercise, too much clothing, that can trigger excessive sweating. Additionally, there are a number of medical conditions that cause hyperhidrosis such as endocrine and metabolic disorders, drug, toxin and substance abuse, respiratory failure, cutaneous disease and spinal cord injury (Leung et al., 1999). Excessive production causes social problems for the sufferer, leading to embarrassment, low self-esteem and social isolation.

Venous disease

Thromboembolic disease

Deep vein thrombosis (DVT) is the abnormal formation of a thrombus within the deep veins of the calf, thigh or pelvis. The thrombus is composed of a fibrin network with erythrocytes, platelets and leukocytes adhering to this surface (Hirsh and Hoak, 1996). The incidence of DVT amongst hospitalised patients increases with age and may be as high as 60% in orthopaedic patients. The incidence in those aged between 65 and 69 years is 1–3 per 1000, rising to 2–8 per 1000 in those aged between 85 and 89 years (Kniffin et al., 1994).

Venous thromboembolism may cause death due to a *pulmonary embolism*. Pulmonary embolism occurs when a fragment of the thrombus becomes detached from its site of origin, usually from the veins proximal to the popliteal vein (Shetty, 1997), from where it is circulated to the pulmonary circulation, causing obstruction of a branch or branches of the pulmonary artery. Pulmonary embolism originating from the calf vein is rare because these thrombi tend to be small and are unlikely to occlude major branches of the pulmonary artery, whilst embolism originating from the proximal vein carries a 40–50% risk of pulmonary embolism (Kakkar et al, 1969). Death may result from pulmonary embolism if 50% or more of the pulmonary artery is occluded by thrombus or there are multiple small thrombi (Moser, 1977). The pulmonary embolism or multiple emboli cause pulmonary hypertension (cor pulmonale), which decreases cardiac output from the right ventricle. The increased pulmonary vascular resistance causes right ventricular failure, which may be acute with a large embolism or may be more a gradual process as the right ventricle gradually enlarges and fails to pump effectively against the increased resistance through the pulmonary circulation. Right ventricular failure compromises systemic cardiac output leading to hypotension and shock (Wilkins and Dexter, 1993).

It is estimated that 1 in 10 000 men, and 1.5 in 10 000 women die each year in the UK from pulmonary embolism and DVT (Hopkins and Wolfe, 1991). Chronic venous leg ulcers are also a complication that may follow DVT (Perkins and Galland, 1999).

Aetiology and pathophysiology of thromboembolism

Abnormal blood clotting can occur due to the following causative factors: venous stasis, hypercoagulation states and vessel trauma (*Virchow's triad*).

Venous stasis commonly occurs during periods of immobility, because of prolonged bedrest in excess of 4 days, limb paralysis, perioperatively and because of heart failure (Perkins and Galland, 1999). Venous stasis may also be caused by any type of travel with a duration in excess of 4 hours (Ferrari et al., 1999). The risk of DVT increases in malignancy and pregnancy (Hirsh and Hoak, 1996).

Venous return is reduced by half in the standing position and by two-thirds in the sitting position, leading to venous stasis in the deep veins (Ferrari et al., 1999). Blood stasis is further increased by any pressure exerted by the edge of a chair or due to sitting with the legs crossed. An hour of quiet sitting causes an increased haematocrit and plasma protein concentration in excess of 25% (Ferrari et al., 1999). Venous stasis impairs clearance of the activated coagulation factors, predisposing the patient to a hypercoaguable state and thrombosis formation (Hirsh and Hoak, 1996). Air travel carries additional risks that can predispose the individual to thrombosis. Dehydration appears to occur more rapidly, despite a fluid intake normally regarded as adequate (Ferrari et al., 1999). Reduced cabin air pressure during air travel decreases haemoglobin saturation and appears to reduce spontaneous endothelial fibrinolysis, a natural process that dissolves thrombus.

Regardless of the causes of DVT, they are frequently undiagnosed because they may cause few or only minor clinical signs and symptoms. When symptoms do exist the affected limb is swollen and tender. If the vein becomes completely occluded by thrombus, the leg becomes pale and may compromise arterial perfusion (*phlegmasia alba dolens*) (Schlant and Alexander, 1994), whereas a massive proximal thrombus leads to a blue leg because of marked swelling and cyanosis (*phlegmasia cerulea dolens*) (Shetty, 1997).

DVT may cause chronic disease in some patients due to persistent leg swelling and pain because of venous valve damage. The thrombotic process responsible for valvular damage leads to venous hypertension, varicose vein formation and possible skin ulceration (Hirsh and Hoak, 1996).

Varicose veins

Varicose veins are the commonest condition affecting the venous circulation. All peripheral veins have valves which prevent the backflow of blood and facilitate venous return to the right atrium of the heart. Dysfunction of these valves allows backflow of blood, resulting in *venous hypertension* and causing the vein to become distended and tortuous.

Varicose veins affect about 20% of the adult population, whilst a greater percentage will develop small thread-like veins (*telangiectasia*) (Murie and Callam, 1999). Varicose veins develop very slowly and may present initially as minor venous telangiectasia in the skin, progressing to chronic venous insufficiency which may be associated with venous ulcers (Murie and Callam, 1999). Telangiectasia are a localised collection of distended capillary vessels, which appear as thin and thread-like and are easily visible under the skin surface. These probably occur due to an increase in local venous pressure resulting from valvular incompetence which causes distension of the capillary circulation.

Varicosities can affect any vein; the commonest veins affected are the long and short saphenous veins of the lower limbs (Chapter 7).

However, varices may develop in the anorectal region causing haemorrhoids, whilst varicose veins affecting the oesophagus are referred to as oesophageal varices.

Pathophysiology of varicose veins

It remains controversial whether varicose veins are due to a primary genetic defect affecting the valves or to an abnormality affecting the vein wall resulting in dilatation which prevents the valve functioning effectively (Murie and Callam, 1999). Regardless of the cause of the underlying pathology, the primary mechanism responsible for varicose veins is incompetence of the valves, which results in retrograde flow (backflow) of blood in the vein. The backflow of blood causes venous hypertension and the vein becomes distorted because of excessive lengthening and dilatation. There are two types of varicose veins: *primary*, where the underlying cause is unknown, and *secondary*, where they occur following DVT, pregnancy or due to pelvic malignancy.

Varices of the lower limbs are easily observed as they may be superficial, lying in the subcutaneous fat causing the skin overlying the affected veins to take on a knotty appearance.

There is a widely held belief that younger women are more commonly affected by varicose veins than men. However, this is not borne out by epidemiological studies that suggest the prevalence of varices is similar in both sexes (Callam, 1994; Murie and Callam, 1999). However, older women who have had children have a higher prevalence of varicose veins, although it is unclear whether pregnancy accelerates the disease process or is an independent risk factor (Murie and Callam, 1999). Other factors such as obesity, occupation and race may play a role in the development of varicose veins, but it is unclear whether these factors are a cause or simply worsen the primary cause.

Deep vein thrombosis is a secondary cause of varicose veins, causing an increase in venous blood pressure distal to the thrombosis which affects the competence of the valve (Murie and Callam, 1999). The dysfunctioning venous valves lead to venous insufficiency and venous hypertension. Longstanding venous hypertension causes haemosiderin deposits to form in the skin, resulting in the formation of brown pigmentation near the ankle, whilst lipodermatosclerosis causes a palpable induration and scarring of the skin which probably reflects severe tissue injury (Coleridge-Smith, 1997). Venous hypertension also causes increased capillary permeability with loss of proteins particularly fibrinogen. This process would appear to favour the formation of fibrin complexes that further compromise the circulation (Langemo, 1999). Additionally, there is increasing evidence that venous hypertension causes white blood cell trapping within the capillaries, and the low blood flow favours leukocyte adhesion to the capillary walls. The inflammatory response mediated by these leukocytes may be responsible for further capillary damage, which further reduces cutaneous blood supply (Coleridge-Smith, 1997). These pathological processes allow the formation of tissue oedema which in normal circumstances is returned to the circulation by the lymphatic system. However, patients with venous hypertension also have reduced lymphatic drainage (Bull et al., 1993). These multiple pathological insults of venous hypertension set the substrate for venous ulcer formation (see Chapter 8).

Venous ulcers are an area of sloughing necrosed skin tissue usually located at the medial malleolus (inner aspect of the ankle) (Langemo, 1999). The cause of venous ulceration is attributed to venous hypertension and the processes described above. However, the exact mechanisms responsible for venous ulceration remain unclear (Coleridge-Smith, 1997).

The clinical manifestation of varicose veins varies. Some individuals are asymptomatic, but may be concerned about the ugly appearance of the veins. Others may experience a range of symptoms such as pain, thrombophlebitis, bleeding and subsequent bruising, lipodermatosclerosis and eczema. Chronic venous insufficiency leads to symptoms of itching, ankle and calf swelling, venous claudication and varicose ulcers (Murie and Callam, 1999).

Lymphoedema

Oedema is the accumulation of tissue fluid within tissues, and is usually caused by the generalised conditions shown in Table 2.2. Lymphoedema is principally due to a problem with the lymphatic system, most commonly affecting the limbs (Figure 2.3), genitalia and face. It can be classified as primary or secondary, the causes of which are shown in Table 2.2.

Table 2.2 Causes of oedema and lymphoedema

Primary lymphoedema	Secondary lymphoedema	Oedema
Idiopathic	Filariasis	Renal, hepatic, cardiac failure
Congenital	Tuberculosis	Low plasma proteins
Familial	Tumour excision and radiotherapy	Idiopathic cyclic oedema
	Lymphoedema artefacta	Post-thrombotic syndrome
		Secondary venous obstruction, e.g. pregnancy, pelvic mass

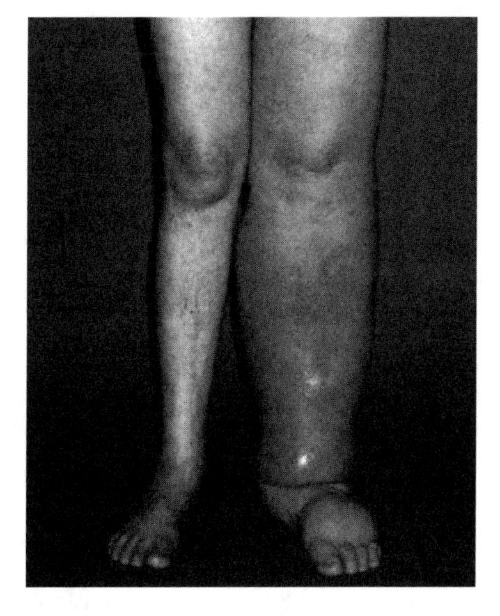

Figure 2.3 Lymphoedema of the left leg. (Courtesy of Professor P. Mortimer, St George's Hospital, London.)

It is usually easy to differentiate with a clinical examination.

The cause of primary lymphoedema is uncertain, but thought to be either increased lymph formation or decreased clearance. Lymphatic vessels have been shown histologically to be abnormal with inflammatory infiltrate, and nodes show evidence of fibrosis. There may be a genetic component, e.g. Milroy's disease responsible for 3% of cases, where it may be that infection or trauma act as a trigger.

Secondary lymphoedema is generally caused by infection, e.g. filarial worms (Williams, 1997) and tuberculosis. However, in the UK, surgical block dissection and radiotherapy, e.g. post-mastectomy, is a more common cause (28% of cases in one health district) (Mortimer et al, 1996). Lymphoedema artefacta is a patient-induced condition caused by restrictive bands around arms or legs that impede lymph drainage.

Acknowledgement

The author would like to thank Stella Vig for helpful discussion and checking the typescript.

References

Anon (1964) Smoking and Health: Report of the Advisory Committee to the Surgeon General of the Public Service. Washington DC: Government Printing Office.

Anon (1998) Cholesterol and coronary heart disease: screening and treatment. Effective Health Care 4(1): 1–15.

Aqel B, Olin JW (1997) Thromboangiitis obliterans (Buerger's disease) Vascular Medicine 2: 61–66.

Atasoy E (1996) Thoracic outlet compression syndrome. Orthopedic Clinics of North America 27(2): 265–288.

Bell P (1996) Leaking abdominal aortic aneurysms. Care of the Critically Ill 12(2): 59–61.

Bull RH, Gane JN, Evans JE, Joseph AE, Mortimer PS (1993) Abnormal lymph drainage in patients with chronic venous ulcers. Journal of the American Academic Dermatology 28: 585–590.

Callam MJ (1994) Epidemiology of varicose veins. British Journal of Surgery 81: 167–173.

Campbell RWF (1998a) Management of unstable coronary artery disease. Clinical Cardiology 21: 314–322.

Campbell R (1998b) Atrial fibrillation. European Heart Journal 19(Suppl E): E41–45.

Chetter IC, Kent PJ, Kester RC (1998) The hand arm vibration syndrome: a review. Cardiovascular Surgery 6(1): 1–9.

Coleridge-Smith PD (1997) The microcirculation in venous disease. Vascular Medicine 2: 203–213.

Cooke JP (1997) The pathophysiology of peripheral arterial disease: rational targets for drug intervention. Vascular Medicine 2: 227–230.

Cosgrove LE (1995) Coronary-subclavian steal after CABG surgery. Critical Care Nurse 15(3): 19–22.

Criqui MH, Deneberg JO, Langer RD, Fronek A (1997) The epidemiology of peripheral arterial disease: importance of identifying the population at risk. Vascular Medicine 2: 221–226.

Davies MJ (1994) Pathology of arterial thrombosis. British Medical Bulletin 50: 789–802.

Davies MJ (1997) The role of plaque pathology in coronary thrombosis. Clinical Cardiology 20(Suppl I): 1–7.

Davis C, Longstreet J, Moscucci M (1997) Vascular complications of coronary interventions. Heart, Lung 26(2): 118–127.

Doering LV (1999) Pathophysiology of acute coronary syndromes leading to acute myocardial infarction. Journal of Cardiovascular Nursing 13(3): 1–20.

Doll R, Peto R (1976) Mortality in relation to smoking: 20 years observation on male British doctors. British Medical Journal ii: 1525–1536.

Dormandy J, Heeck L, Vig S (1999a) Predicting which patients will develop chronic critical leg ischaemia. Seminars in Vascular Surgery 12(2): 138–141.

Dormandy J, Heeck L, Vig S (1999b) Acute limb ischaemia. Seminars in Vascular Surgery 12(2): 148–153.

Dormandy J, Heeck L, Vig S (1999c) Lower-extremity arteriosclerosis as a reflection of a systemic process: Implications for concomitant coronary and carotid disease. Seminars in Vascular Surgery 12(2): 118–122.

Fahey VA (1994) Vascular Nursing. Philadelphia: WB Saunders.

Ferrari E, Chevallier T, Chapelier A, Baudouy M (1999) Travel as a risk factor for venous thromboembolic disease. Chest 115: 440–444.

Furberg C, Hennekens C, Hulley S, Manolio T, Psaty B, Whelton PK (1996) Task Force 2. Clinical epidemiology: The conceptual basis for interpreting risk factors. Journal of the American College of Cardiology 27(5): 976–978.

Fuster V, Gotto A, Libby P, Loscalzo J, McGill H (1996) Task Force 1. Pathogenesis of coronary disease: The biological role of risk factors. Journal of the American College of Cardiology 27(5): 964–1047.

Gensini GF, Comeglio M, Colella A (1998) Classical risk factors and emerging elements in the risk profile for coronary artery disease. European Heart Journal 19(Suppl A): A53–61.

Gordon C (1998) Large vessel vasculitides. Medicine 26(4): 18–19.

Greenberg R, Risher W (1998) Clinical decision making and operative approach to thoracic aortic aneurysms. Surgical Clinics of North America 78(5): 805–826.

Gronholdt M-LM, Dalager-Pedersen S, Falk E (1998). Coronary atherosclerosis: determinants of plaque rupture. European Heart Journal 19(Suppl C): C24–29.

Grubb NR, Fox AA (1999) Pathophysiology, pharmacology and medical treatment of angina. Trends in Cardiology and Vascular Disease 1(4): 39–45.

Gurfinkel E, Bozoviich G Daroca A, Beck E, Mautner B (1997) Randomised trial of roxithromycin in non-Q-wave coronary syndromes: ROXIS pilot study. Lancet 350: 404–407.

Hankey GJ, Elkeboom J (1999) Homocysteine and vascular disease. Lancet 354: 407–413.

Hirsh J, Hoak J (1996) AHA Medical/Scientific Statement: Management of deep vein thrombosis and pulmonary embolism. Circulation 93: 2212–2245.

Ho M, Belch JJ (1998) Raynaud's Phenomenon: State of the Art 1998. Scandinavian Journal of Rheumatology 27: 319–322.

Hopkins NFG, Wolfe JHN (1991) Thrombosis and pulmonary embolism. British Medical Journal 303: 1260–1261.

Ierardi RP, Shuman CR (1998) Control of vascular disease in patients with diabetes mellitus. Surgical Clinics of North America 78(3): 385–392.

Izzat MB, Jones AJ, Angelini GD (1994) Acute aortic dissection. British Journal of Hospital Medicine 52(10): 523–528.

Jennette JC, Falk RJ, Andrassy K et al. (1994) Nomenclature of systemic vasculitides: The Proposal of an International Consensus Conference. Arthritis and Rheumatism 37: 187–192.

Kakkar VV, Flank C, Howe CT, Clarke MB (1969) Natural history of deep vein thrombosis. Lancet ii: 230–232.

Kannel WB, Skinner JJ, Schwartz MJ, Shirtless D (1970) Intermittent claudication: incidence in the Framingham study. Circulation 41: 875–883.

Kassianos G (1999) Dallas: Short news from the AHA: Homocysteine and the heart. Trends in Cardiology and Vascular Disease 1(3): 18.

Kester RC, Leveson SHE (1981) A Practice of Vascular Surgery. London: Pitman.

Khan F (1999) Vascular abnormalities in Raynaud's phenomenon. Scottish Medical Journal 44(1): 4–5.

Kniffin WD, Baron JA, Barrett J, Birkmeyer JD, Anderson FA (1994) The epidemiology of diagnosed pulmonary embolism and deep venous thrombosis in the elderly. Archives of Internal Medicine 154: 861–866.

Knight CJ (1999) New insights into the pathophysiology of acute coronary occlusion. European Heart Journal 1(Suppl F): F3–6.

Kumar PJ, Clark ML (1998) Clinical Medicine. London: WB Saunders.

Kuo CC, Grayston JT, Campbell LA, Goo YA, Wissler RW, Benditt EP (1995) Chlamydia pneumoniae (TWAR) in coronary arteries of young adults (15–34 years old). Proceedings of the National Academy of Sciences, USA 92: 6911–6914.

Langemo K (1999) Venous ulcers: Etiology and care of patients treated with human skin equivalent grafts. Journal of Vascular Nursing 17(1): 6–11.

Leung A, Chan PYH, Choi ACK (1999) Hyperhidrosis. International Journal of Dermatology 38: 561–567.

Levien L, Veller MG (1999) Popliteal artery entrapment syndrome: More common than previously recognised. Journal of Vascular Surgery 30(4): 587–598.

Libby P (1996) Atheroma: More than mush. Lancet 348(Suppl 1): 4–7.

Lilly LS (ed.) (1992) Pathophysiology of Heart Disease. Philadelphia: Lea & Febiger.

Macfarlane JR, Thorbjarnarson B (1966) Rupture of splenic artery aneurysm during pregnancy. American Journal of Obstetrics and Gynecology 95(7): 1025–1037.

Maitland JM (1999) Primary care of stroke patients. Trends in Cardiology and Vascular Disease 1(6): 25–28.

McBride P (1992) The health consequences of smoking: Cardiovascular diseases. Medical Clinics of North America 76: 333–353.

McGrae-McDermott M, McCarthy W (1995) Intermittent claudication: The natural history. Surgical Clinics of North America 75(4): 581–591.

McCollum CH, De Bakey ME, Myhre MO (1983) Popliteal aneurysms: Results of 87 operations performed between 1957–1977. Cardiovascular Research 21(4): 93–100.

Mills JL, Porter JM (1993) Buerger's disease: a review and update. Seminars in Vascular Surgery 6: 14–23.

Mishima Y (1996) Thromboangiitis obliterans (Buerger's disease) International Journal of Cardiology 54(Suppl): S185–187.

Mortimer PS, Bates DO, Brassington HD (1996) The prevalence of arm oedema following treatment for breast cancer. Quarterly Journal of Medicine 89: 377–380.

Moser KM (1977) Pulmonary embolism. American Review of Respiratory Disease 115: 829.

Murie J, Callam MJ (1999) Causes, risks and assessment of varicose veins. Trends in Cardiology and Vascular Disease 1(3): 35–39.

Novak C, Mackinnon SE (1996) Thoracic outlet syndrome. Orthopedic Clinics of North America 27(4): 747–757.

O'Brien SP, Mureebe L, Lossing A, Kertein MD (1998) Epidemiology, risk factors and management of peripheral vascular disease. Ostomy/Wound Management 44(9): 68–75.

Overell JR (1999) Cardiac causes of stroke. Trends in Cardiology and Vascular Disease 1(4): 13–14.

Pasternak R, Grundy S, Levy D, Thompson P (1996) Task Force 3. Spectrum of risk factors for coronary artery disease. Journal of the American College of Cardiology 27(5): 978–1047.

Perkins J, Galland B (1999) Venous thrombosis and pulmonary embolism: Part 1. Prevention. Care of the Critically Ill 15(4): 140–143.

Rivard A, Fabre J, Silver M, Chen D, Murohara T, Kearney M, Magner M, Asahara T, Isner J (1999) Age-dependent impairment of angiogenesis. Circulation 99: 111–120.

Robertson WB (1967) International atherosclerosis project. Pathologia Microbiologia 30(5): 810–816.

Sans S, Kesteloot H, Kromout D (1997) The burden of cardiovascular disease mortality in Europe. European Heart Journal 18: 1231–1248.

Savage CO (1998a) Systemic vasculitides: An overview. Medicine 26(4): 12–13.

Savage CO (1998b) Medium vessel vasculitides. Medicine 26(4): 14–15.

Schlant R, Alexander RW (1994) Hurst's – The Heart: Companion Handbook. New York: McGraw Hill.

Shah P (1997) New insights into the pathogenesis and prevention of acute coronary syndromes. American Journal of Cardiology 70(12B): 17–23.

Shetty HG (1997) Management of deep vein thrombosis. Prescribers' Journal 37(3): 166–172.

Stary HC, Chandler B, Dinsmore RE, Fuster V, Glagov S, Insull W, Rosenfeld M, Schwartz CJ, Wagner W, Wissler R (1995) A definition of advanced types of atherosclerotic lesions and a histological classification of atherosclerosis. Circulation 92(5): 1355–1374.

Sternbergh WC, Gonze MD, Garrard CL, Money S (1998) Abdominal and thoracicoabdominal aortic aneurysm. Surgical Clinics of North America 78(5): 827–834.

Sunthareswaran R, Horton-Szar D (1998) Cardiovascular System. London: Mosby.

Terry ML, Berkowitz HD, Kerstein MD (1998) Tobacco: its impact on vascular disease. Surgical Clinics of North America 78(3): 409–427.

Toutouzas PC, Tousoulis D, Davies GJ (1998) Nitric oxide synthesis in atherosclerosis. European Heart Journal 19: 1504–1511.

Turton EPL, Kent PJ, Kester RC (1998) The aetiology of Raynaud's phenomenon. Cardiovascular Surgery 6(5): 431–440.

Wilkins RL, Dexter JR (1993) Respiratory Disease: Principles of Patient Care. Philadelphia: FA Davis Company.

Williams A (1997) Lymphoedema. Professional Nurse 12(9): 645–648.

Wood D, De Backer G, Faergeman O, Grahm I, Mancia G, Pyorala K et al. (1998) Prevention of coronary heart disease in clinical practice: Recommendations of the second Joint Task Force of European and other Societies on Coronary Prevention. European Heart Journal 19: 1434–1503.

Wolf PA, Clagett GP, Easton JD, Goldstein LB, Gorelick PB, Kelly-Hayes M, Sacco RL, Whisnant JP (1999) Preventing ischaemic stroke in patients with prior stroke and transient ischaemic attack. Stroke 30: 1991–1994.

CHAPTER 3

Promoting Health in Vascular Nursing

BELINDA LITCHFIELD

Introduction

The promotion of health in vascular nursing is a pivotal and ongoing responsibility of the nurse. Whether a patient has no overt vascular problems, little or very serious vascular pathology, the prevention of disease is of paramount importance for the best possible health outcome. The nurse will need to assist patients to make lifestyle changes from the earliest stages of disease, for example, from the time that claudication is first diagnosed through to the period when aiding patient recovery following surgery.

Interventions will involve working with patients to improve health in a number of different aspects of lifestyle including diet, smoking behaviour, exercise, blood pressure and stress management. It is up to the nurse to assess a patient's health promotion needs, and to plan, implement and evaluate interventions that are appropriate and realistic and that incorporate a holistic appreciation of the uniqueness of each patient's circumstances.

This chapter is divided into four sections. The first section considers the concepts of health and health promotion and looks at health promotion policy that is of relevance in vascular nursing. Then attention turns to examine the main risk factors for vascular disease. We then explore some of the main psychological theories that help to explain health behaviour before examining in some detail the nurse's role in planning and delivering health education.

Health and health promotion

What is health?

The holistic view of health taken in this chapter views it as a multidimensional concept involving physical, mental, emotional, spiritual, social and sexual dimensions influenced by both societal health (which involves the basic infrastructure of society) and environmental health (involving the physical environment in which we live) (Aggleton and Homans, 1987). Health is therefore a complex concept which each person may perceive differently and to which a different value may be ascribed.

One view of health may be found in the WHO definition of 1948 which states that health is a state of complete physical, mental and social wellbeing and not merely the absence of disease. It is hard, however, to define wellbeing and the definition suggests that health is a state which may be hard to reach and difficult to recognise when achieved. It is difficult too to have all aspects of wellbeing in a good state at all times; for example, is a patient who has undergone a below-knee amputation but not yet able to walk in a state of 'complete physical, mental and social wellbeing'?

A more elaborate concept of health is posed by Seedhouse (1994) who views health as a foundation for achievement, enabling a person to achieve their realistic chosen and biological potentials. This theory may be applied to situations in vascular nursing, for example, patients with critical leg ischaemia who experience mobility restrictions, pain, non-healing ulcers and psychological distress. These patients may view a necessary amputation as offering a new lease of life with a new opening for enjoying life's opportunities.

What is health promotion?

Health promotion is 'the process of helping people to increase control over and improve their health', (WHO, 1984). It is an umbrella term for many activities that enhance good health and prevent ill-health. This may include any activity that encourages wellbeing for individual or communities, and will include the development and use of local/national/international policies and campaigns, mass media and preventive health activities. Health promotion may involve many individuals at all levels of social organisation.

What is health education?

Health education, on the other hand, is one health promotion activity which involves giving information and advice to patients (McBride, 1995) and is the kind of activity nurses are involved in day by day. It is fundamental to the work of a nurse in a vascular care setting since much ill-health and distress can be avoided by the implementation of health advice into daily lifestyles. Particularly relevant to vascular nursing is advice for quitting smoking, weight reduction, salt or lipid lowering dietary advice, suitable exercise, preventative foot care and diabetes control.

Empowerment

The concept of empowerment is integral to promoting health. It enables people to take control over their lives and the factors that affect their health. At an individual level self-empowerment helps people identify why they persist in self-destructive behaviours (for example, overeating or smoking) and helps them develop the skills and confidence needed to make choices. Empowerment is a reflexive activity – that is no one can give power to another. One can merely help individuals to attain and keep their own sense of power over their own health; achieving this will raise their self-esteem (Forster, 1995).

An overview of the development of national health promotion initiatives related to vascular nursing

The qualities which are enshrined in health promotion are illustrated in the aims of the World Health Organisation (WHO, 1985) and the five elements of the Ottawa Charter (WHO, 1986). WHO has been enormously influential in widening health promotion policy from a focus upon specific health promotion programmes to a focus upon regional, national and international health promotion strategies and initiatives.

In 1974 a report by Lalonde, in Ottawa, Canada, called for a redirection of health promotion initiatives away from the emphasis upon the personal approach to health to a new public approach which recognised the responsibility played by all sectors of social organisation. The Alma Ata Declaration of the World Health Organisation (WHO, 1978) influenced governments to recognise the role of primary healthcare in preventing disease and maintaining health. The main goal of this Declaration has been the improvement of health and health-related problems by the year 2000 (MacKintosh, 1996). A document entitled 'Health for All by the Year 2000' (WHO, 1985) was drawn up (revised by WHO, 1993) in order to put the goals of the Alma Ata Declaration into practice. The central purpose of the document was to promote healthy lifestyles, reduce preventable diseases (such as vascular disease) and provide full health coverage for the population. However, it was found to be somewhat over-idealistic. The Ottawa Charter (WHO, 1986) recommended more precise mechanisms for the implementation of the goals of the Alma Ata Declaration (WHO, 1978). In essence these promoted personal and community involvement in health promotion, public involvement in decision-making as well as personal control, skills acquisition and also individual and community empowerment.

In 1992 the Health of the Nation document (DOH, 1992) sought to 'add years to life and life to years'. Influenced by the Health for All by the Year 2000 document (WHO, 1985), it complemented these concepts by focusing upon five main health problems, the first of which is relevant to vascular nursing:

- heart disease and stroke
- cancer
- mental illness
- HIV/AIDS and sexual health
- accidents

Specific health problems were chosen because each one was a major cause of premature death or avoidable ill-health, effective interventions were seen to be achievable and it was thought to be possible to monitor progress towards each target. The document set targets for reductions in morbidity and death rates in these key areas which mostly expired by year 2000.

In relation to vascular disease targets were set in CHD/strokes, smoking, blood pressure and diet with nutrition (Table 3.1). It is notable that none were set for physical activity, however.

There has been a movement towards targets in most cases. However, three relevant areas remain in which achievement has been poor. Instead of a drop there has been a rise in the number of

Table 3.1 The Health of the Nation targets for coronary heart disease/strokes, blood pressure, diet, nutrition and smoking

CHD and stroke
1. To reduce death rate for both in people under 65 years by at least 40% by year 2000.
2. To reduce death rate for CHD in people aged 65-74 by at least 30% by year 2000.
3. To reduce death rate for stroke in people aged 65–74 by at least 40% by year 2000.

Smoking
1. To reduce prevalence of smoking to no more than 20% by year 2000.
2. At least 33% of women smokers to stop at start of pregnancy by the year 2000.
3. To reduce smoking prevalence of 11–15 year olds by 33% by 1994.

Diet and nutrition
1. To reduce average food energy derived from saturated fatty acids by at least 35% by 2005.
2. To reduce total fat intake by at least 12% by year 2005.
3. To reduce proportion of men and women who are obese by at least 25% and 33% respectively by 2005.

Blood pressure
1. To reduce mean systolic BP by at least 5 mmHg by 2005.

The Health of the Nation – A Strategy for Health in England – July 1992, Department of Health, London.

obese people, a rise too in cancer of the lung in women under 75 years as well as an increase in smoking in school age children (Latter, 1998), and these will have implications for planners of vascular care services.

Our Healthier Nation (DOH, 1999), produced by the Labour Government, aims to take the work of the Health of the Nation (DOH, 1992) document further. Its focus is upon those aged up to 65 years. Its overall aims are to increase both length of life and freedom from disease, and also to narrow the gap between rich and poor of the UK. This paper acknowledges that all inequalities need to be addressed in order to tackle health inequalities. The paper urges the collaboration of key government policy-makers such as environmental/social and economic policy-makers to assess the impact on their individual policies upon health.

Our Healthier Nation (DOH, 1999) has identified four priority areas (coronary heart disease, cancer, sexual health and accidents) for health promotion activity. There is one main target set related to heart disease and stroke prevention from which separate strategies for smoking and alcohol consumption and other risk factors may be set (Table 3.2).

Table 3.2 Targets for heart disease and stroke

To reduce the death rate from coronary heart disease and stroke and related diseases in people under 75 years by at least two-fifths by 2010, saving up to 200 000 lives in total. Department of Health (1999) Our Healthier Nation, White Paper. London: Department of Health.

The major risk factors for vascular disease

This section will consider the major risk factors for vascular disease already discussed in the previous chapter and will consider the nurse's health promotion role in relation to each. These are listed in Table 3.3.

Table 3.3 Risk factors for vascular disease

Cigarette smoking
Hyperlipidaemia
Obesity
Alcohol intake over recommended limits
Diabetes
Hypertension
Clotting disorders
Other risk factors:
Stress
Lack of exercise
Lack of foot care

Smoking

It is well known that tobacco use is strongly linked to heart disease and lung cancer. However, it is less commonly appreciated by patients that it is also strongly linked to the onset and progression of vascular disease, including lower extremity ischaemia, claudication, graft failure and amputation (Hart, 1993) as well as aortic aneurysm (Tooke and Lowe, 1996). Smoking is also the single most preventable cause of premature morbidity and mortality and as such provides a unique challenge to patients and health professionals.

Smoke contains more than 4000 active compounds and affects blood vessels in several ways. Nicotine causes vasoconstriction, reducing blood to the extremities. It causes the release of catecholamines, which raise heart rate and blood pressure, alters myocardial contractibility and stroke volume, and cause increased resistance to blood flow and platelet aggregation. Inhaled carbon dioxide reduces oxygen transport to the tissues, increases blood viscosity and increases fibrinogen levels (Hart, 1993). In relation to any kind of surgery smoking increases the complications that may be experienced during the wound healing process (Netscher and Clamon, 1994).

The prevalence of smoking in the UK is generally declining. However, concern remains over the numbers of young people, especially girls, who smoke (Hart, 1993).

Quitting permanently, however, is difficult and Fisher et al. (1990) state that an individual needs five to six serious quit attempts to be successful.

Interventions include individual or group counselling and support groups, hypnotherapy, nicotine replacement therapy, aversion therapy as well as identified strategies between the individual and the patient.

A favourable opportunity to quit smoking occurs when admitted to hospital. This is because smoking in hospital is discouraged, being ill can reduce craving and illness makes the pursuit of the behaviour more difficult (Wewers and Ahijevych, 1996). Admission to hospital for a vascular procedure such as a diagnostic angiogram or angioplasty and the realisation of the threat smoking plays in compromising health may also provide the patient with a period of time for self-reflection that is contextually relevant. Patients will not give up, however, unless they are motivated to do so and nurses need to be actively alert in recognising the patient who may use hospital admission as a catalyst to reduce or quit smoking.

Hyperlipidaemia

Abnormal fat levels in the blood result in atherosclerosis from both hypercholesterolaemia and hypertriglyceridaemia. Both are known as hyperlipidaemias. Fatty acids and glycerol derive from molecules of fat and are called triglycerides. Cholesterol derives from saturated fat breakdown.

Hypercholesterolaemia (and also hypertriglyceridaemia) is a significant risk factor for the development of vascular disease. The normal cholesterol level is 6.5 mmol/l but patient cholesterols are often maintained at much lower levels (for example, less than 5 mmol/l), particularly in those who are in a high risk category because they have vascular disease or diabetes. It is estimated however that 9–23% of elderly men and 18–40% of elderly women have cholesterol levels in excess of recommended levels (Williams, 1996).

Lipids consist of low density lipoproteins (LDL) which contain more cholesterol than other lipid proteins and have a high affinity for arterial walls. Very low density lipoproteins (VLDL) contain high levels of triglycerides and are associated with premature atherosclerosis. Conversely, high density lipoproteins (HDL) contain fewer lipids and actively carry lipids away from arterial walls to the liver for metabolism. HDLs are therefore seen as protective to health.

Patients with vascular disease who have hyperlipidaemia may be treated with a low cholesterol diet. Specific advice about this diet is given in Table 3.4.

Drugs (statins) may be used to lower lipid levels but this decision should be made jointly between the doctor and the patient. Their benefit is not clearly established and side effects can occur. Types available include reductase inhibitors, nicotinic acid and bile acid

Table 3.4 Daily dietary recommendations for the treatment of hyperlipidaemia

Limit fat to 30% of total daily intake with only 10% of calories taken from saturated fat
Carbohydrate to make up at least 50% of calorie intake
Protein to make up 20% of calories
Two 3 oz servings of meat daily
Three servings of vegetables daily
Three servings of fruit daily
Six servings of bread and pasta daily
Two servings of milk daily; only three egg yolks per week where cholesterol is to be limited
Patients should seek personally tailored advice from a dietician.

American Heart Association's diet (source: Cahall and Spence, 1995).

sequestrants, simvastatin, lovastatin, cholestyramine and colestipol (Williams, 1996).

Obesity

Obesity is a growing problem in the UK. In 1993 13% of men and 16% of women were overweight and it is forecast that by the year 2005 this will rise to 18% of men and 24% of women (DOH, 1995). Obesity has a multifactorial causation including sedentary lifestyle, eating habits and other factors such as the high fat and sugar content of modern day food products. Obesity may act as a promoter of diabetes and chronic venous disease (such as varicose veins) (Callam and Ruckley, 1996). In the presence of peripheral vascular disease it may impede mobility and wound healing. Its risks are greater in the presence of hypertension, pre-existing diabetes and smoking.

Obesity is notoriously difficult to correct on a permanent basis. Dietary recommendations need to be taught to a patient using appropriate adult learning strategies. All advice needs to be tailored to each individual, taking account of gender, age, and food preferences and the patient's lifestyle. Goals set should be modest and measurable, and they should permit gradual change. Dieticians are invaluable in the assessment and planning stage but nursing interventions are needed for the implementation and evaluation of dietary advice (Grace et al., 1994). The quality of the relationship therefore between the patient and the dietician and the patient and the health professional (nurse), is vital to ensure free communication and the best possible outcome for the patient.

Alcohol intake over recommended limits

Current low risk ranges for alcohol consumption are 21 units for a man and 14 units for a woman per week. One unit can be described as half a pint of beer, a single measure of spirits or a small glass of wine. One person in five, however, currently drinks over this limit.

Drinking alcohol is not an independent risk factor for the development of vascular disease (Smith and Jacobson, 1988). Indeed, there is some evidence to suggest that drinking small amounts of alcohol has a health protective action in preventing vascular disease. This protective value is lost, however, when more than 2 units a day are consumed (Tooke and Lowe, 1996). Overconsumption of alcohol is responsible for a wide variety of circulatory, neurological and digestive conditions including cancer (Kemm and Close, 1995).

Diabetes

Diabetes is associated with vascular disease. Both type 1 (insulin-dependent) and type 2 (non-insulin-dependent) diabetes involve defects in the metabolism of carbohydrate, protein and fat resulting in impairment in the production or utilisation of insulin (Rosenberg, 1990). Both types can lead to macrovascular and microvascular disease. Macrovascular disease is associated with accelerated atherosclerosis of arteries and diabetics have a three times higher rate of coronary heart disease death than non-diabetics (UKPDS Group, 1998). Microvascular disease includes both small vessel disease and microangiopathy involving capillary basement membrane thickening and increased capillary permeability. This is commonly seen in the eye as retinopathy and in the kidney as nephropathy as well as the lower limb extremities (including peripheral vascular disease). In addition, diabetics also experience sensory and motor neuropathy which contribute to the development of leg/foot ulcers. The seriousness of poorly controlled diabetes in causing chronic complications needs to be appreciated by health professionals and patients alike as the incidence of lower limb amputations is 11–14 times higher in those with diabetes than in non-diabetic populations (Siitonen et al., 1993).

There is no doubt that people with diabetes having any kind of surgery experience a significantly higher incidence of wound complications and delayed healing. This is especially true for people with diabetes having vascular surgery. Indeed in the presence of microvascular disease associated hypoxia and resulting tissue malnutrition adds to the risk of wound complications (Rosenberg, 1990). Crucial in these patients is the need to maintain good glycaemic control both pre- and postoperatively in order to minimise these complications.

Hypertension

Hypertension is a significant risk factor for vascular disease and is associated with the development of atherosclerosis in the coronary and cerebral circulations and also in the peripheral circulation where it doubles the risk of claudication (Regensteiner and Hiatt, 1994).

Hypertension exists when the systolic pressure is greater than 140 mmHg and the diastolic pressure is greater than 90 mmHg. However, in diabetes a diagnosis of hypertension should be made when levels as low as 135/80 are detected (UKPDS Group, 1998) so that treatment can be initiated. The incidence of hypertension rises with age – by 64–75 years 75% of men and 74% of women have a systolic blood pressure greater than 140 mmHg.

Non-pharmacological interventions to prevent and treat hypertension include adequate exercise, weight reduction, alcohol reduction and reduced sodium intake. The recommended sodium intake is about 6 grams per day. There is much potential for the reduction of sodium in diets and public awareness raising by the media and health education would assist in bringing pressure to bear on the food manufacturing industry, where salt is valued for its preservative properties in modern food preparation techniques (McAbee, 1995).

Pharmacological interventions include use of drugs such as diuretics, beta and alpha blockers, calcium channel blockers and angiotensin-converting enzyme (ACE) inhibitors.

Clotting disorders

Certain abnormalities of the clotting mechanism are associated with an increased risk of peripheral vascular disease (Regensteiner and Hiatt, 1994). Work done with patients who have lower limb atherosclerosis has detected an increased thrombotic tendency. Platelet function is adversely affected, including a tendency for these to aggregate more readily. Blood viscosity and plasma fibrinogen levels are generally elevated and this is not accounted for by smoking or other risk factors. What needs further investigation, however, is the role this plays in the aetiology of peripheral vascular disease (Callam and Ruckley, 1996).

Other risk factors

Stress

The experience of stress affects the body and the mind. Physiologically stimulation of the sympathetic nervous system causes peripheral vasoconstriction (Herbert, 1997). It also increases cholesterol and platelet levels, decreases clotting time and sustains high blood pressure. It mobilises catecholamines (such as adrenaline and noradrenaline), which in turn stimulate the release of glucose, fatty acids and cholesterol into the circulation. This contributes towards the development of atherosclerotic plaque, which is undesirable in the presence of vascular disease.

Stressors abound in contemporary society. What is crucial is the individual's perception of the stress that is experienced. Inability to control perceived stress increases the experience. Individuals need to take steps to avoid stressors whenever they can and to cope with stressors they cannot avoid. This will require the nurse to use both her counselling and communications skills to help the patient develop problem-solving coping mechanisms.

Lack of exercise

Exercise has a beneficial effect on the heart and lungs, increasing capacity and function as well as strengthening bones. In peripheral vascular disease exercise has a unique role, enhancing the development of needed collateral circulation, strengthening muscles and providing a general sense of wellbeing (Cahall and Spence, 1995). Exercise also prevents venous stasis and promotes venous return. It is a useful tool to aid the reduction of high blood pressure and is a vital adjunct to dietary control for weight loss and hyperlipidaemia.

Exercise in peripheral vascular disease is particularly beneficial and can include walking, running, stair climbing and cycling. Patients with cardiopulmonary disease will need individual assessment as those with uncontrolled hypertension or early heart failure will need stabilisation before commencing exercise. Exercise programmes need to be chosen so that they can be incorporated into the patient's lifestyle and level of fitness. To this end, patients should be referred where possible to a vascular rehabilitation programme. Chapter 9 gives details of an exercise programme for those with claudication.

Lack of foot care

Those with peripheral arterial disease have an increased need to avoid foot trauma because even mild infections can cause problems with serious consequences resulting in amputation. Vulnerability to these problems is increased if the patient has diabetes. Patients need to be educated about this and advised to fit foot care and inspection into their daily routine so that their early observations may be reported and thus retard the progress of disease (Cookingham, 1995). Health professionals should not hesitate to refer patients to a chiropodist and to advocate regular use of this valuable member of the healthcare team. A list of main foot care points is given in Table 3.5.

Table 3.5 Main foot care points for patient education

Daily inspection of feet
Check pedal pulses (if appropriate)
Use magnifying mirrors if necessary
Check each toe for cracks or blisters
Feet and legs to be cleansed daily with mild soap and warm water
Do not soak feet for more than 10 minutes
Use lubricants to feet and legs but not between toes
Diabetics to have toenails trimmed by chiropodist
Do not use over-the-counter corn and callus removers
Prevent callus with pumice stone
Never go barefoot
Wear socks with shoes
Buy only comfortable shoes
Do not wear sandals, thongs or heels

Source: Cahall and Spence (1995).

The psychology of behaviour change

An increase in knowledge alone does not necessarily lead to an alteration in patients' behaviour and nurses cannot afford to make this assumption. Behaviour change is also influenced by personal, psychological and social variables. The psychological literature offers a number of useful models which help us to understand the contribution of these factors. This section will now focus upon some of the psychological models but will not consider sociological material in any depth.

People's behaviour is informed by their beliefs and values. These inform their attitudes and in turn their intention to behave in a particular way. A belief is defined as the knowledge we have about the world; a value represents ethical codes as well as social and cultural norms.

People strive to keep consistency between their beliefs, values, attitudes and behaviour. This is a powerful force and inconsistency in these provides uncomfortable feelings known as cognitive dissonance (Festinger, 1957; cited in Pennington, 1986). This is the feeling that arises when an individual has two cognitions (ideas, beliefs, attitudes) that are inconsistent with each other. In decision-making Festinger (1957) claims that we aim to reduce our discomfort by taking steps to suppress the negative feelings that are at odds with our behaviour, for example smoking and its role in causing vascular problems.

However, people have different tolerance levels for dissonance. Festinger (1957) says that experienced dissonance can be reduced by bolstering the alternative decided upon and downgrading the alternative that is rejected. For example, patients may decide that smoking is unlikely to affect them personally and that the health professional is being unnecessarily pessimistic. This will serve to reduce the discomfort of having two inconsistent cognitions.

The stages of change model

Prochaska and DiClemente (1984) identified that an individual needs to negotiate several stages in the achievement of a behavioural change until it is attained (Figure 3.1). The first stage is precontemplation, when individuals are not thinking about nor intending to change behaviour because they are unaware or unwilling to do so. In the stage of contemplation the individuals are now thinking of changing but not in the immediate future. Preparation follows this and actual change becomes imminent. The fourth stage is action and involves the changes being actively attempted. Maintenance follows in which sustained changes occur that need conscious effort. Lastly, built into the model is the stage of relapse, when changes did occur in the past but do so no longer. This model highlights the importance of maintenance and relapse. Relapse is not an end-point in itself but better viewed as one stage on the road to change and permits an individual who relapses not to be deemed 'a failure'.

Prochaska and DiClemente (1984) claim that individuals will have different beliefs, attitudes, values and motivation at each different stage and that they may stay in the precontemplation and contemplation stages for extended periods. It is important to identify the stage individuals may be in because different interventions will

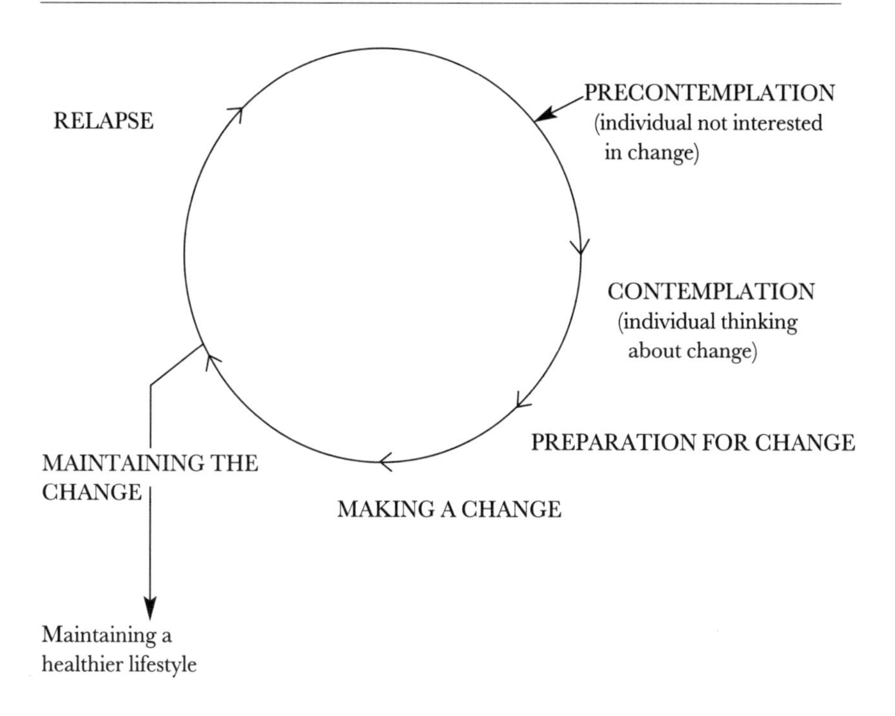

Figure 3.1 The stages of change model (Prochaska and DiClemente, 1984; Naidoo and Wills, 1994).

be appropriate at different stages. This is imperative in nursing patients with chronic illnesses such as vascular diseases because adopting an intervention that is inappropriate may harm the patient/health professional relationship and negatively influence the individual's attitude towards the needed change that is desirable for long-term health.

The model has been usefully measured and applied to a number of health behaviours, in particular to smoking (Prochaska et al., 1991), dietary change (Brownell and Cohen, 1995), exercise (McDowell et al., 1997) and treatment for alcohol misuse, all of which are risk factors for vascular disease.

Locus of control

The concept of control is important to both health and wellbeing. Health locus of control theory states that those who consider health and recovery to be determined by their own actions have an internal locus of control as a personality trait. By contrast, those who believe that their health and recovery is not within their own power are likely to be passive in response to health professionals (Rotter, 1966). Closely linked to locus of control is the concept of self-efficacy which Bandura (1977a) defined as the certainty of conviction that one can successfully perform the behaviour that will produce the desired outcome.

Factors that affect both locus of control and self-efficacy include being able to master an activity, observing others performing it and being persuaded by a credible authority (Carroll, 1995). Both concepts appear logical and are closely linked with self-esteem. Achievement of health goals for which individuals perceive themselves responsible increases personal confidence and the expectation that the success will be repeated. The nurse needs to assess patients' locus of control and work to positively influence self-efficacy expectations by assessing patient needs, building up patient self-confidence and providing continuous support.

The concept of self-efficacy has also been successfully linked to smoking cessation (De Vries and Backbier, 1994) and to recovery from coronary artery bypass graft in the elderly (Carroll, 1995). De Vries and Backbier (1994) studied individuals at different stages of change and stated that boosting self-efficacy is particularly relevant during the contemplation stage within the stages of change model.

The health belief model

The health belief model (Figure 3.2; Becker, 1974) is based upon two types of beliefs that motivate people to take preventive health measures. The individual needs to make two subconscious assessments of the feasibility of the proposed health behaviour plus an analysis of the benefits versus the cost of adopting a new health behaviour. The assessment of feasibility includes individuals' judgements of the perceived threat of the health problem itself and how susceptible they are to the particular condition if the behaviour is not adopted and the degree of severity of organic, psychological or social consequences that may result from it. The cost/benefit analysis includes sociodemographic influences such as those of peers, age, gender, social class and cues received from health professionals and others as well as the media.

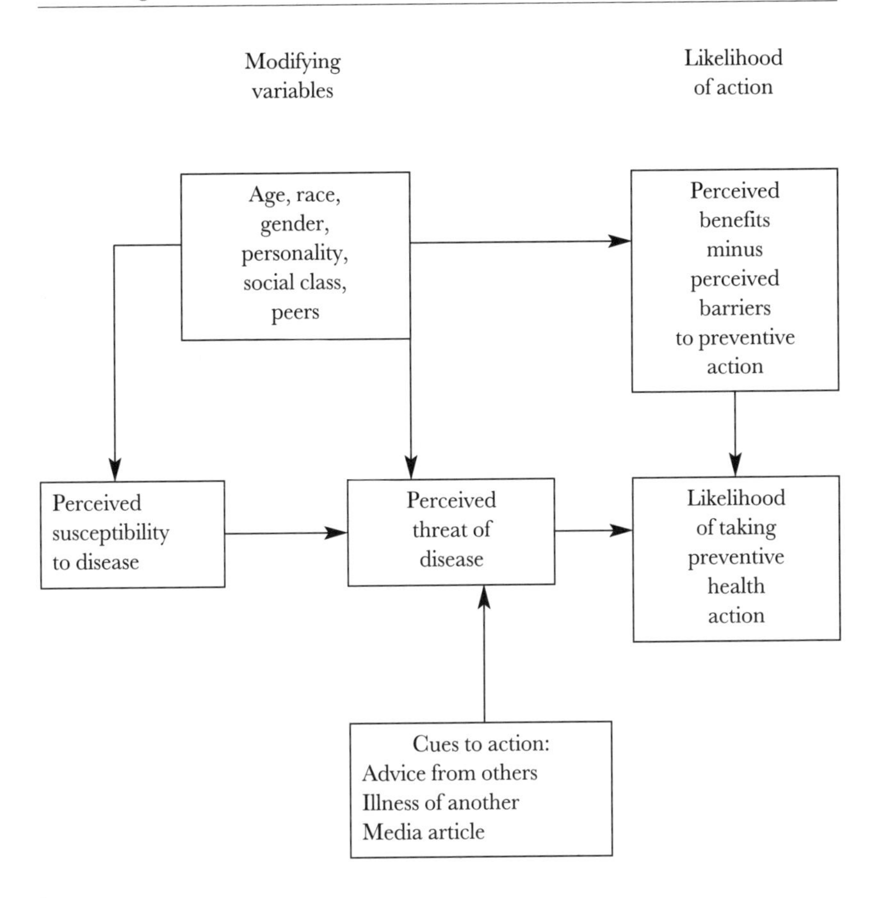

Figure 3.2. The health belief model (Becker, 1974; Sarafino, 1994).

The health belief model has been successfully applied in dietary change, especially weight loss (Sarafino, 1994), and in diabetes self-care behaviour (Maldonato et al., 1995) and smoking (Flay, 1985).

Application to vascular nursing

These theories will now be discussed in application to the nurse's health promotion management of patients who show risk factors for vascular disease.

In relation to any behavioural change the most important initial step is in the assessments the nurse makes of various patient factors such as his/her health beliefs, values, attitudes, locus of control, self-efficacy, perceptions of susceptibility, intention and what stage they have reached in the stages of change model. This information needs to be recorded and communicated to other staff. Combined with information about health status it will enable realistic plans to be drawn up in discussion with the patient and for both patient and health professional to share these expectations.

Having created a plan of care the nurse will then need to adopt many different roles including those of counsellor/adviser/facilitator in order to aid the patient's own self-empowerment. This involves focusing upon the patient's own network of personal resources such as self-esteem, self-efficacy and internality of locus of control in order to boost these and the patient's own confidence.

Some initial education may be necessary for baseline knowledge. Monitoring tools such as diaries or record cards for food intake, smoking behaviour, exercise patterns, walking distances and blood pressure recording may be valuable to record behaviours (Brownell and Cohen, 1995), but should be used cooperatively together by patient and health professional to analyse behaviour – they should not be used as a means by which to rebuke. It is important too that goals set should be modest so that patients may be encouraged by their achievement. It is still quite common for health professionals to strive for complete cessation of adverse behaviours (since this will bring the best health outcome) but this may not be a realistic goal and failure to achieve these will undermine patient confidence and self-esteem.

The patient/health professional relationship is also important. Vital too is detailed referral to the community nursing and care services upon discharge from acute hospital care to ensure continuity of all health-promoting initiatives.

Health professionals have obligations too. Continuing professional development allows for the updating and increase of knowledge about the benefits of changing poor health habits, the difficulties involved and the best means to do so. Practitioners who have had recent training are more likely to promote the good health behaviour as well as display it themselves (McDowell et al., 1997). For the sake of their own credibility as a role model it is obvious that staff should ensure they lead healthy lifestyles themselves.

Many health professionals have insufficient skills and techniques to effectively communicate and deliver patient education strategies.

This is due as much to the emphasis in hospital settings upon hands-on care and cure as it is to the lack of opportunity and time to practise these skills. The dominance of the medical model and the mechanics of current hospital organisational power systems ensure that only lip service can be offered to ensuring patients' beliefs, opinions and difficulties are readily taken into account. Patients are then given passive roles in promoting their own health and are not actively enlisted in helping themselves. This results in an underestimation by the health professional of the tasks involved for the patient in altering their health behaviour and gives rise, upon occasion, to victim-blaming attitudes when results desired by health professionals are not achieved.

Nurses caring for vascular patients should not therefore be complacent in seeking to further promote their understanding of behaviour change and the best practice for helping to bring it about.

Teaching and learning

The multifactorial causation of vascular disease places education for its prevention at the top of the nurse's agenda whether working in an acute vascular or community setting. Frequently, however, despite information and advice being given to patients it is clear from patients' continued poor health that this advice is unheeded. The tendency in practice, however, is often to repeat giving the same advice to the patient.

The traditional medical model has relied hitherto on its authoritarian position – exhorting patients to comply with medical and nursing advice. Such an approach is doomed in gaining permanent health behaviour change simply because not all the important influences on the patient's health are being taken into consideration. These include social, mental, emotional, spiritual and physical dimensions (Forster, 1995).

The main aim of health education is to enable individuals to be free to make their own health choices according to their own needs. The purpose of health education initiatives then is to help patients become aware of the constraining influences upon their personal health and to become empowered to take action upon these. In this way, as well as understanding information, patients may actually be able to use it to their own advantage.

Adult learning

So how do adults learn? This needs to be understood so that appropriate plans for teaching can be drawn up in order to facilitate learning in patients with vascular disease.

The concept of modelling from social learning theory (Bandura, 1977b) suggests that we learn by observing the behaviour of another person. As children we were exposed daily to adult teachers whom we observed and from whom we learned teaching strategies and techniques that were suitable for us as children. It is quite natural then that we should bring our preconceived ideas about teaching and learning into our interactions with our patients. However, most patients with vascular disease are adults and differ from children in the way they learn and therefore in the teaching strategies that adult teachers should use with them. Hinchliff (1995) states that adults' readiness to learn is related to what they need to know in order to be able to perform activities for themselves, that learned material is used to solve problems and that adults are highly motivated by their need to maintain their own self-esteem.

This then implies that the nurse who attempts to teach adults will need to practise teaching techniques that are appropriate for adult learners.

The process of health education

Like the nursing process there are four main spheres of activity to consider when undertaking health education. These include assessment and planning of the education as well as its implementation and evaluation (Ewles and Simnett, 1996).

Identification of the characteristics of the patient

Assessment needs to take account of the unique characteristics of the individual who is to be taught. All individuals vary in their experience and knowledge about a health issue as well as in their cultural needs, attitudes, motivation, expectations, receptivity and mental abilities; variables such as age, gender and the presence of any disease processes are also important (Ewles and Simnett, 1996).

Identification of the learning need

Assessment will allow the nurse to identify some areas of need where health education may benefit the patient (for example, smoking cessation, foot care or diabetes control). It is important, however, that this need is identified by the patient as being important too. If a patient does not recognise this then the education is less likely to be remembered and less likely to be incorporated into daily behaviour. If, on the other hand, the patient recognises the need and expresses a desire for the education then the teaching is likely to be welcomed and responded to positively (Bradshaw, 1972).

Planning aims and objectives

The next task is to define the focus of the aims of the teaching session – that is to draw up broad statements of what is being attempted. From these the objectives can be defined – these are carefully worded statements identifying what it is hoped the patient will achieve by the end of the health education session, in other words, what the results will be.

These could be broken down for convenience into three types of learning as identified by Bloom (1956; cited in Jarvis, 1988). These are categorised as cognitive (related to knowledge and thought), affective (related to attitudes, beliefs and values and their change) and psychomotor (related to attainment of skills). Objectives should be specific, realistic, achievable (within the resources available) and measurable (using important indicators which allow their achievement to be detected). An example of these objectives written for a health promotion session aimed at helping patients to stop smoking is found in Table 3.6.

Planning teaching methods

The three types of learning lend themselves best to the use of different teaching methods. For example, an objective that requires the patient to learn new knowledge may require the use of a method that will impart knowledge such as direct information-giving, use of written information to back this up or a video. An affective objective will be best achieved by using methods that allow patients to talk to others and gain different perspectives such as discussion with

Table 3.6 Example of objectives written for teaching session to a patient who has expressed the need to stop smoking

Cognitive objective: That by the end of the session the patient should know what support is available to him/her to stop smoking.
Affective objective: That by the end of the session the patient should express greater confidence towards his/her ability to stop smoking.
Psychomotor objective: That by the end of the session the patient should be able to show cigarette refusal strategies.

another individual (health professional or suitable other patient), group discussion or role play. An objective related to the acquisition of psychomotor skills may need the demonstration of that skill, with repetition and practice. An example here, depending on resources, could be supervised exercise groups and teaching programmes for patients with intermittent claudication achieved in hospital or community settings.

Detailed planning of all health promotion sessions is desirable in order to have a logical and progressive outline of any session's content and the teaching methods and materials that will be used. Planning also involves consideration of evaluation strategies. These are discussed below.

Implement the health education

After careful assessment of health education needs and planning to meet these, the teaching is now ready to be implemented. Some general principles of teaching are listed in Table 3.7.

Evaluation

Evaluation of any health promotion session involves critical assessment of what has been achieved and how it has been achieved. This allows recognition of the need to change or improve methods, material and resources used and to improve health promotion practice. Evaluation provides evidence to support the delivery of repeated health promotion sessions (Simnett, 1997) and is vital to provide evidence of clinical effectiveness.

Table 3.7 Teaching principles

Points to consider:
Take time to plan your teaching
Use suitable language that the patient can understand
Deliver a suitable amount of information for the patient's concentration span
Choose a suitable length of time for the session
Make sure your session has an introduction, a body and a conclusion
Find out what the client already knows
Keep advice precise and specific
Key points should be repeated and explained
Use visual aids, diagrams and leaflets
Ensure that the venue is private, there are no interruptions
Ensure that the patient does not have pain, is not hungry or unduly anxious nor tired
Use communication skills appropriately
The use of praise is likely to motivate
Use eye contact
Listen to your own voice and ensure it is pleasant to listen to with variety of tone, expression and lilt
Include relatives where possible
Evaluate what you have done

Evaluation can be undertaken at two levels: process evaluation looks at what happened during the health promotion session and makes some judgements about it. This looks at the finer points related to the actual delivery and the reception of the message. Information may be gained by reflection upon one's own performance, from feedback from peers or the patient taught, and takes place from the beginning of the delivery of the health promotion session itself (Naidoo and Wills, 1994).

Impact and outcome evaluation are concerned with the results of the session. Impact evaluation is seen to be the short-term change in cognition, psychomotor skills or affect. Outcome evaluation is an assessment of whether or not the planned objectives of the session have been achieved and therefore takes a longer-term view (Naidoo and Wills, 1994).

For example, in a session about healthy eating for weight loss, examination of the process may involve an evaluation of the adequacy (or not) of the length of the session, the amount of information given and the visual aids used. Impact evaluation would involve an evaluation of the patients' understanding as demonstrated by their changed behaviour over food choices and outcome evaluation would be shown by the actual weight loss that occurs over time (Simnett, 1997).

The use of written materials

Written materials are commonly used in order to promote a health promotion message. Many kinds are available in relationship to vascular disease health risks and can be given to patients in order to reinforce verbal health messages.

Leaflets are often given to patients following interventions such as angioplasty, arterial bypass surgery, aortic aneurysm or carotid surgery and they should include advice about mobility, wound care, returning to work, driving and flying as well as pain relief. Health promotion advice related to smoking, exercise, medication compliance (including antiplatelet treatment, antihypertensive, diabetic and lipid lowering drugs) should also be included.

However, leaflets should be used with caution since patients' receptivity to them will depend upon the timeliness and perceived relevance for them of the advice given. The content of leaflets should be explained by the nurse and should be chosen with great care for their suitability for each patient. Other considerations include the readability and legibility of material, the use of clear language, short sentences; advice should be specific and there should be follow-up names and addresses for further information provided on the leaflet. Leaflets can of course be home-made but unless sophisticated and expensive IT packages are used, the end result can sometimes be amateur in appearance and offputting to read (Ewles and Simnett, 1996).

Posters are useful to provide broad and brief health promotion messages and information regarding angiograms/angioplasty and reconstructive bypass surgery, the content of which can be supplemented by a leaflet.

Summary

This chapter has offered a view of health and health promotion, health education and empowerment, and has outlined the major reports that have influenced health promotion's evolution as they relate to vascular disease. It has identified the main risk factors for vascular disease, the main health education advice that patients need and the nurse's role in this. It has then considered some of the important and influential psychological models of behaviour change and has suggested some areas in which practice could usefully be sharpened in order to promote behaviour change. Finally, the chapter has looked at the main aim and purpose of health education, the unique qualities of the adult learner and the process of planning health education as well as specific teaching principles that should be utilised.

What is clear is that to a large extent (but not exclusively) individuals with vascular disease hold their health in their own hands. The risk factors perpetuated by lifestyle can only be amenable to change if all the patient's influences on health are recognised. Nurses have a responsibility to acknowledge and work with these in order to reduce the distress, physical and psychological costs of vascular disease.

References

Aggleton P, Homans H (1987) Educating about AIDS. NHS Training Authority.

Bandura A (1997a) Towards a unifying theory of behaviour change. Psychological Review 84: 191–215.

Bandura A (1977b) Social Learning Theory. Englewood Cliffs, NJ: Prentice Hall.

Becker MH (1974) The Health Belief Model and Personal Health Behaviour. Health Education Monographs 2: 324–508.

Bloom B (ed.) (1956) Taxonomy of Educational Objectives – Book I, The Cognitive Domain. London: Longman.

Bradshaw J (1972) The concept of social need. New Society 19: 640–643.

Brownell K, Cohen L (1995) Adherence to dietary regimes 1: an overview of research. Behavioural Medicine 20(4): 149–169.

Cahall E, Spence R (1995) Practical nursing measures for vascular compromise in the lower leg. Ostomy/Wound Management 41(9): 16–32.

Callam M, Ruckley C (1996) The epidemiology of chronic venous disease. In: Tooke J, Lowe G (eds) A Textbook of Vascular Medicine, chapter 34. London: Arnold.

Carroll D (1995) The importance of self-efficacy expectations in elderly patients recovering from coronary artery bypass surgery. Heart and Lung 24(1): 50–59.

Cookingham A (1995) Peripheral vascular disease: educational concerns for patients with a chronic disease in a changing health-care environment. AACN Clinical Issues 6(4): 670–676.

De Vries H, Backbier E (1994) Self-efficacy as an important determinant of quitting among pregnant women who smoke: the pattern. Preventive Medicine 23: 167–174.

Department of Health (1992) The Health of the Nation: a Strategy for England and Wales. London: HMSO.

Department of Health (1995) Obesity – Reversing the Increasing Problem of Obesity in England – A Report from the Nutrition and Physical Activity Task Force. London: DOH.

Department of Health (1999) Our Healthier Nation. White Paper. London: DOH.
Ewles L, Simnett I (1996) Promoting Health – A Practical Guide. London: Baillière Tindall.
Festinger L (1957) A Theory of Cognitive Dissonance. Stanford, CA: Stanford University Press.
Fisher E, Haire-Joshu D, Morgan G, Rehberg H, Rost K (1990) Smoking and smoking cessation. American Review of Respiratory Disease 9: 702–720.
Flay B (1985) Psychosocial approaches to smoking prevention. Health Psychology 4: 449–488.
Forster D (1995) Education for health. In: Pike S, Forster D. Health Promotion for All, chapter 9. London: Churchill Livingstone.
Grace M, Crosby F, Ventura M (1994) Nutritional education for patients with peripheral vascular disease. Journal of Health Education 25(3): 142–146.
Hart B (1993) Vascular consequences of smoking and benefits of smoking cessation. Journal of Vascular Nursing 6(2): 48–51.
Herbert L (1997) Caring for the Vascular Patient. Edinburgh: Churchill Livingstone.
Hinchliff S (1995) The Practitioner as Teacher. London: Scutari Press.
Jarvis P (1988) Adult and Continuing Education – Theory and Practice. London: Routledge.
Kemm J, Close A (1995) Health Promotion – Theory and Practice, London: Macmillan Press.
Lalonde M (1974) A New Perspective on the Health of Canadians – A Working Document. Ottawa: Canada.
Latter S (1998) HP in the acute setting: the case for empowering nurses. In: Kendall S, Health and Empowerment – Research in Practice, chapter 1. London: Arnold.
MacKintosh N (1996) Promoting Health – An Issue for Nursing. Wilts: Quay Books.
Maldonato A, Bloise D, Ceci M, Fraticelli E, Fallucca F (1995) Diabetes mellitus: lessons for patient education. Patient Education and Counselling 26: 57–66.
McAbee R (1995) Primary prevention of hypertension. AAOHN Journal 43(6): 306–312.
McBride A (1995) Health Promotion in Hospital – A Practical Handbook for Nurses. London: Scutari Press.
McDowell N, McKenna J, Naylor P (1997) Factors that influence practice nurses to promote physical activity. British Journal of Sports Medicine 31: 308–313.
Naidoo J, Wills J (1994) Health Promotion – Foundations for Practice. London: Baillière Tindall.
Netscher D, Clamon J (1994) Smoking: adverse effects on outcomes for plastic surgery patients. Plastic Surgical Nursing 14(4): 205–219.
Pennington D (1986) Essential Social Psychology. London: Arnold.
Prochaska J, DiClemente C (1984) A Transtheoretical Approach: Crossing Traditional Boundaries of Change. Harnewood: Dpon Jones/Irwin.
Prochaska J, Vilicer W, Guadagnoli E, Rossi J, DiClemente C (1991) Patterns of change: dynamic typology applied to smoking. Multivariate Behavioural Research 26: 83–107.
Regensteiner J, Hiatt W (1994) Medical management of peripheral arterial disease. Journal of Vascular and Interventional Radiology 5(5): 669–677.
Rosenberg C (1990) Wound healing in the patient with diabetes mellitus. Nursing Clinics of North America 25(1): 247–261.

Rotter J (1966) Generalised expectancies for internal versus external control of reinforcements. Psychological Monographs 80: 609.
Sarafino E (1994) Health Psychology – Biopsychosocial Interactions. Chichester: Wiley.
Seedhouse D (1994) Health the Foundations for Achievement. Chichester: Wiley.
Siitonen O, Siitonen J, Niskanen L, Laasko M, Pyorala K (1993) Lower extremity amputations in diabetic and non-diabetic patients. Diabetes Care 16: 16–20.
Simnett I (1997) Setting goals and objectives and measuring achievements of health promotion. Managing Health Promotion – Developing Healthy Organisations and Communities, chapter 6. Chichester: Wiley.
Smith A, Jacobson B (1988) The Nation's Health – A Strategy for the 1990s. London: Kings Fund Publishing Office.
Tooke J, Lowe G (1996) A Textbook of Vascular Medicine. London: Arnold.
UKPDS Group (1998) Intensive blood glucose control with sulphonylureas or insulin compared with conventional treatment and risk of complications in patients with type 2 diabetes – United Kingdom Prospective Diabetes Study. Lancet 352: 837–853.
Wewers M, Ahijevych K (1996) Smoking cessation interventions in chronic illness. Annual Review of Nursing Research 14: 73–93.
Wilkinson J (1999) Understanding patients' health beliefs. Professional Nurse 14(5): 320–322.
Williams A (1996) Cardiovascular risk-factor reduction in elderly patients with cardiac disease. Physical Therapy 76(5): 469–480.
World Health Organisation (1948) World Health Organisation Constitution. Geneva: WHO.
World Health Organisation (1978) Report on the International Conference on Primary Health Care. Alma Ata, Copenhagen: WHO.
World Health Organisation (1984) Health Promotion: A WHO Discussion Document on the Concepts and Principles. Geneva: WHO.
World Health Organisation (1985) Health for All. European Health for All series. Copenhagen: WHO Regional Office for Europe.
World Health Organisation (1986) The Ottawa Charter for Health Promotion, An International Conference of Health Promotion – The Move towards a New Public Health. Canada.
World Health Organisation (1993) Health for All Targets: The Health Policy for Europe, updated edition. Copenhagen: WHO Regional Office for Europe.

CHAPTER 4

Assessment of Patients with Vascular Disease

NICOLA STUBBING AND JANET CHESWORTH

The aim of this chapter is to give insight into the assessment of patients with vascular disease.

The basis of a good assessment is the ability to undertake a thorough history and physical examination of the patient.

By undertaking a careful assessment, a plan of care and the interventions required will be developed, which will allow the patient to receive optimal care. It is at this stage that a positive relationship between the nurse and patient may be developed.

The assessment of the patient with vascular disease covers more than just a physical assessment; a functional, spiritual and cultural assessment will also need to be undertaken (Peterson, 1999). It is important to assess the patient's knowledge, understanding and attitude towards the disease, since psychological factors will influence the patient's ability to adapt to vascular illness. Incorporating all of the above in a patient assessment ensures that a holistic approach to their management will be accomplished. A detailed assessment assists in providing seamless care if close links are forged with the community, and allows vital information to be passed freely between professionals both in the community and in hospital. This will also improve the standard of care for clients in the pre- and postoperative stages.

This chapter will not incorporate every symptom and sign of vascular disease; these specific aspects will be covered by individual chapters within the book.

Preparation required prior to assessment

It is important when undertaking a health history that external factors have been given some thought prior to any interview taking place. These factors may include ensuring that the physical environment is suitable, privacy for the patient is maintained and interruptions are kept to a minimum or refused.

An explanation of the procedure for taking a history and physical examination should be given prior to starting.

Any equipment that is likely to be used should be easily accessible. Items that may be required for assessment of a patient with vascular disease include a stethoscope, sphygmomanometer, blood sugar measuring equipment, Doppler ultrasound, weighing scales, tape measure, urinalysis equipment and oximeter. A patella hammer, tuning fork, pen torch and items to enable assessment of sensitivity to pain, touch, heat and cold will also be required.

History taking and initial assessments

Documentation

The medical records contain all data relating to the patient, from all disciplines that have patient involvement. All documentation should be in accordance within the UKCC (1998) guidelines and must be concise, legible, accurate, dated, timed and signed. Abbreviations should be discouraged.

Demographic details

It is important to obtain name, address, birth date, age, sex, marital status, dependants, ethnic origin, religion, occupation, significant life events and hobbies in order to gain a true picture of the patient's lifestyle. An important aspect is to note who supplies the information, is it the patient, a relative or a friend? All this information will help staff to be realistic in their goals for management of the patient at home.

Reason for visiting a medical practitioner

The medical/nurse practitioner will normally ask the patient why they have presented. The patient will usually reply in a short statement, which should be documented in their exact words, e.g. 'pain in my legs every night'; this shows the exact reason why the patient feels a consultation is necessary.

History of presenting condition

This should be a chronological record of the presenting symptoms. Each symptom the patient gives in the history of the presenting condition should be looked at independently. The patient should be asked to describe the 'pain in the legs at night', from the time it commenced until the consultation visit. For conditions that may have lasted months or years, the medical practitioner should find out why the patient is seeking a consultation now. When taking a history of the presenting condition, Jarvis (1996) suggests that the final summary should include eight critical characteristics:

1. The exact location of the pain, identified by pointing to the exact spot by the patient.
2. The character of the pain: is the pain a dull ache, vice like, throbbing etc.
3. The severity of the pain.
4. How the condition has affected the patient's daily activities; the onset, duration and frequency of the symptoms. Be specific in times and dates if possible.
5. The place that the symptoms appear; is the patient undertaking any specific activity to bring on the symptoms?
6. Any factors that may relieve or aggravate the condition?
7. Associating factors; are there any other symptoms associated with the primary symptom?
8. The patient's perception of the condition and how daily activities may be affected.

Past medical history

The information gained from the past medical history (PMH) is important, as it may be relevant to the current state of health. The PMH may be broken down into several categories:

- General health.
- Childhood illnesses – here conditions should be identified that may have sequelae for the client, i.e. poliomyelitis, scarlet fever,

rheumatic fever. Illnesses such as rubella, chickenpox, measles, mumps should also be identified.
- Adult illnesses – conditions such as diabetes, tuberculosis, hypertension, epilepsy, previous myocardial infarction, jaundice, cerebrovascular event and any respiratory problems should all be identified.
- Hospitalisations – why was the patient in hospital and for how long?
- Operations – when and what operations has the patient undergone? It is also important to ask if the patient suffered any anaesthetic problems.
- Trauma history – has the client suffered any accidents? How long ago? Were there any injuries such as fractures or head injury?
- Obstetric history – how many pregnancies has the patient had? How many were complete deliveries and how many were incomplete pregnancies?

Allergies

When asking questions about allergies, food, medication and contact agents should all be discussed. Questions regarding the nature of the reaction and identification of what exactly happens to the patient should be asked. In order to maintain safe practice, it is vital that good communication channels allow information about allergies to be passed between healthcare professionals.

Medication

Within this aspect of assessment the patient should be asked to give details of all medications taken; this includes prescription medicines and over-the-counter medicines such as aspirin, vitamins etc. Many patients do not consider over-the-counter medicines to be ‘true’ medicines and therefore may not realise their relevance to their care management.

Family history

The family history of a patient is extremely important, as information regarding the cause and age of death of relatives may have genetic relevance to the patient. Questions should be asked regarding any family history of hypertension, diabetes, peripheral vascular disease, cerebrovascular event, coronary heart disease, renal problems, cancer and mental health problems.

Psychosocial history

The nurse may be able to obtain a greater understanding of the patient's feelings, fears and any cultural beliefs associated with their illness by undertaking a psychological assessment. Contributing factors towards the patient's illness may be identified.

Risk factor assessment

Three major factors that have been identified as contributing to the atherosclerotic process are smoking cigarettes, hypertension and hypercholesterolaemia (see Chapter 3). Other risk factors that must be taken into consideration are previous pulmonary embolism or deep vein thrombosis and known concurrent diseases such as respiratory, cerebrovascular or cardiac disease and diabetes.

Factors such as obesity, immoderate alcohol usage, sedentary lifestyle, drug use, poor nutritional status and poor social provision should also be considered when undertaking an assessment.

Neurological assessment

When undertaking a neurological assessment it is vital to obtain an accurate history. If the patient is unable to communicate for himself, relatives and friends may help to provide this information. Factors that should be reviewed in the history include the characteristics of the complaint, the onset of the condition, the time scale and pattern of the condition and the extent of any deficit. Within the history the practitioner should identify any treatments or investigations previously undertaken, any factors that precipitate or relieve the condition, the present neurological state and any other neurological symptoms.

Neurological assessment is divided into two levels. For patients who have no significant symptoms, a screening neurological examination should be performed. A complete neurological examination should be undertaken on patients who have neurological symptoms, e.g. loss of coordination, weakness, or who have signs of neurological dysfunction. Patients with peripheral vascular disease often give a history of a cerebrovascular event (CVE) or transient ischaemic attacks (TIA) which may be evident with neurological deficits (see Chapter 13). The neurological system will also be affected by ischaemia, particularly in the feet, which could lead to a reduction or loss of sensation. Reduced motor control will lead to an alteration in gait and loss of autonomic neurological activity.

Nutritional assessment

Within this assessment, factors such as eating problems, gastrointestinal disorders, recent weight loss/gain, musculoskeletal problems and weakness should all be considered (Fahey, 1999). Many problems occur if the patient is malnourished, including electrolyte imbalance, delayed wound healing and sepsis. These risk factors will have an influence on the morbidity and mortality of vascular patients.

The nurse should identify the type of diet the patient eats, the type of fluids and the amount consumed. The texture of the skin should be examined for dryness, presence of a rash and any skin breaks or wounds. Within the assessment the nurse should also consider the condition of the patient's mouth. Ill-fitting dentures or poor dentition will contribute to a poor nutritional intake. A full nutritional assessment by the dietetic department should be undertaken if malnutrition is suspected.

Pain assessment

The description of the pain should lead the assessor to consider if the patient is suffering from either arterial or venous disease. Ulcers may cause considerable pain. However, pain is subjective and the patient should be given the opportunity to explain the severity and type of pain. This may be helped by the use of a visual analogue scale and many hospitals now incorporate these scales into their pain assessment chart or medication sheet.

Intermittent claudication or rest pain may be the presenting complaint made by a patient suffering from arterial ischaemia. The patient with intermittent claudication may describe a sharp pain, aching, weakness or heaviness brought on by walking, which is relieved when the patient rests for a few minutes. The patient suffering from more severe arterial ischaemia may also describe pain being relieved in their limbs if they sleep in a chair with their legs down, or if they hang their legs outside the bed when lying down. If the patient's pain is not treated effectively they may suffer from reduced mobility. Further details of pain management can be found in Chapter 6.

Pressure sore risk assessment

This is a vital undertaking in any vascular patient and ideally a standardised scale such as the Waterlow scale should be utilised immediately on admission. Patients suffering from arterial disease frequently have pressure sores prior to admission, or have a high risk of developing a pressure sore while in hospital due to their arterial insufficiency and immobility. Following initial assessment the nurse should always consider whether pressure-relieving aids are appropriate and re-evaluate the patient regularly following interventions and changes in the patient's condition. Vascular patients should always be given a high priority for pressure-relieving devices. Factors discussed in the nutritional assessment should also be considered and treated in order to decrease the risk of pressure sore formation (see Chapter 5).

Leg ulcer assessment

Chronic leg ulceration will affect at least 1% of the population during their lifetime (Dale and Gibson, 1993). The incidence of leg ulceration increases with age.

Leg ulcers are debilitating and painful. Sufferers are affected not only physically but also psychologically, causing anxiety and depression, and may result in social isolation.

The accurate and timely assessment of patients with leg ulceration is fundamental to their effective management. A holistic approach to assessment is vital.

The determination of the underlying aetiology is essential and correction of these factors should be the main aim in leg ulcer management. The differentiation between venous and arterial disease is important in determining the aetiology of leg ulcers.

Doppler ultrasound is an accurate and convenient method of assessing the arterial and venous systems in the legs. It can provide objective information in addition to that obtained by clinical examination and history taking, enhancing the differential diagnosis of leg ulceration. This is discussed in detail in Chapter 8.

Social circumstances

A thorough understanding of the patient's social circumstances is important. Social isolation is a frequent problem for many patients with peripheral vascular disease, affecting their quality of life. When planning care the nurse should be aware that factors such as pain, mobility, depression, stress and anxiety, smoking and drinking habits could contribute to social isolation. Alternatively these factors may be present as a result of social isolation itself.

Activities of daily living

With any vascular patient it is vital that a functional assessment is undertaken. This will measure a person's self-care ability and lifestyle handicap. There are many problems associated with vascular conditions. These include decreased mobility, inadequate pain relief and insomnia. All of these may interfere with activities of daily living, threatening the patient's independence. The effects of these problems may not be purely physical since they may also be detrimental to social relationships. It is therefore important that the nurse has a full understanding of these problems. It must be remembered, however, that this information need not necessarily be gained during the preliminary interview; much of the information will be obtained while the nurse or other care disciplines are caring for the patient. If a holistic approach is used when assessing a patient, it will ensure that all the patient's needs are met on discharge by the multidisciplinary team.

Patients' understanding

The nurse should be certain the patient understands their problem and the treatment required. The patient's consent will be required for any invasive procedure that they undergo during their treatment.

Advice regarding causes and management of their condition should be discussed in terms that the patient understands (see Chapter 3). Verbal information should be reiterated and reinforced with written advice. National and local vascular groups can provide useful sources of information covering a wide range of vascular conditions to which the patient can refer.

The nurse should ensure that the information is consistent with any guidelines from their own area and that the information is regularly reviewed and updated.

Physical examination

Measurement of weight and height

By undertaking baseline measurements of weight and height the patient's body mass index can be calculated. These measurements are also of value to physiotherapists and occupational therapists when assessing patients for wheelchairs. Weight change is a useful indicator for measuring fluid retention.

Pulse rate

The rhythm, rate and volume should be ascertained. The rhythm should be assessed to see if it is regular or irregular. If there is an irregularity, identify if there is any pattern occurring, i.e. does the volume change on every alternate beat – bigeminy, is the pulse regular then irregular. Any rhythm other than the normal regular rhythm should have an electrocardiogram recorded to ascertain the true rhythm.

The rate should be assessed to identify if a patient has a bradycardia – below 60 beats per minute (bpm), normal rate – 60 to 100 bpm or tachycardia – above 100 bpm.

Respiration

Respiration should be recorded observing the rate, pattern, effort and depth.

The rate is usually between 10 and 20 breaths per minute.

A respiratory rate below 10 breaths per minute is known as bradypnoea. Increased intracranial pressure or depression of the respiratory centre in the medulla, which may be drug induced, are some of the reasons for bradypnoea.

A respiratory rate greater than 24 breaths per minute with shallow respiration is known as tachypnoea. This is a usual response to exercise, fever or fear. However, an increase in respiratory rate may also identify some conditions such as pneumonia, alkalosis, respiratory insufficiency and pleurisy (Jarvis, 1996).

The pattern of breathing should be assessed to see if it is even or uneven.

The effort the patient is using to breathe should be observed, i.e. is the patient breathing quietly with ease or is great effort required?

The depth of breathing should be observed to see if the breathing is deep or shallow; at the same time the expansion of the chest should be observed to identify symmetry or asymmetry in movement of the chest wall. The normal depth of respiration is considered to be between 500 and 800 ml per respiration (Jarvis, 1996).

Blood pressure

Blood pressure should be taken in both arms on the initial assessment of the patient. Infrequently readings have a 5–10 mmHg difference; the higher value should be recorded. If, however the difference is between 10 and 15 mmHg, arterial obstruction may be indicated on the side of the lower reading. The blood pressure in a young healthy adult is approximately 120/80 mmHg, although there are many factors such as weight, age, sex, amount of exercise taken that will cause variations to these readings.

Peripheral pulse palpation

Peripheral pulse site palpation will give valuable information about the location and severity of arterial disease.

An absent or diminished pulse indicates an arterial stenosis or occlusion proximal to the pulse site.

Pulses can be graded in strength from absent to normal. However, an abnormal bounding pulse will be detected in an aneurysmal vessel and its inclusion in a grading system is useful. One example is as follows (Fahey, 1999):

- absent (0)
- diminished (1)
- normal (2)
- aneurysmal (3)

Some centres may use other symbols, i.e. +/– for present or absent pulses, using ++ for normal, and + for a reduced volume pulse.

An assessment of pulses from upper to lower limbs allows the examiner to determine the presence, rate and strength of blood flow in a systematic manner. Examination of the arms with palpation of brachial and radial pulses enables a comparison with the lower limbs to be made.

The abdominal aorta should be examined for evidence of aneurysm. When examining a patient, inspect the contours of the abdomen, note any abdominal distension, visible mass, bulging or asymmetry in the shape of the abdomen. Observe the position of the umbilicus: is it midline, is there any discoloration and is it inverted? Note the colour of the skin. Observe for any pulsation of the aorta, in a thin person this may frequently be seen in the epigastric region. However, marked pulsation with widened pulse pressure will occur with aortic aneurysm, hypertension and aortic insufficiency (Jarvis, 1996). According to Bernstein (1993) the size of an aortic aneurysm is considered to be above 3 cm in diameter. In some centres patients with an aorta of more than 3 cm will be recalled for ultrasound screening on a regular basis (Scott et al., 1988; O'Kelly and Heather, 1989). Percussion of the abdomen is undertaken to identify location of the organs and any abnormal mass or fluid. Auscultation should be undertaken to check for vascular and bowel sounds. Palpation is undertaken to assess the location and size of organs, and any abnormal texture or tenderness is noted. Palpation is undertaken in two stages, the first stage being light palpation and the second being deep palpation. Palpation should be undertaken in a clockwise manner, with areas of tenderness left until last. Deep palpation is frequently undertaken using the bi-manual technique. This is performed by placing one hand on top of the other. The lower hand is relaxed and palpates, the top hand pushes down on the lower hand and the abdomen may be pushed down by 5–8 cm. The aorta may be examined slightly to the left of the midline using opposing thumb and fingers (Jarvis, 1996).

Both legs should be examined at the femoral, popliteal, posterior tibial (PT) and dorsalis pedis (DP) pulse sites. Comparison between limbs can be helpful.

The femoral pulse can be located by externally rotating the hips and palpating just below the inguinal ligament, 2–3 cm laterally from the pubis (Figure 4.1a).

To assess the popliteal artery, partially flex the knees of a supine patient, place thumbs on the knee and fingertips in the fossa pushing towards the tibial bone. Use gentle pressure to locate the artery. Alternatively, the patient can be placed in the prone position with the knee partially flexed, although elderly patients with vascular disease may find this position uncomfortable.

The popliteal pulse is often difficult to palpate (Figure 4.1b), if easily palpated it may indicate a popliteal aneurysm (Rutherford, 1995).

The posterior tibial pulse is located in the groove behind the medial malleolus (Figure 4.1c). The dorsalis pedis is a continuation of the anterior tibial (AT) artery and can be palpated along the dorsum of the foot, between the first and second metatarsal bones (Figure 4.1d and e). In 10% of the population the dorsalis pedis pulse is absent. The peroneal pulse should be assessed (Rutherford, 1995). This is located laterally above the lateral malleolus (Figure 4.1f).

(a)

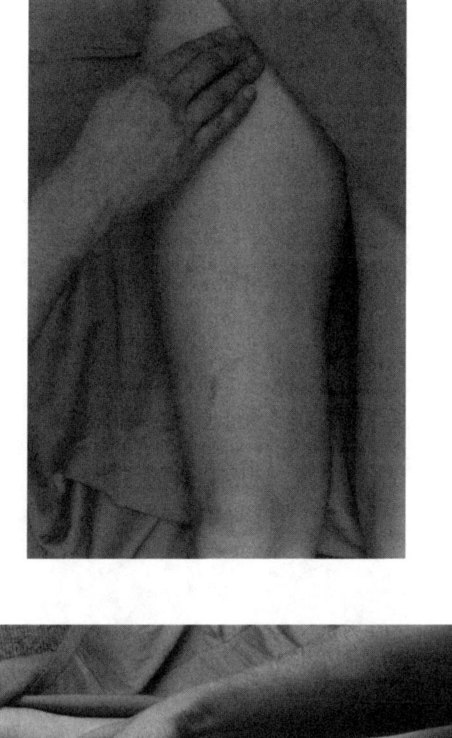

(b)

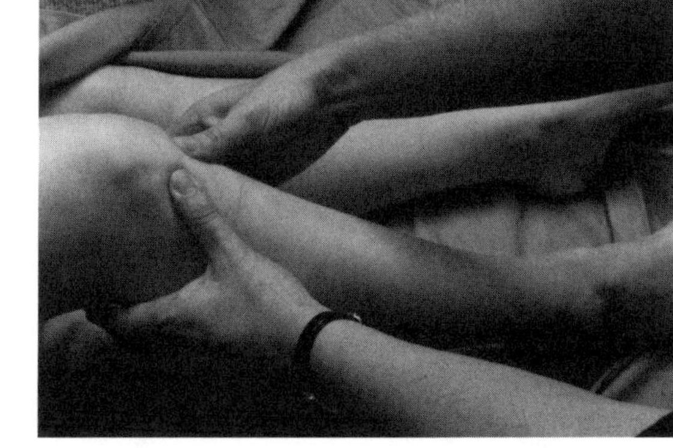

Figure 4.1(a–b). Pulse palpation sites. (a) Femoral. (b) Popliteal.

(contd)

(c)

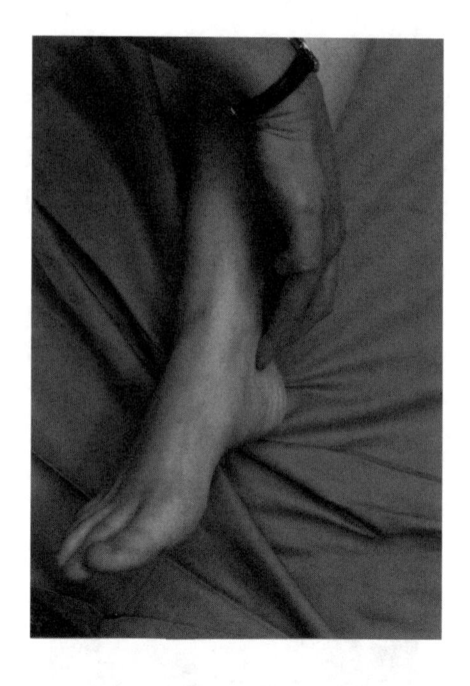

(d)

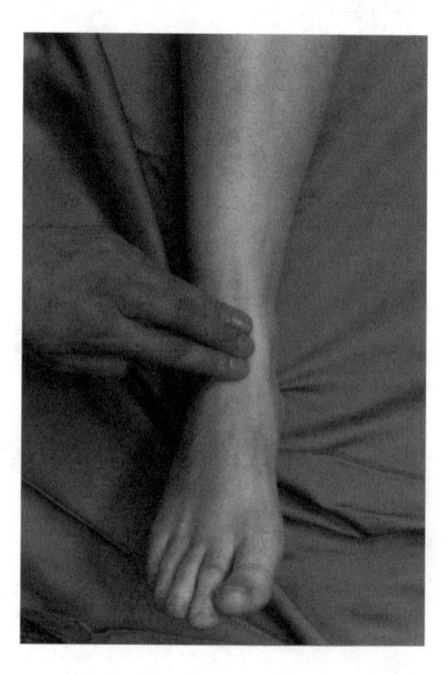

Figure 4.1(c–d). Pulse palpation sites. (c) Posterior tibial. (d) Anterior tibial.

(e)

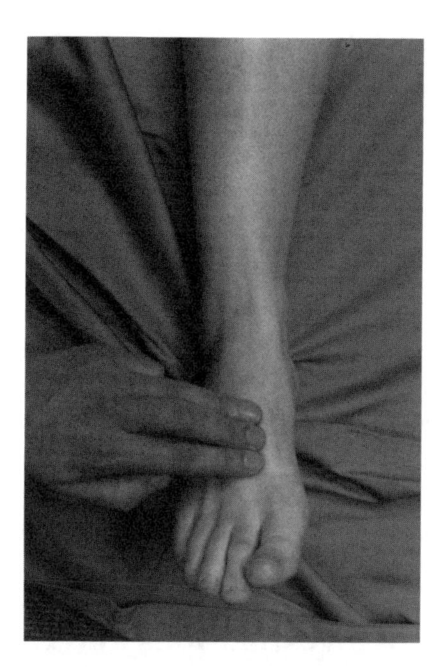

(f)

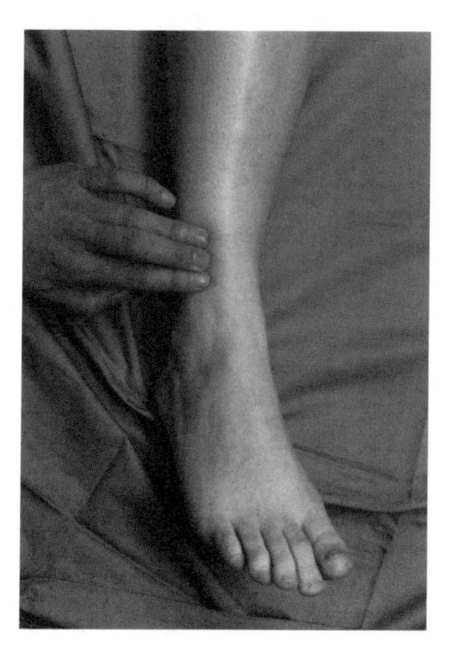

Figure 4.1(e–f). Pulse palpation sites. (e) Dorsalis pedis. (f) Peroneal.

Oedema, woody indurated skin and ulceration may make pulse palpation difficult in the distal arteries, reducing the reliability of the examination (Callum, 1987).

The palpation of pulses is a subjective assessment and should be used as a first line of investigation and followed by more objective methods of non-invasive assessment such as Doppler pressures.

Auscultation

Sounds from the heart, lungs, blood vessels and abdomen may be heard by auscultation using a stethoscope. Auscultation should be undertaken to identify arrhythmias, cardiac murmurs and bruits. Turbulent blood flow caused by a change in diameter of arterial lumen is known as a bruit (noise). This may be heard as a murmur or abnormal sound. Bruits may be found in the carotid, aorta, femoral, renal or iliac vessels. In the young healthy adult bruits are found infrequently.

Description of investigations and rationale

Urinalysis

This should be undertaken on all patients to detect glycosuria, normal and abnormal components of urine, and may aid in the diagnosis of renal disorders.

Blood glucose testing

The frequency of this investigation will be determined on an individual basis dependent upon patient need.

A raised blood glucose may indicate a pre-diabetic state or diabetes mellitus and a fasting venous blood glucose may be required to confirm diagnosis.

An elevation or a decrease in the blood glucose level may make the practitioner aware of other illnesses.

For diabetic patients taking medications such as insulin or oral hypoglycaemic agents, assessment of blood glucose level will allow the professionals to see how effective their medication is.

Blood screening

Red cell disorders, white cell disorders and clotting disorders are three of the main groups into which diseases of the blood fall. Before undertaking major surgery it is important to carry out many of the tests listed below in order to identify any disorders and to form a baseline for future blood investigations following surgery.

Blood tests that may be required:

- Haemoglobin (Hb) – haemoglobin in the erythrocyte is the oxygen transport mechanism, carrying oxygen to the tissues from the lungs. If there is inadequate oxygen transport the patient will not be able to endure a lengthy anaesthetic. Wound healing will also be affected if the haemoglobin level is low. Cancers, anaemias, diseases of the kidney, excess intravenous fluids are some of the conditions that may be detected. A raised haemoglobin level may indicate the presence of a body fluid deficit.
- Erythrocyte sedimentation rate (ESR) – raised sedimentation rates indicate inflammation and are not specific to any disorder. There is alteration of blood proteins causing red blood cells to aggregate, causing them to become heavier than normal. The degree of inflammation corresponds to the rate red blood cells fall to the bottom of the tube.
- Liver function test (LFT) – various functions of the liver may be evaluated by this test, examples being filtration, excretion, metabolism and storage.
- White blood cell count (WBC) – WBC values are useful for diagnosing health problems and ascertaining the presence of infection. The practitioner must be aware that many drugs may increase or decrease the WBC value.
- Platelet count – platelets (thrombocytes) are essential elements of blood that promote coagulation and maintain haemostasis. It must be remembered that many drugs may cause a decrease in the platelet count. Examples are aspirin, thiazide diuretics, sulphonamides and chemotherapeutic agents.
- Lipoproteins – cholesterol, triglycerides and phospholipids are the three main lipoproteins. Electrophoresis separates the two fractions of lipoproteins – alpha, high density lipoproteins (HDL) and beta, low density/very low density lipoproteins (LDL, VLDL). The beta group are the main contributors to coronary artery disease and atherosclerosis. The high density lipoproteins, consisting of 50% protein, aid in lessening plaque

deposits in blood vessels. Increased lipoproteins are phenotyped into five types – I, II (A and B), III, IV and V. The reason for measuring lipoproteins is to identify patients with hyperlipoproteinaemia, differentiate the phenotypes of lipidaemias and monitor lipid counts in patients with hyperlipidaemia.

For an accurate result the nurse should ensure where possible that prior to blood sampling, a regular diet is taken for 3 days, no alcohol is taken for 24 hours and water only is taken for 12 hours (LeFever Kee, 1998).

Cardiovascular investigations

Investigations to assess the heart's ability to cope with increased stress perioperatively may be undertaken. These may include:

- An electrocardiogram (ECG) – this is usually performed on all patients requiring surgery or invasive radiological intervention for peripheral vascular disease. It records the electrical activity of the heart using electrodes and a galvanometer (ECG machine). It may identify cardiac dysrhythmias and electrolyte imbalance. It may also be used to monitor any ECG changes occurring whilst stress and exercise tests are being undertaken.
- Treadmill electrocardiography – ECG monitoring is continuously undertaken whilst the patient is walking on the treadmill. Blood pressure measurement should also be recorded during an exercise test, as a fall in blood pressure may signify myocardial ischaemia. Conduction abnormalities or exercise-induced arrhythmias may also reflect ischaemia. However, arrhythmias that disappear are usually benign (Jones and Thompson, 1998).
- Echocardiography – by using a handheld ultrasound scanning transducer and moving it over the chest wall in the area of the heart, structure, size, function and valvular disease may all be identified by this non-invasive investigation in a two-dimensional (2-D) way. This test shows the movements and motions of structures within the heart and gives a cross-sectional view.
- Isotope scanning – myocardial perfusion scanning may be used in patients who are unable to exercise, such as patients

with claudication. Following administration of an intravenous isotope such as thallium, scintiscans of the myocardium during stress and at rest are taken. This test may be used in conjunction with traditional exercise testing or when using pharmacological stressors such as dobutamine. A perfusion defect during stress and rest usually indicates a previous myocardial infarction. If a perfusion defect occurs during stress only, this usually indicates reversible myocardial ischaemia.

Information regarding ventricular function may be obtained by measurement of the ejection fraction by radionuclide blood-pool scanning.

Pulmonary investigations

A chest X-ray is usually taken on all vascular patients undergoing surgery. Bone and tissue structure is observed, which may help to identify any cardiac or respiratory abnormalities in the chest.

Pulmonary function tests may be undertaken in order to differentiate between obstructive and restrictive lung disease and to identify the severity of the disorder. There are many pulmonary physiological tests that may be performed. The readings taken are compared with standard values. These may include:

- Tidal volume (TV) – the amount of air inhaled and exhaled during normal breathing.
- Vital capacity (VC) – the maximum amount of air exhaled following maximal inhalation.
- Functional residual capacity (FRC) – following normal expiration this is the amount of air left in the lungs.
- Forced expiratory volume in one second (FEV^{1}) – the greatest amount of air exhaled in one second.

Significant abnormalities in the above may mean there is a high risk of pulmonary complications postoperatively. Further tests such as identifying the response rate to bronchodilators may be indicated.

Oximetry may be undertaken preoperatively to identify a baseline. If the reading is abnormal, arterial blood gases should be undertaken. This will then allow for decisions to be made regarding the oxygen requirement of the patient and the possible need for assisted ventilation postoperatively.

Capillary refill

This test is also known as the blanch test. It is designed to measure circulation of blood in the fingers and toes. To perform the test, pressure is applied to the nail of a digit until the digit loses colour. On release of pressure, if the patient has good cardiac output and digital perfusion, the refill time should be less than 3 seconds. A capillary refill time of more than 5 seconds is considered abnormal and indicates poor peripheral perfusion.

Allen test

This test is performed to determine patency of the radial and ulnar artery distal to the wrist. The patient should be sitting with hands resting with palms uppermost. The radial artery is compressed manually by the observer. The patient repeatedly makes a fist causing blanching and then opens their hand.

If colour returns immediately while radial artery is compressed, then the ulnar artery is patent. Pallor persists if the ulnar artery or its arch is occluded (MacVittie, 1998).

Doppler ultrasound

The Doppler principle is the change in frequency of sound waves reflected off a moving object. As the object approaches the observer the frequency of the sound waves increases, and as it moves away from the source the frequency decreases (Gerlock et al, 1988).

Doppler ultrasound can be used to determine the velocity of blood using this principle. The change in frequency of the sound emitted and received is converted to an audible signal or seen as a waveform on a chart recorder.

Bi-directional continuous wave Doppler can be used to assess blood flow in both the venous and arterial systems.

Doppler probes of varying frequencies can be used to obtain signals from vessels at different depths. The lower the frequency of probe the deeper the penetration of the signal. Generally probes of 5 MHz and 8 MHz are used for vascular assessment, the 5 MHz giving deeper penetration.

Limb inspection for arterial disease

Oedema

The lower limb should be examined for size, symmetry and presence of oedema. Pitting oedema may indicate congestive cardiac failure, renal failure or hepatic cirrhosis. Ischaemic rest pain may cause the patient to hold the limb dependent with associated oedema in the leg. The patient may sleep in a chair or hang their leg out of bed to gain relief.

Pressing the skin firmly over the tibia for 5 seconds will identify pretibial oedema. If pitting occurs it should be graded 1+ mild to 4+ severe, although this is a subjective scale (Jarvis, 1996).

Skin changes

Poor tissue nutrition caused by chronic reduction in arterial blood supply will result in a range of skin changes including loss of hair from the limb, scaling of the skin, atrophy of the subcutaneous tissue, thickening of nails and slow nail growth.

The skin is vulnerable to breakdown, particularly from injury. Ulceration or gangrene may be present, particularly over pressure points such as the heels, the dorsum of the foot and metatarsal heads.

Colour

Both limbs should be examined to determine any differences in colour.

With the patient supine, elevate the leg and note any colour changes. If the limb becomes pale within 30 seconds, this is indicative of severe chronic arterial insufficiency. When ischaemic the dependent limb becomes red due to the chronic dilatation of the microcirculation distal to the arterial occlusion. Pallor on elevation and dependent rubor (Figure 4.2) is known as Buerger's sign (Rutherford, 1995). Healthy limbs maintain their colour on elevation.

Movement and mobility

A common complaint of patients with peripheral arterial disease is intermittent claudication, described as pain in the calf, thigh or buttock that is brought on by exercise and relieved with rest.

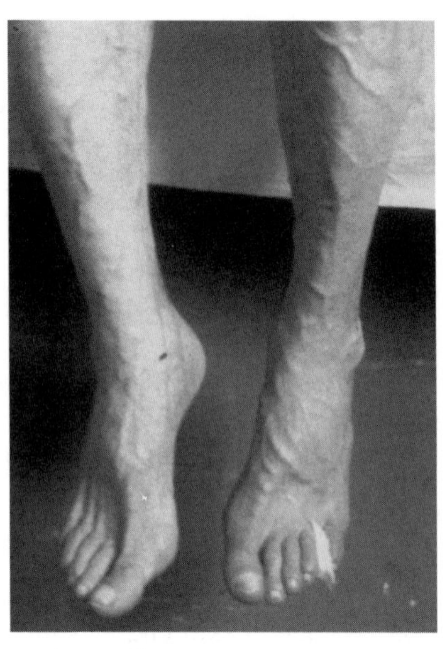

Figure 4.2 Dependent rubor see Plate 1.

Muscle groups distal to the arterial obstruction will become painful with a cramp-like sensation, usually affecting the calf muscles first.

Generally pain comes on after the same degree of exercise, but walking quickly or up a gradient will bring on the pain more rapidly.

Pain on walking may be non-vascular in origin. Osteoarthritis of the hip or knee may bring on pain with walking, but its intensity may be variable and is often worse in the morning and improves during the day. Foot pain on walking may also be caused by pes planus (flat feet).

Lumbar disc disease may cause tingling and numbness in the legs, affecting mobility.

Spinal stenosis is a degenerative condition and may cause neurogenic claudication. Symptoms include pain, numbness and weakness in the back and legs, which is relieved with rest or changing position (Dilley, 1993).

It is important to differentiate these symptoms from those caused by arterial disease.

Rest pain caused by chronic arterial occlusion will limit mobility due to the severity of the pain. Sitting and sleeping in a chair at night may relieve discomfort, as gravity will assist the perfusion of blood into the foot.

In acute arterial occlusion the limb may be numb and virtually paralysed. This is an indication of severe advanced ischaemia and rapid intervention is required. Classic features of acute or acute on chronic occlusion are known as the 6 p's:

- pain
- pallor
- pulselessness
- paraesthesia
- paralysis
- perishing cold

In chronic arterial insufficiency muscle group function may be reduced by a compromised arterial blood supply. The ability to flex and extend the toes may be diminished. Movement of the ankle may be limited by dependency oedema.

Muscle weakness caused by progressive atrophy may occur as a result of disuse.

Joint stiffness at the hip and knee can result when the patient keeps their hip joints flexed in an attempt to relieve the pain of chronic arterial insufficiency. Physical exercise should be encouraged to maintain joint mobility (Olin and Krajewski, 1996).

Mobility assessment

Mobility may be limited by coexisting pathologies such as arthritis of the hip, knee or spine. Cardiac ischaemia may cause angina, preventing the patient from exercising to a sufficient level to cause claudication. Chronic lung conditions and congestive cardiac failure may cause breathlessness, limiting ability to mobilise.

It is important to assess the patient for all potential mobility-limiting conditions, as they may mask symptoms of worsening ischaemia.

Assessment of the patient's mobility should involve physiotherapists and occupational therapists. A care pathway should be developed from admission to their return to the community.

Temperature

Ensure that the room temperature is not too cool.

Check both the limbs for skin temperature – both limbs should be warm.

Start with the toes and work up the legs feeling symmetrically. Severe arterial insufficiency will result in a cool limb. Note any changes in temperature and whether there is a gradual or abrupt change. There may be an obvious demarcation in temperature.

Arterial investigations

Continuous wave Doppler can be used to locate a diseased segment of the arterial system in the leg by assessing the common femoral, popliteal, posterior tibial (PT) and dorsalis pedis (DP) arteries.

A healthy arterial signal has a sharp positive wave peak during systole, followed by a negative wave during the early diastolic phase as a result of the elastic recoil of the artery walls (dicrotic notch). A further positive wave is seen in late diastole, as blood moves from the arteries into the arterioles and venous circulation. The normal waveform is triphasic (Figure 4.3a).

In a diseased vessel the diastolic component is gradually lost (Figure 4.3b). In an occluded vessel the pulse wave will be of low amplitude (monophasic) or may be absent (Figure 4.3c).

Signals distal to the diseased arterial segment will be abnormal whilst proximal to the diseased segment they will exhibit normal multiphasic flow patterns.

If no signals can be obtained at the ankle pulse sites with the patient lying supine, the legs may be hung dependently and pulses checked in this position. Gravity may restore flow to some of the vessels indicating patency. This should be documented.

Ankle brachial pressure index

The ankle brachial pressure index (ABPI) is an objective method of assessing the arterial blood supply to the legs.

The patient should rest in the supine position for 20 minutes if possible. If the patient is breathless they should be supported with pillows. The altered test position should be documented, as pressure recordings may be altered.

An explanation of the procedure should be given to relieve anxiety.

An appropriately sized cuff should be placed over the upper arm. A cuff that is too short or narrow will give an overestimation of blood pressure (O'Brien et al., 1997).

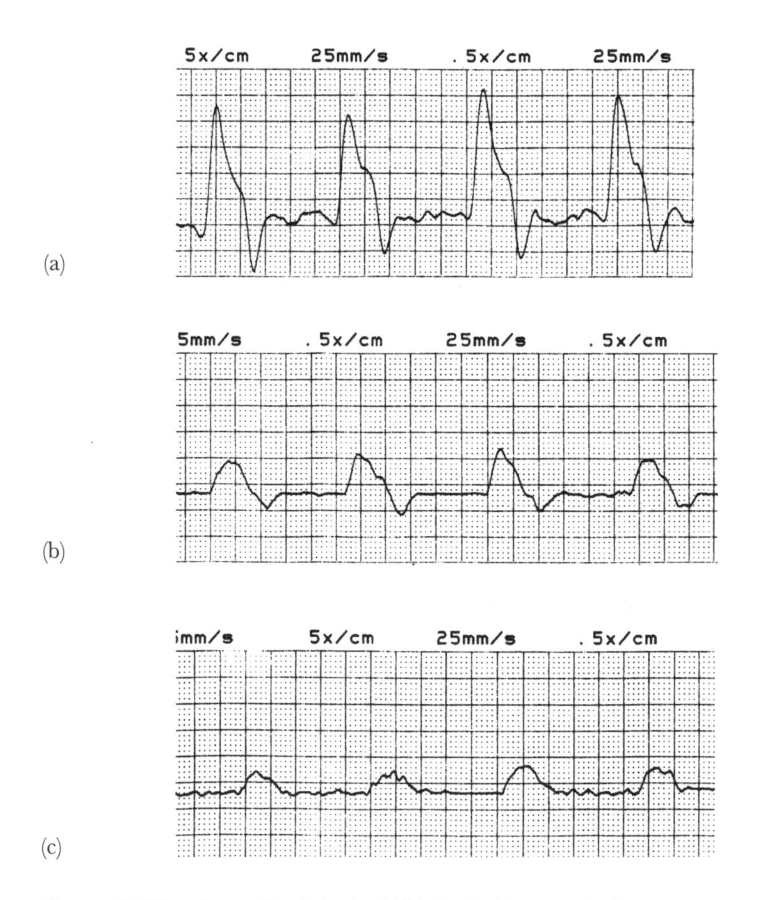

Figure 4.3 Waveforms, (a) triphasic; (b) biphasic; (c) monophasic.

The brachial pressure should be measured using a Doppler probe angled at between 45° and 60° to the vessel to obtain the best signal. The procedure should be repeated for the other arm. The highest pressure should be used in the calculation of the pressure index (Stubbing et al., 1997).

An appropriately sized cuff should then be placed around the ankle above the malleoli. The systolic pressures in the posterior tibial (PT) (Figure 4.4), anterior tibial (AT) and peroneal (PER) arteries should be obtained. The DP is more commonly used than the AT or PER. The other leg should then be assessed.

To assess patients with ulceration above the malleoli, a thin waterproof layer such as Op-site or clingfilm should be placed between the covered ulcer and the cuff to prevent contamination.

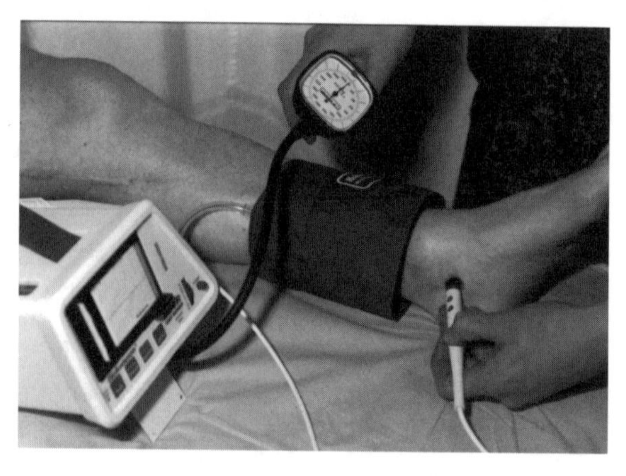

Figure 4.4 Measurement of posterior tibial artery pressure using Doppler ultrasound for ankle brachial pressure index measurement.

The highest ankle pressure is used in the calculation of the pressure index. The ABPI is calculated as shown in Figure 4.5.

Pitfalls in obtaining ABPI

Ankle pressures of more than 300 mmHg (Blackburn and Kennedy, 1999) or an ankle pressure measurement 5–10% too high indicates calcification of the medial wall of the artery, increasing its rigidity (Zierler and Sumner, 1995). This is more commonly found in patients with diabetes and renal failure. Therefore toe pressures are a more reliable measure of flow, as discussed later. In this instance the ABPI will not be a suitable test to assess the blood supply to the foot.

$$\text{Ankle brachial pressure index} = \frac{\text{Highest ankle systolic pressure (mmHg)}}{\text{Highest brachial systolic pressure (mmHg)}}$$

Interpretation

0.9–1.3: Normal (at rest)
0.35–0.9: Intermittent claudication
0.4 or less: Rest pain
0.25 or less: Ischaemic ulceration or impending gangrene

Figure 4.5 Ankle brachial pressure index and interpretation. Source: Olin and Krajewski (1996).

Wave form analysis gives an indication of the quality of the blood supply. It is important to check all ankle pulses.

Patients with thickened, woody ankles may have elevated pressure readings as a result of the increased resistance to compression of the fibrosed tissue above the malleoli.

A 5 MHz probe may be required to assess large or lymphoedematous limbs to ensure an adequate signal.

Exercise test

Exercise tests may be indicated in patients with a history of intermittent claudication who have normal resting ankle pressures with no evidence of arterial disease; also in patients who are being assessed for disease progression or treatment efficacy following radiological intervention, surgery or exercise therapy.

Stressing the blood supply to the calf muscle by exercising can demonstrate a stenosis previously masked in a resting pressure test.

Some exercise tests require the patient to walk on a treadmill to the point of claudication. This is referred to as claudication distance (CD). This test may give some indication of the patient's disability, but may not relate to the patient's ability to walk at their own pace, which may be of more relevance. A corridor walk test can be used along a measured distance if the patient is unable to tolerate the treadmill.

Before exercise is undertaken by the patient, the nurse should ensure that the patient can tolerate the degree of exercise required to perform the test adequately. The patient should not perform an exercise test if they have symptomatic cardiac disease such as unstable angina, or a recent history of myocardial infarction, severe breathlessness, hypertension, or orthopaedic problems which limit mobility (Demasi et al., 1994).

A 1-minute exercise test (Laing and Greenhalgh, 1980) may be used as it limits the amount of exercise that the patient is required to perform while providing sensitive and objective information about the patient's condition. Following baseline ankle pressures, the patient walks on the treadmill for 1 minute at a 10% incline at 4 km/h. The pressure at the ankle is then measured straight after exercise. A pressure drop of more than 30 mmHg from the baseline resting pressure is significant and indicates arterial narrowing. The greater the drop in pressure the more severe the stenosis.

Tiptoe exercises (Harris et al, 1995) or mechanical aids may be used to exercise the leg muscles if the patient is unable to tolerate walking.

Reactive hyperaemia

This test can be used for patients who are unable to perform an exercise test, due to disability or breathing difficulties.

Blood flow is occluded at the upper thigh level, using an appropriately sized pneumatic cuff and inflating it to 50 mmHg above the thigh systolic pressure. The pressure is maintained for 3 minutes then released and ankle pressures assessed every 30 seconds for 4 minutes, then every minute up to 10 minutes after cuff release or until the pressure returns to pre-test level. A normal limb will return to pre-test level within 1 minute. In the presence of arterial disease a pressure drop of 35% will be noted and the recovery time will be in excess of 1 minute (Gerlock et al., 1988). Some patients may find this test uncomfortable.

Toe pressures

In patients such as diabetics, with medial calcification of their tibial and peroneal vessels, ABPIs will be falsely elevated. Arterial calcification seldom occurs in the toe. Toe pressures can be measured using either photoplethysmography or strain gauge plethysmography and a small pneumatic cuff (Figure 4.6).

Toe pressures are usually lower than brachial pressures. A brachial/toe pressure index greater than 0.6 is normal. A haemodynamically significant lesion is present if the index is less than 0.6. Rest pain is usually present in patients with an index less than 0.15 (Strandness, 1996). In some centres absolute pressures only are recorded. Absolute pressure in the toes of 20-30 mmHg is usually associated with rest pain.

Pole test

An alternative test to assess for severe leg ischaemia in the presence of medial calcification of the distal arteries is the Pole test or limb elevation.

A Doppler signal is obtained at the ankle in a rested supine patient. The limb is elevated until the Doppler signal disappears.

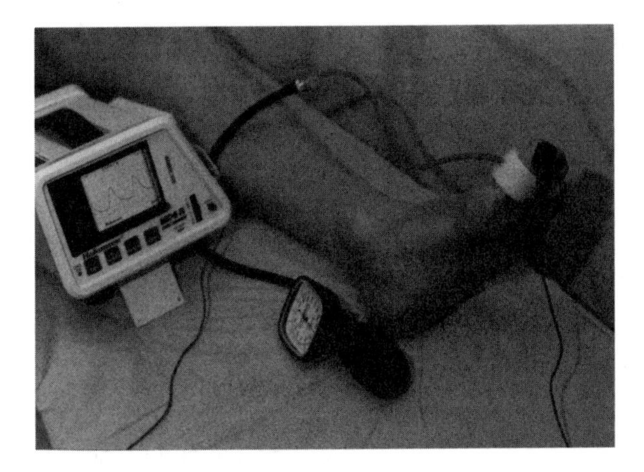

Figure 4.6 Toe pressure measurement using photoplethysmography.

The height at which the signal disappears can be measured with a calibrated pole (Smith et al., 1994) or measured in centimetres and converted to mmHg by multiplying by 0.735 (Goss et al., 1991).

This test can be useful in determining patients with critical ischaemia.

Colour duplex scanning

Ultrasound imaging uses a probe, which emits short pulses of ultrasound into the body. The signals are reflected from tissues allowing an image to be built up, showing tissue density and boundaries.

Duplex scanners are able to display blood velocities in addition to an image. Colour duplex scanners detect the movement of blood and display it as colour. The direction of the blood flow is colour coded, usually to blue or red. Velocity is shown as the hue of the colour (Lunt, 1999). This allows rapid assessment of blood flow patterns and stenosis within a vessel.

Using colour duplex scanning the arterial tree from the aorta to the tibial vessels can be imaged. Stenoses and occlusions can be demonstrated, providing a useful 'roadmap' for planning future procedures. Techniques such as angioplasty or stenting (Chapter 9), may be used in vessels with suitable stenoses whilst surgery may be offered to patients with more complex or extensive stenosis or occlusive disease (Chapter 10).

Colour duplex imaging can be used to assess the size, location and quality of saphenous veins for use in femoro distal bypass surgery. This will greatly assist in the planning of the surgery.

Regular *graft surveillance* using colour duplex imaging can demonstrate potential graft failure by detecting stenosis, particularly at anastomosis sites. Patients are assessed at 6-weekly to 3-monthly intervals during the first 18 months following surgery.

Magnetic resonance imaging

Magnetic resonance imaging (MRI) relies on protons aligning with a magnetic force in a strong magnetic field. During the realignment phase weak radio signals are emitted, which can be detected by coils placed around the patient. The source of the signal can then be mapped, allowing an overall image to be built up (Armstrong and Wastie, 1987).

MRI can be used to give useful images of the vascular system, particularly aortic aneurysms and visceral branches. Images can be obtained without using contrast media.

The patient lies within a large circular magnet housed in a gantry. The imaging process is slow but allows images to be reconstructed in any plane. The patient needs to keep still during the procedure. For these reasons patients with a suspicion of rupture or transection of the aorta may not be assessed safely due to difficulty in resuscitation. This is also the case for ventilated patients.

Benefits of this imaging technique include no ionising radiation and no known adverse effects.

MRI cannot be undertaken with some metal surgical clips and cardiac pacemakers because of the strong magnetic fields.

Claustrophobia and holding still for 4–8 minutes at a time can pose difficulties for some patients; images may be degraded if patients cannot hold still.

MRI can provide better images than computerised tomography (CT) for some postoperative patients, giving clearer images of perigraft collections and aneurysms at the graft anastomosis site (Isherwood and Jenkins, 1993).

Magnetic resonance angiography

Magnetic resonance angiography (MRA) is used to study blood vessels and blood flow. Different techniques can demonstrate not only the vessels of interest but also their surrounding tissues and end organ. Images are not limited by overlying bone, body fat, bowel gas, or vessel calcification. Images can be viewed in three dimensions from any angle.

Patients with compromised renal function may be assessed using this technique as contrast media need not be used. The risk of emboli from catheter insertion is also removed, as no catheter is required.

Assessment of the thoracic aorta using MRA is of particular use as other imaging modalities are limited in this area.

MRA has been shown to provide reliable images of normal or occluded peripheral vessels to the popliteal level. However, stenosis has not been assessed with consistent accuracy.

Computerised tomography

Conventional computerised tomography (CT) scanning uses a rotating X-ray source with a series of detectors collecting data. This allows individual slices to be obtained, which may be positioned as close or distant to each other as the operator requires.

Spiral CT allows a continuous rotation of the gantry while the patient moves through the X-ray beam. This process is very fast and avoids artefact caused by respiration (Pearce et al., 1995).

The data collected are linked to the previous set and can generate a three-dimensional image.

Injection of an intravenous contrast medium can create a CT angiogram. This technique has been shown to be valuable in the diagnosis of abdominal aortic aneurysms, renal artery stenoses and carotid artery stenoses.

Advances in MRI and CT mean that both modalities can provide similar information. However, there may be benefits to using one or other test in different situations.

The contrast media used in CT can cause problems in patients with impaired renal function and allergic reactions. It also subjects the patient to ionising radiation. Metallic objects may cause artefacts with CT, but this is a greater problem with MRI. Patients with pacemakers cannot be given MRI.

The time taken for tests to be completed may be of importance. Generally MRI is slower than CT, which may cause difficulties for some patients.

The cost of tests is also a contributing factor in their use and currently MRI is more expensive than CT.

Angiography (arteriography)

This is frequently known as arteriography and is an invasive technique. Despite introduction of CT and MRI scanning, arteriography continues to be the ideal investigation to identify the condition of the vessels and to allow for intravascular therapy. The investigation allows a clear and definitive diagnosis to made. It can be used more selectively if performed following non-invasive tests.

Radio-opaque contrast is injected via an artery, usually the femoral, and a series of timed X-rays taken to demonstrate the lumen of the vessels distally. This may provide information about the quality of vessels proximal and distal to a stenosis.

Venous arteriography is obtained by injecting contrast into the veins.

Subtraction films of the area are taken to give images of the aorta and great vessels. This technique does not give as good images as direct arterial cannulation (Sutton, 1993).

Digital subtraction angiography (DSA)

This technique involves storing images on a computer and transferring them to digital information. Stationary background such as bowel, bones and other tissues is then subtracted from the image to give an enhanced view of the vessels (Figure 4.7).

DSA has a number of advantages. Better images of blood vessels are obtained. A lower dose of contrast media is required and can be given through a smaller gauge catheter, which is safer. The degree of stenosis is estimated by the density of contrast. On-table angiography can be useful to check graft patency, anastomosis and run off vessels during surgical procedures.

The disadvantages are that contrast media may be detrimental for patients with renal disease and the insertion of catheters may also cause embolisation. Withdrawal of a catheter may cause a false aneurysm.

Care of the patient prior to arteriography

Patient education incorporating the reasons why the procedure is being performed and what the procedure will entail is vital prior to any procedure.

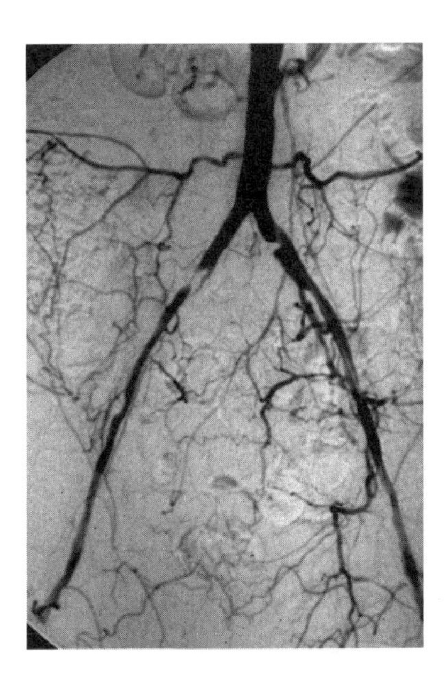

Figure 4.7 Digital subtraction angiogram.

The patient should be warned that injection of the contrast causes a sensation of heat and some discomfort.

Different centres use different procedures in preparation for arteriography; these may include: the patient being kept on fluids only, shaving the groins, and intravenous (IV) access obtained prior to arrival in the radiological department.

Prior to the investigation, renal function should be assessed because the contrast medium has the potential to be nephrotoxic (Fahey, 1999). This will allow any changes in renal function to be identified following examination. To prevent renal problems occurring it is advisable for the patient to be well hydrated before commencement of the procedure. The following care guidelines are also recommended:

- Diabetic patients who take metformin should have this omitted for 48 hours after arteriography as it may increase the risk of renal impairment.
- Patients known to have renal impairment require intravenous fluids 12–24 hours prior to arteriography to prevent dehydration.

- Insulin-dependent diabetics may require a sliding scale insulin regime until they are eating normally.
- Clotting studies should be undertaken, to ensure they are within normal limits before the procedure. If the patient is taking warfarin this is usually changed to intravenous heparin prior to examination and may be temporarily stopped immediately prior to arteriography.
- The bladder should be emptied before the investigation as the patient will need to lie very still during the procedure.
- Intravenous prophylactic antibiotics will need to be given immediately prior to the procedure to prevent infection in patients with previous synthetic grafts or stents, or those having a stent inserted.
- Informed consent should be obtained.

Care of the patient – post arteriography

Careful monitoring of the patient is vital in order to identify any complications following arteriography. This may include the following measures:

- Monitoring of vital signs every 15 minutes for one hour, then at 30 minute intervals for a further hour, then decreasing the frequency of observations as the patient's condition allows.
- Depending on the size of the catheter used the patient should be on bed rest for a minimum of 4 hours.
- The puncture site should be assessed for haemorrhage, the formation of a haematoma or false aneurysm, which should be reported immediately.
- The patient should be encouraged to drink at least 2 litres of fluid to flush out contrast medium from the kidneys.
- The patient should be nursed relatively flat in bed and instructed to keep the affected limb straight for 4–6 hours after the procedure, depending upon the size of the catheter used.
- Limb and foot perfusion should be assessed hourly.
- The monitoring of distal pulses using a handheld Doppler is vital, and should be performed not less than hourly. Any alteration in pulses may identify complications such as arterial thrombosis or embolism. If the nurse detects occlusions swiftly, further complications may be lessened.

- Pressure relief for sacrum and heels will be required during the bedrest period for patients with critical ischaemia.
- If intravenous hydration is not continued after the investigation, IV cannulation must be maintained to allow ease of access should any complications occur.
- If the patient has been on a heparin infusion, this is usually restarted following the procedure.
- Urea and electrolyte levels and full blood counts are usually taken on the day following the investigation.

Limb inspection for venous disease

Oedema

Oedema is the result of chronic venous hypertension, which itself is caused by incompetence of the valves in the deep, superficial and perforating veins. This results in a failure of the calf muscle pump to effectively return blood up the leg. The increased pressure in the venous system causes capillary dilatation and increased capillary permeability, which results in engorgement of the tissues of the lower leg.

Standing for long periods of time or sitting with legs dependent with little opportunity to mobilise, such as long haul flights or bus journeys, may worsen symptoms. Some relief may be offered by elevating the legs or performing ankle exercises or walking.

A painful, swollen leg may indicate an acute venous thrombosis. The degree of swelling will depend on the location of the thrombus. Calf vein thrombus may result in minimal swelling whilst thrombus in the iliac or femoral veins may cause the entire leg to become swollen.

Obstruction of lymph drainage results in spongy diffuse swelling of the limb.

Skin changes

Lipodermatosclerosis describes the altered skin condition that occurs as a result of chronic venous hypertension.

The thickened and woody texture of the skin of the lower leg is thought to occur as a result of fibrin which is deposited around the capillaries and acts as a diffusion barrier, depleting the surrounding tissues of oxygen and nutrients (Browse, 1986).

Varicose eczema is the result of increased levels of proteolytic enzymes, which pass through distended capillary walls and act as irritants. Bacteria present on the skin surface may contribute to skin irritation.

Colour

Staining around the lower calf can occur with chronic venous hypertension as a result of leakage of red blood cells into the tissues. Breakdown products of the haemoglobin called haemosiderin cause typical brown discoloration of the skin (Morison and Moffatt, 1994).

Movement and mobility

Limited mobility in elderly patients with venous disease may be worsened by a variety of coexisting conditions causing restricted joint movement and muscle weakness as a result of disuse and cardiac and respiratory problems.

Inactivity of the calf muscle pump will aggravate the symptoms of venous hypertension and may also increase the risk of deep vein thrombosis.

Mobility should be encouraged; walking and ankle exercises such as extension, flexion and rotation may be of particular use, even in chairbound patients (Morison and Moffatt, 1994).

Venous investigations

Manual compression test

This test can be performed to determine valve competence.

The patient stands still while the examiner's hand is placed over the lower part of the varicose vein. The other hand compresses the vein at a higher level. If valves in the vein are competent, the wave will not be transmitted to the lower level. If the wave is palpable at the lower level, the valves are incompetent (Jarvis, 1996).

Trendelenburg test

This test is performed to determine the origin of varicose veins (Macvittie, 1998).

The patient is placed in the supine position. The leg is elevated to empty the veins of blood. A tourniquet is applied to the upper thigh to occlude the long saphenous vein (LSV).

The patient is then stood upright and the veins observed for filling. If refilling occurs rapidly the perforator valves are shown to be incompetent. When pressure is released, if refilling occurs gradually, the valves in the LSV are shown to be competent. If rapid refilling occurs the valves are incompetent.

The test can be repeated occluding the short saphenous vein (SSV) by applying the tourniquet below the knee.

This test can also be used to assess the competency of valves in the perforating veins (Rutherford, 1995).

Homan's sign

This is a clinical assessment to detect deep vein thrombosis (DVT). The patient should lie in the supine position with legs straight. The foot is sharply dorsiflexed, exerting pressure on the posterior tibial vein (PTV). If pain is felt with this manoeuvre the test is positive. This occurs in 35% of cases of DVT (Jarvis, 1996).

Alternatively, the knee can be slightly flexed and the gastrocnemius muscle compressed against the tibia. Normally no pain is felt.

This test is now of limited value due to the improved degree of accuracy in current diagnostic techniques.

Continuous wave Doppler

This is used to assess valve competence in the deep and superficial veins and vein obstruction. The equipment provides a useful screening tool but requires a level of expertise in its use.

Flow in the vein is demonstrated by augmentation, using the hand to compress the distal calf while holding the Doppler probe over the vein. If a signal is obtained when flow is augmented, the vein is shown to be patent. Reflux on release of the calf indicates valve incompetence at that level. The absence of a signal following calf compression may indicate vein obstruction.

The presence of collateral vessels, recanalised veins and duplicate veins creates difficulties in interpretation of findings. Further investigation using imaging techniques may be required to clarify results.

Venous duplex

Colour duplex imaging of the venous system is used to identify deep vein thrombosis with high specificity and sensitivity, particularly in the proximal vessels (MacVittie, 1998). The technique involves compressing the veins of a supine patient using gentle probe pressure. Failure to compress the vein indicates the presence of thrombus. The extent of thrombus can be measured from anatomical landmarks to give a useful reference for future assessments.

The efficacy of treatment is assessed, by comparing measurements before and after therapy.

The use of colour duplex imaging can provide a rapid demonstration of flow direction in the deep, superficial and perforating veins. The exact location of vein junctions, collateral vessels, perforating and duplicate veins may be helpful in planning surgery. This information will help to determine the most appropriate management of the patient's condition.

Veins used for arterial bypass surgery can be *mapped*. Diameter measurements can be of use to the surgeon in determining suitability of the vein as a conduit for bypass surgery.

Plethysmography

Plethysmography assesses changes in blood volume and provides an indirect method of assessing the venous system for valve incompetence and calf pump malfunction (Fahey, 1999).

A variety of methods can be used to measure volume changes, including electrical impedance, air, strain gauge, water and photoplethysmography.

Photoplethysmography (PPG) uses an infrared light sensor to assess the relative changes in blood volume caused by venous emptying following a standardised foot exercise test.

The light source is placed above the ankle and emits infrared light into the tissue beneath and the receiver measures the light intensity reflected by the tissue. A large blood volume reduces the light signal while less blood volume increases the signal intensity.

Following exercise, veins refill slowly as a result of arterial inflow across the capillary bed. Rapid refilling is caused by valve incompetence and is demonstrated by a reduction in the reflected light signal.

Venous refill time (VRT) is assessed. A VRT of 25 seconds or more is normal. A VRT of less than 20 seconds is abnormal and indicates valve incompetence. A cuff may be applied to occlude the superficial veins. If the VRT improves to greater than 25 seconds, following cuff application, superficial vein incompetence is demonstrated. If the VRT remains below 20 seconds, deep or perforating vein incompetence is indicated.

This test can provide functional information about the benefits of superficial vein surgery and may aid decision-making about the use of compression hosiery.

The equipment can be used in the community in the assessment of patients with leg ulcers.

Venography

This test has long been used to demonstrate venous abnormalities.

Contrast media is injected into the veins and a series of X-rays taken to show venous filling. Ascending venography is used to diagnose thrombus. Descending venography can be used to assess valve incompetence.

Contrast media may cause allergic reaction in some patients. The procedure may actually cause thrombophlebitis and is often painful. For these reasons non-invasive tests such as colour duplex scanning are preferred.

Care management

Patients with peripheral vascular disease are managed in many different ways. In order to ensure continuity for all patients, a suggested care management pathway is demonstrated in Figure 4.8 which practitioners may wish to adopt.

Conclusion

The examinations described in this chapter provide a guideline for the practitioner. Many tests are subjective and this should be considered in their interpretation and the limitations understood. Practitioners should work within the resources and constraints of their environment, and regularly review and update their practice.

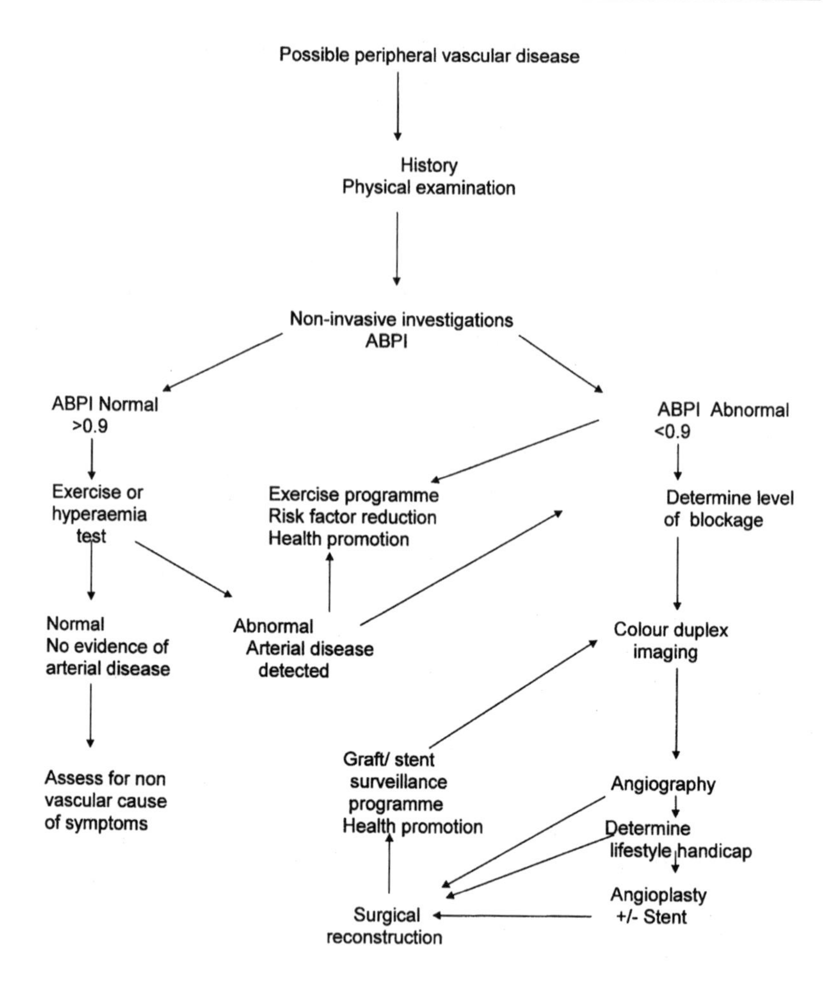

Figure 4.8 Management pathway of patient with peripheral vascular disease.

References

Armstrong P, Wastie ML (1987) Diagnostic Imaging, 2nd edn. Oxford: Blackwell Scientific Publications.

Bernstein EF (1993) Vascular Diagnosis, 4th edn. St Louis: Mosby.

Blackburn DR, Kennedy L (1999) Non Invasive Vascular Testing. In: Fahey V (ed.) Vascular Nursing, 3rd edn. Philadelphia: WB Saunders.

Browse NL (1986) The aetiology of venous ulceration. World Journal of Surgery 10: 938–943.

Callum MJ (1987) Hazards of compression treatment of the leg: an estimate from Scottish surgeons. British Medical Journal 295: 1382.

Dale JJ, Gibson B (1993) Leg ulcer management. Professional Nurse 8(5): 3.

Demasi RJ, Gregory RT, Wheeler JR, Snyder SO, Gayle RG, Parent FN, Brandt D (1994) Exercise testing diagnosis and follow-up. Journal of Vascular Technology 18(5): 257–261.

Dilley, R (1993) The history and physical examination in vascular disease. In: Bernstein EF (ed.) Vascular Diagnosis, 4th edn. St Louis: Mosby.

Fahey V (1999) Vascular Nursing, 3rd edn. Philadelphia: WB Saunders.

Gerlock AJ, Giyanani VL, Krebs C (1988) Applications of Noninvasive Vascular Techniques. Philadelphia: WB Saunders.

Goss DE, Stevens M, Watkins PJ, Baskerville PA (1991) Falsely raised Ankle/ Brachial Pressure Index: A method to determine tibial artery compressibility. European Journal of Vascular Surgery 5: 23–26.

Harris LM, Koerner NA, Curl GR, Ricotta JJ (1995) Active pedal plantarflexion: a haemodynamic measurement of claudication. Journal of Vascular Technology 19(3): 115–118.

Isherwood I, Jenkins JPR (1993) MR angiography. In: Sutton D (1993) A Textbook of Radiology and Imaging, vol. 1. London: Churchill Livingstone.

Jarvis C (1996) Physical Examination and Health Assessment, 2nd edn. Philadelphia: WB Saunders.

Jones J, Thomson CRV (1998) Essential Medicine, 2nd edn. New York: Churchill Livingstone.

Laing SP, Greenhalgh RM (1980) Standard exercise test to assess peripheral arterial disease. British Medical Journal 280 (6206): 13–16.

LeFever Kee J (1998) Handbook of Laboratory and Diagnostic Tests with Nursing Implications, 3rd edn. Connecticut: Appleton and Lange.

Lunt M (1999) Review of duplex and colour Doppler imaging of lower limb arteries and veins. Journal of Tissue Viability 9(2): 45–55.

MacVittie BA (1998) Vascular Surgery. St Louis: Mosby.

Morison M, Moffatt C (1994) A Colour Guide to the Assessment and Management of Leg Ulcers, 2nd edn. London: Mosby.

O'Brien ET, Petrie JC, Littler WA, de Swiet M, Padfield PD, Dillon MJ, Coats A, Mee F (1997) Blood Pressure Measurement. Recommendation of the British Hypertension Society, 3rd edn. London: British Medical Journal Publishing Group.

O'Kelly TJ, Heather BP (1989) General practice-based population screening for abdominal aortic aneurysms: a pilot study. British Journal of Surgery 76(5): 479–480.

Olin G, Krajewski LP (1996) Atherosclerosis of the aorta and lower extremity arteries. In: Young GR, Olin G, Bartholomew JR (eds) Peripheral Vascular Diseases, 2nd edn. St Louis: Mosby.

Pearce WH, Salyapongse AN, Fitzgerald S (1995) Computed tomography and magnetic resonance imaging in vascular disease. In: Rutherford RB (ed.) (1995) Vascular Surgery, 4th edn. Philadelphia: WB Saunders.

Peterson V (1999) Just the Facts. A Pocket Guide to Basic Nursing. St Louis: Mosby.

Rutherford RB (1995) Vascular Surgery, 4th edn. Philadelphia: WB Saunders.

Scott RAP, Ashton HA, Kay DN (1988) Routine ultrasound screening in management of abdominal aortic aneurysm. British Medical Journal 296(6638): 1709–1710.

Smith FCT, Shearman CP, Simms MH, Gwynn BR (1994) Falsely elevated ankle pressures in severe leg ischaemia. The Pole Test – an alternative approach. European Journal of Vascular Surgery 8(4): 408–412.

Strandness DE (1996) Non-invasive vascular laboratory and vascular imaging. In: Young GR, Olin G, Bartholomew JR (eds) Peripheral Vascular Diseases, 2nd edn. St Louis: Mosby.

Stubbing N, Bailey P, Poole M (1997) Putting research into practice in community leg ulcer assessment. Journal of Wound Care 6(9): 417–418.

Sutton D (1993) A Textbook of Radiology and Imaging, vol 1. London: Churchill Livingstone.

UKCC (1998) Guidelines for Records and Record Keeping. London: United Kingdom Central Council for Nursing, Midwifery and Health Visiting.

Zierler RE, Sumner DS (1995) Physiologic assessment of peripheral arterial occlusive disease. In: Rutherford RB (ed.) Vascular Surgery, 4th edn. Philadelphia: WB Saunders.

CHAPTER 5

Challenges of Pressure Ulcer Prevention in Peripheral Vascular Disease

KRZYSZTOF S. GEBHARDT

Introduction - is there a problem?

Pressure ulcers occur mainly during acute illness. They are an acute trauma which is a result of compressive and shearing forces applied to the body causing tissue distortion. Distortion of the tissues occludes blood vessels running through them. Tissues supported by those blood vessels become ischaemic. If the ischaemia persists for a sufficient period of time, the ischaemic tissues die and a pressure ulcer is formed. The healthy body avoids pressure ulceration by the sensory nervous system detecting ischaemia, and the motor nervous system altering body position or initiating activity to remove the distorting forces. To restore ischaemic cells to normal function, a healthy hyperaemic response is necessary to make up lost tissue perfusion (Bliss, 1998).

In patients with peripheral vascular disease (PVD), reactive hyperaemia is likely to be compromised due to a disturbed peripheral blood flow and suboptimal microcirculatory mechanisms. It appears reasonable to suppose that such patients would be at risk of pressure ulceration of the affected areas. Some evidence appears to support this view. Bliss and Schofield (1996), for example, report that pressure was an important aetiological factor in the development of leg ulcers in a series of patients with vascular disease. Impaired sensation appears to be the main factor predisposing to foot ulcers in diabetics (Boulton, 1992), a serious and common complication. However, since diabetics are likely to have some degree of PVD

(Pecoraro et al., 1990), vascular incompetence cannot be discounted as a contributing factor. Similarly, spinally injured patients are particularly prone to developing recurrent pressure ulcers if they have unrecognised vascular disease (Yokoo et al., 1996).

Furthermore, patients with PVD may have to endure lengthy radiological and/or surgical procedures which require anaesthesia and periods of immobilisation. Complex wound care procedures such as skin grafting and vacuum dressings cause further periods of immobility. To maintain a level of independence, amputees may spend prolonged periods of time in wheelchairs with poor pressure relief. All these factors increase the likelihood of potentially vulnerable patients spending a lot of time with their pressure areas at risk.

In advanced PVD, the arterial supply may be so poor that following even a short period of distortion ischaemia, reactive hyperaemia is insufficient to restore tissues to their pre-ischaemic state quickly or at all. In some cases the white patches which appear on light finger pressure and rapidly recolour on healthy skin (similar to the blanching test used by plastic surgeons to assess the viability of skin flaps) take a very long time to disappear (Lee and Thoden, 1985). Even a relatively short period of distortion ischaemia or frequent re-application of pressure to such an area is very likely to result in a pressure ulcer. When it does occur, such an ulcer tends to be severe and difficult or impossible to heal (Figure 5.1). Great care, therefore, must be taken to prevent damage to such limbs.

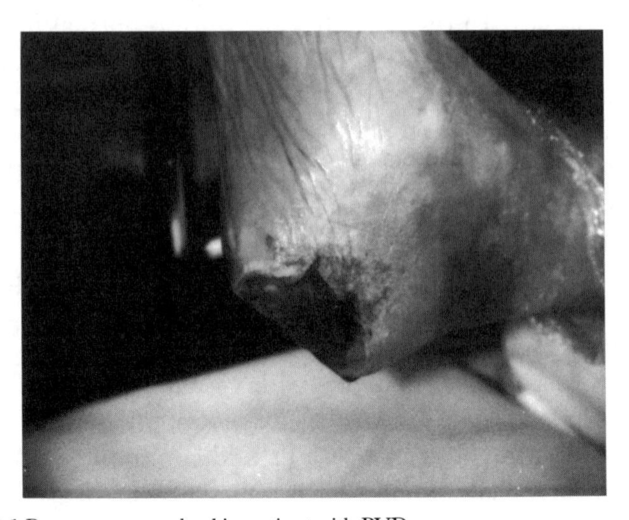

Figure 5.1 Pressure sore on heel in patient with PVD.

Although many clinicians agree that pressure ulcers are a common complication of PVD there is little epidemiological data on incidence in this group, or data to show that the presence of PVD is an independent risk factor for pressure ulcers. Patients admitted to specialist hospital vascular units have been found to have a relatively high incidence. The author found that of 1730 patients with PVD admitted to one unit over a $3^1/_4$ year period, an estimated 69 (4%) developed pressure ulcers. In another unit, similar results were observed by Gray (1998). However, incidence of pressure ulcers on limbs was lower than expected in both studies. In the author's study, for example, no patients developed pressure ulcers on their limbs other than those who already had sacral ulcers. In both study areas, the incidence rate changed little despite the introduction of equipment and education which has resulted in significant reductions in the incidence of pressure sores in local orthopaedic wards.

The principles of pressure ulcer prevention

There are numerous guidelines (NPUAP, 1992; EPUAP, 1998) and texts (Dealey, 1997; Bader, 1990) available that describe general principles of pressure area care in some depth and scope. Therefore, this chapter will limit itself to the potential problems specific to PVD sufferers. The approach to pressure ulcer prevention needs to be different depending on whether the susceptibility to ulcer formation is acute or chronic (Table 5.1).

Table 5.1 The principles of pressure sore prevention

Patients acutely susceptible
Assessment of risk within 2 hours
Positioning
Pressure-relieving devices
Treatment of underlying illness/trauma

Patients chronically susceptible
In conjunction with the patients and/or carer(s):
- Assessment of risk activities
- Planning of daily routine
- Clothing/footwear
- Support furniture (bed, chair etc.)
- Pressure-relieving devices where appropriate
- Skin examination
- Written information

The acutely susceptible patient

Acute susceptibility arises due to sudden illness or trauma, or due to an operative procedure. It is likely to be of relatively short duration and once the underlying causes are resolved, the patient will usually no longer be susceptible. For example, a patient admitted for carotid surgery may only require high dependency care for a short period on the day of the operation and overnight but will no longer be susceptible the following day. Following an acute episode, however, the patient may remain chronically susceptible if the acute episode causes permanent damage to the body's defence mechanisms against pressure damage. This situation is not uncommon in PVD where an acute thrombosis or embolus may lead to permanent damage of the blood vessels and a resultant chronic reduction in vascular efficiency – for example where a patient with acute femoral embolism requires embolectomy/thrombectomy or clot lysis.

All patients admitted to acute care should be assessed for pressure sore risk (Audit Commission, 1995). While the use of risk assessment scales such as Norton (Norton et al., 1962), Waterlow (Waterlow, 1988) and Braden (Bergstrom and Braden, 1992) has been heavily advocated, there is little evidence that using such a scale is better than clinical judgement or that it improves outcomes (Cullum et al., 1995). Patients with PVD with 'at risk' limbs may not be identified if they have few other 'risk factors'. So even if a risk score is used, this must never be a substitute for sound clinical assessment and judgement. If a patient is deemed to be susceptible, a comprehensive care plan needs to be developed which covers areas such as positioning, pressure-relieving devices and the reduction of risk factors where possible. This preventive regime must continue until the patient is sufficiently recovered to no longer be at risk.

The chronically susceptible patient

Chronic susceptibility will last for a prolonged period of time, often for the remainder of the patient's life, due to permanent damage caused by trauma or by degenerative disease. Many PVD sufferers will come into this category, for example patients with varying degrees of ischaemia for whom there is no cure and who require palliative care. Chronic susceptibility can be exacerbated by acute episodes. For example, an intercurrent illness such as a chest or urinary tract infection may reduce tissue tolerance to pressure and thus acutely increase susceptibility for the duration of the illness.

Before he or she is discharged into the community, any patient susceptible to pressure sores (and/or their carers) must be aware of the existing pressure ulcer risk, how to prevent development, what the early signs of pressure damage are and what to do if those signs appear. A discharge plan should be developed in conjunction with the patient, their carers and the community services – occupational therapy and district nursing. Following discussion of high-risk activities such as sitting on chairs or hard surfaces and how to minimise them, a plan of daily activity should be developed which:

- minimises time spent in one position;
- ensures adequate furniture is available with appropriate pressure-relieving equipment;
- ensures adequate back-up in case of equipment failure;
- provides training for the patient and/or carer(s) on inspection of the skin for pressure damage on a regular basis;
- makes sure the patient and/or carers have access to immediate help should skin damage occur.

All information given orally should be reinforced with written information and (where available) videos.

Specific problems of patients with PVD

Chair nursing

Sitting is a high-risk activity for anyone who is susceptible to pressure ulcers. Many surveys of pressure ulcers have found that chairbound patients are more likely to have ulcers than bedbound patients with the same degree of perceived risk (St Clair, 1992; Nyquist and Hawthorn, 1987; Barbenel et al., 1977). It has been shown that the high incidence of pressure ulcers in elderly, postoperative, orthopaedic patients can be significantly reduced if they are not permitted to sit for more than 3 hours at a time (Gebhardt and Bliss, 1994).

There are several reasons why this should be so. The combined effects of gravity and immobility (which reduces venous return, particularly from the legs as the calf muscle pump is inactivated) (Ashby et al., 1995) lead to a pooling of blood in the legs (Gauer and Thron, 1965). To prevent ischaemia in vital organs such as the brain and heart, blood is diverted from inessential activities, one of these being the circulation of the skin. This is likely to make the skin more susceptible to pressure damage than that of, for example, a recumbent individual.

At the same time, most of the body weight is concentrated on a small area generating large compressive forces (Staas and Cioschi, 1991). Also, compared to lying, there are significant shearing forces applied, as gravity tends to pull the skeleton forwards and downwards, while frictional forces between the skin and chair surface tend to resist the forward motion. Where the sitting posture is not ideal (Figure 5.2), these forces can be significantly increased (Medical Devices Agency, 1997).

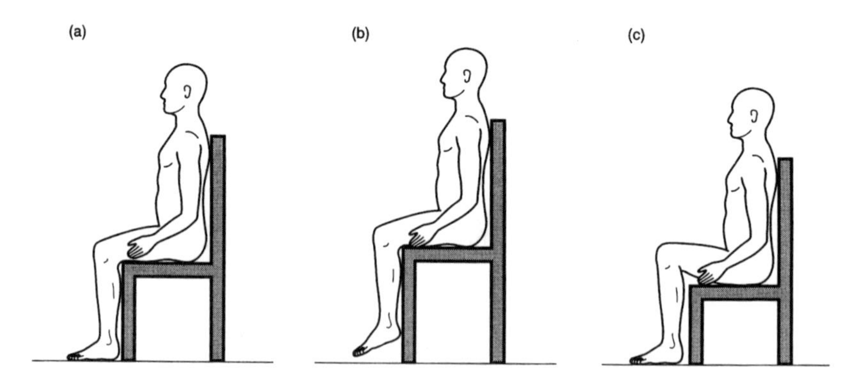

Figure 5.2 Sitting postures: (a) Optimal (b) Seat too high. (c) Seat too low.

Patients with severe PVD of the legs usually suffer rest pain due to ischaemia (see Chapter 6). However, this pain is usually least when sitting with legs dependent. This is probably because with arterial disease, blood flow into the legs improves when assisted by gravity while in venous disease, the improvement in blood flow in the legs which follows lying down possibly releases cytokines (Ferreira, 1972) which can cause severe pain. Patients with severe PVD, therefore, sometimes prefer to spend as much time as possible sitting and are resistant to bedrest or may sit on the edge of the bed with their affected leg or legs hanging over the edge in a dependent position. Prior to hospital admission for treatment, a patient with ischaemic rest pain may have spent days or weeks sleeping in an armchair at home and have severe mobility problems. These long periods of time spent sitting may, at least partially, explain the high incidence of buttock and sacral sores found in this diagnostic group.

To prevent pressure sores in patients with PVD, therefore, as much if not more attention needs to be paid to seating as to bedrest. Whilst use of pressure-reducing/relieving cushions is heavily advocated, there is little evidence of their efficacy. The main nursing effort should be directed towards reducing the time spent in a chair to not more than 2 hours at a time. This can only be achieved if rest pain is reduced or eliminated by regular, adequate analgesia (including opiates if necessary). Every effort should be made to ensure that the patient can sit in the optimal position (Figure 5.2a). In a patient who is very resistant to going back to bed, it may be helpful to use a profiling chair, combined with a pressure-relieving/reducing overlay so that they can gradually become reaccustomed to the horizontal position. They will also have the security of knowing that they can get their legs down immediately (via the patient control panel) should the pain of leg elevation become unbearable, without having to wait for a carer to help.

Choice of pressure-relieving supports

The provision of pressure-relieving/reducing support surfaces for patients to lie on is considered one of the central planks of pressure sore prevention strategy. Alternating pressure mattress replacements and overlays has been shown to be effective for pressure sore prevention (Bliss et al., 1967; Gebhardt et al., 1996) and are relatively inexpensive. However, they should be used with great care in this patient group as they depend on the patient having adequate reactive hyperaemia for their effect. Supports which have high inflation pressures should probably be avoided. In patients with critical ischaemia, flotation devices such as low airloss mattresses and beds may be a better option. Heel elevators have also been advocated but little is known about their efficacy or safety.

Compression bandaging and hosiery

When patients develop leg ulcers due to venous disease, applying high compression to the limb has been found to be an effective treatment (Baker et al., 1997). However, application of this therapy to a patient with any degree of arterial disease (and this includes patients with mixed arterial and venous disease – which Callam et al. (1987a) showed to be a common condition) may result in disastrous pressure ulceration (Figure 5.3) (Callam et al., 1987b) which can lead to amputation. Even in the absence of arterial disease, an inexpertly applied bandage can cause trauma due to ridges and troughs of pressure causing tissue distortion. Therefore, high compression therapies should only be applied by specially trained practitioners after a thorough assessment of the state of the patient's vasculature including Doppler to exclude arterial disease (Royal College of Nursing and Midwifery, 1998).

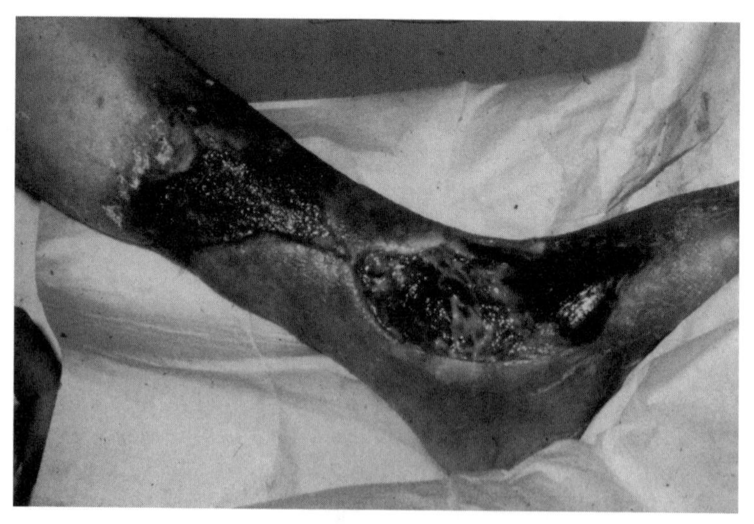

Figure 5.3 Pressure ulceration caused by compression bandaging. (Courtesy of M Bliss.) See Plate 2.

Although usually applying less pressure than compression bandaging, compression hosiery such as that used for leg ulcer prevention, or anti-embolic stockings often used postoperatively for the prevention of deep vein thrombosis are also prone to causing limb trauma (Callam et al., 1987b; Bak-Christensen et al., 1989). In some cases this can be severe. Particularly damaging injuries can be caused when thigh-length stockings are rolled down. Again, patients with PVD are likely to be particularly susceptible to this type of trauma. Compression hosiery is contraindicated in patients with an ankle/brachial pressure index (ABPI) of less than 0.8, should be applied with caution and only if ordered by vascular surgeons.

When applying anti-embolic stockings, the legs must be measured and only the correct size of stocking applied. Legs should be re-measured as legs can swell significantly despite the wearing of compression hosiery, especially when a patient sits in a chair. The hosiery should be removed daily and the skin inspected for any signs of damage, particularly over bony prominences such as shins, ankles and bunions. There is some evidence that the worst injuries occur in patients whose limbs have not been regularly inspected while wearing compression hosiery (Newton, 1998).

Patients with PVD should only have lightweight conforming bandages applied to secure wound dressings. If the patient does not tolerate even these types of bandages, dressings can be secured with a loose application of non-elasticated tubular bandage. The bandaged limbs should be checked regularly and the bandaging loosened if swelling occurs. This is particularly important for patients suffering from compartment syndrome (see Chapter 10) who have had fasciotomy incisions in the calf performed to reduce compartmental pressure.

Foot ulceration

Inappropriate footwear can cause significant damage to feet. Patients who have both sensory loss and ischaemia are particularly vulnerable, as has previously been noted in the case of patients with diabetes. There is an extensive literature on foot ulceration in diabetes and its management (e.g. Tunbridge and Hare, 1990) as well as numerous guidelines (e.g. Scottish Intercollegiate Guidelines Network, 1997). Management is best carried out by specialist podiatrists in specialised clinics (Edmonds et al., 1986). However, non-diabetics with similar problems are less likely to receive care from podiatrists. Patients with early symptoms of chronic ischaemia such as intermittent claudication and those with more advanced, limb-threatening disease, particularly if they have any associated sensory loss, should be given verbal and written advice on foot care and suitable footwear. Although this is best given by a podiatrist specialising in neuropathic feet, often this is not possible and such advice may need to be given by nurses in both acute and community settings. Where patients require bulky wound dressings to feet and toes, it may be better to provide surgical footwear to avoid foot compression.

Amputation

Despite national and international efforts to preserve limbs in patients with PVD (e.g. Krans et al., 1992), amputation remains a common outcome for many patients with PVD (Golledge, 1997). Although there is little data on the incidence of pressure sores among amputees, it is thought that they are likely to be susceptible, either because the altered statics of sitting caused by changes in weight distribution create unusual pressure gradients and shearing or, if prostheses are used, because these can cause pressure ulceration of the stump directly.

Where the amputee requires a wheelchair, this should be provided by occupational therapists or wheelchair service. The occupational therapist or wheelchair service will assess whether the patient requires a pressure-reducing or pressure-relieving cushion. Cushions should not be changed without reference to the provider service as even minor changes in the height or depth of the cushion can have significant (and usually detrimental) effects on the posture and comfort of the patient. It should be noted that the length of time the patient may be able to tolerate in a wheelchair, when otherwise in good health, may be much reduced during an episode of acute illness. It is probably best to reduce wheelchair use to no more than 2 hours at a time in such circumstances and then gradually allow longer periods as the patient's condition improves.

Likewise, limb prostheses should be provided and maintained in specialist centres, and should not, under any circumstances, be altered by non-specialists. Patient education in stump care is essential and particular care must be taken during acute illness, as with wheelchair use.

Conclusions

Patients with PVD appear to suffer from a relatively high incidence of pressure ulcers although there is little hard data on incidence and anatomical distribution. Apart from usual pressure area care, particular attention needs to be paid to reducing time spent sitting if this is excessive, taking great care with any compression of the limb (i.e. bandaging, hosiery) and to foot care. In the acutely ill, care needs to be exercised in selecting pressure-relieving surfaces, as in cases of critical ischaemia, surfaces which rely on the presence of adequate reactive hyperaemia may prove ineffective.

As is usual with pressure ulcers, there are more questions than answers. More research is needed to guide pressure area care of patients with PVD. In the first instance knowledge needs to be gained of the incidence and distribution of pressure ulcers in patients with PVD and why some acutely ill patients with vascular disease are so susceptible to ulceration of the buttocks and sacrum. Preventative strategies could then be designed, which themselves will need to be subjected to controlled studies to identify the most effective. Justification for such a research effort lies in the large numbers of individuals that are affected, and in the assumption that in the presence of vascular disease, wound healing is likely to be a protracted and costly business for the individual who sustains the ulcer and for the health service. Pressure damage in limbs with compromised vasculature often leads to amputation, with devastating consequences for the quality of life of the patient and significant expense for the health and social services.

References

Ashby EC, Ashford NS, Campbell MJ (1995) Posture, blood velocity in common femoral vein and prophylaxis of venous thromboembolism. Lancet 345: 419-421.

Audit Commission (1995) United They Stand. Coordinating Care for Elderly Patients with Hip Fracture. London: Her Majesty's Stationery Office.

Bader DL (ed.) (1990) Pressure Sores: Clinical Practice and Scientific Approach. Basingstoke: Maemillans Press.

Bak-Christensen A, Dimo B, Samson D, Wille-Jorgensen P (1989) Cutaneous reactions in relation to the use of 'TED'-stockings. Lancet December 2: 1346.

Baker S, Fletcher A, Glanville J, Press P, Sharp F, Sheldon T et al. (1997) Compression therapy for venous leg ulcers. Effective Health Care 3(4).

Barbenel JC, Jordan MM, Nicol SM, Clark MO (1977) Incidence of pressure sores in the Greater Glasgow Health Board area. Lancet ii: 548-550.

Bergstrom N, Braden B (1992) A prospective study of pressure sore risk among institutional elderly, Journal of the American Geriatrics Society 40: 747-758.

Bliss MR (1998) Hyperaemia. Journal of Tissue Viability 8(4): 4-13.

Bliss MR, Schofield M (1996) Leg ulcers caused by pressure and oedema. Journal of Tissue Viability 6(l): 17-19.

Bliss MR, McLaren R, Exton-Smith AN (1967) Preventing pressure sores in hospital: controlled trial of a large-celled ripple mattress. British Medical Journal i: 394-397.

Boulton ABM (1992) Peripheral neuropathy and the diabetic foot. The Foot 2: 67-72
Callam MJ, Harper DR, Dale JJ, Ruckley CV (1987a) Arterial disease in chronic leg ulceration: an underestimated hazard? Lothian and Forth Valley leg ulcer study. British Medical Journal 297: 929-931.
Callam MJ, Harper DR, Dale JJ, Ruckley CV (1987b) Hazards of compression treatment of the leg: an estimate from Scottish surgeons. British Medical Journal 297: 929-931.
Cullum N, Deeks J, Fletcher A, Long A, Mouneimne H, Sheldon T et al. (1995) The prevention and treatment of pressure sores: how effective are pressure-relieving interventions and risk assessment for the prevention and treatment of pressure sores. Effective Health Care 2(1).
Dealey C (1997) Managing Pressure Sore Prevention. Dinton: Quay Books.
Edmonds ME, Blundell MP, Moores ME et al. (1986) Improved survival of the diabetic foot: the role of the specialised foot clinic. Quarterly Journal of Medicine 60: 763-777.
European Pressure Ulcer Advisory Panel (1998) Pressure Ulcer Prevention Guidelines EPUAP Review 1(l): 7-8.
Ferreira SH (1972) Prostaglandins, aspirin-like drugs and analgesia. Nature New Biology 240: 200-203.
Gauer OH, Thron HL (1965) Postural changes in the circulation. In: Hamilton WF (ed.) Handbook of Physiology. Circulation, pp 2409-2439 Washington: American Physiological Society.
Gebhardt KS, Bliss MR (1994) Prevention of pressure sores in orthopaedic patients - is prolonged chairnursing detrimental? Journal of Tissue Viability 4: 51-54.
Gebhardt KS, Bliss MR, Winwright PL, Thomas J (1996) Pressure relieving supports in an ICU. Journal of Wound Care 5(3): 116-121.
Golledge (1997) Outcome of patients with claudication at 5 years in Edinburgh Artery Study. Lancet 350(9089): 1459-1465.
Gray D (1998) An evaluation of pressure sore prevention strategies in an acute NHS trust. Oral presentation, Tissue Viability. Society's 31st Conference, Edinburgh: 16/17 September 1998.
Krans HM, Porta M, Keen H (eds) (1992). Eurodiabcare. Diabetes Care and Research in Europe: the St Vincent Declaration Action Programme. Copenhagen: World Health Organisation.
Lee BY, Thoden WR (1985) Surgical management of pressure sores. In: Lee BY (ed.) Chronic Ulcers of the Skin. New York: McGraw-Hill.
Medical Devices Agency (1997) Wheelchair cushions static and dynamic. Evaluation PS4; June.
National Pressure Ulcer Advisory Panel (1992) Pressure Ulcers in Adults: Prediction and Prevention. Clinical Practice Guideline, Number 3. Rockville: Agency for Health Care Policy and Research, US Department of Health and Human Services.
Newton H (1998) Anti-embolism stockings: assessing the patient's risk, planning the intervention and evaluating the outcomes. Oral presentation, European Wound Management Association and Journal of Wound Care Autumn Conference. Harrogate International Centre, 17-19 November.
Norton D, MeLaren R, Exton-Smith AN (1962) An Investigation of Geriatric Nursing Problems in Hospitals. London: National Corporation for the Care of Old People.

Nyquist R, Hawthorn PJ (1987) The prevalence of pressure sores within an area health authority. Journal of Advanced Nursing 12: 183-187.

Pecoraro RE, Reaber GE, Burgess EM (1990) Pathways to diabetic limb amputation: bases for prevention. Diabetes Care 7: 852-858.

Royal College of Nursing and Midwifery (1998) Clinical Practice Guidelines. The Management of Patients with Venous Leg Ulcers. Oxford: RCN Institute.

Scottish Intercollegiate Guidelines Network (1997) Management of Diabetic Foot Disease, pilot edition. Edinburgh: The Network.

Staas WE, Cioschi HM (1991) Pressure sores: a multifaceted approach to prevention and treatment. Western Journal of Medicine 154: 539-544.

St Clair M (1992) Descriptive study of the use of a specialty bed in the United Kingdom. Decubitus 5(3): 28-38.

Tunbridge WM, Hare PP (1990) Diabetes and Endocrinology in Clinical Practice, 1st edn, pp 56-57 London: Edward Arnold.

Waterlow J (1988) The Waterlow card for the prevention and management of pressure sores: towards a pocket policy. Care - Science and Practice 6: 8-12.

Yokoo KM, Kronon M, Lewis VL Jr, McCarthy WL, McMillan WD, Meyer PR Jr (1996) Peripheral vascular disease in spinal injury patients: a difficult diagnosis. Annals of Plastic Surzery 370: 495-499.

CHAPTER 6

Pain Management in Vascular Disease

LYN WARD

Pain management is a high priority in caring for patients with vascular disease. The complex nature of the disease makes this a difficult challenge. The most common presenting symptom in lower extremity vascular disease is pain. The character of the pain, and its severity, location, frequency, duration and temporal pattern, are of great importance in treating the problem. Ascertaining what precipitates or aggravates the pain, or makes it subside, often allows a nurse or doctor to diagnose or exclude arterial or venous disease with over 90% certainty (Rutherford, 1995).

Pain is an unpleasant sensory and emotional experience arising from actual or potential tissue damage (Ready and Edwards, 1992). Acute pain is of recent onset and limited duration and is usually related causally and temporally to injury or disease (Carr et al., 1992). Acute pain is a symptom; it should be treated only if an underlying cause is known, if there is a plan to find its cause, or if all possible causes have been ruled out (Ready and Edwards, 1992). One of the typical pain patterns of chronic ischaemia is the persistence of pain, numbness or weakness or both, which may indicate that the patient has severe limb-threatening disease.

This chapter will consider the nature of acute and chronic pain problems facing nurses caring for patients with vascular disease. Pain assessment methods and monitoring of analgesic effectiveness will be discussed. The chapter is intended to provide basic guidelines in pain management and the reader will be directed to further reading.

Acute pain

Acute pain begins with organ damage which releases pain-causing substances. These stimulate local nociceptor nerve fibres, generating impulses which are conducted to the dorsal horn cells of the spinal cord (Woolf, 1994). Here, modulation of the impulses may occur before they are projected into pain-specific areas of the cerebral cortex.

In addition to the major stress of trauma and pain, the substances released from injured tissues evoke 'stress hormone' responses in the patient. These promote the breakdown of body tissue, increase in metabolic rate, blood pressure, blood clotting and water retention, impair immune function and trigger 'fight or flight' responses with autonomic features such as rapid pulse and negative emotions. Inevitably all surgical operations produce trauma and release potent mediators of inflammation and pain.

Acute postoperative pain in peripheral vascular disease arises, albeit hopefully briefly, when curative or palliative surgical procedures are undertaken such as aortic aneurysm repair or arterial bypass surgery. This pain may be controlled by specific modalities such as patient controlled analgesia or epidural analgesia.

Chronic pain

Chronic pain is long-standing, of more than six months duration, and is more of a 'situation' than an explained symptom with a cause and foreseeable end (Bushnell and Justins, 1993). Chronic pain is encountered in hospital and also during home care and its management presents many problems, particularly because of the effect it has on the lifestyle of its sufferers. It is important to distinguish between chronic pain of non-malignant origin and cancer pain. Chronic pain may be accompanied by sleep disturbance, loss of appetite and libido, constipation, preoccupation with illness, personality changes, depression and inability to work. The approach to managing this pain has to be symptomatic, flexible and involve combinations of several treatments. It is important to consider that chronic pain can be extremely debilitating both for the patient and for the whole family or carers.

Occlusion pain

Acute, or acute on chronic arterial occlusion pain is characteristic in that it begins suddenly and reaches a peak rapidly. In cases of arterial occlusion due to embolus or thrombosis of native vessel, or a blocked bypass graft, the patient may describe the pain as being struck down by a severe shocking pain that makes the limb weak. They may be forced to sit down as the extremity gives way. The pain may quickly subside, and depending on the severity of the ischaemia that remains after the initial occlusion, it may either resolve immediately or settle into one of the typical pain patterns of chronic numbness, weakness, or both, which indicates that the patient has severe limb-threatening ischaemia.

Classic features of acute limb-threatening disease known as the 'six p's' are as follows:

- pain
- pallor
- pulselessness
- paralysis
- paraesthesia
- perishing cold

It is important for the nurse to consider these features when assessing pain as these patients require urgent revascularisation for limb-threatening disease.

Insufficiency pain

Chronic arterial insufficiency of the lower extremity causes two characteristic types of pain; intermittent claudication and ischaemic rest pain.

Intermittent claudication has come to mean discomfort or disability associated with exercise. Depending on the site and extent of the arterial occlusion the patient may present with buttock, thigh, calf or foot claudication either singly or in combination. The most common is calf claudication which is recognised by cramping pain in the calf that can be reproduced by the same amount of exercise.

Claudication is completely relieved by a minute or so of rest and rarely needs analgesia. Patients often describe claudication pain as a dull ache or heaviness of the limb. Patients with intermittent claudication do not usually have pain at rest, although night cramps can occur as the disease progresses.

Ischaemic rest pain is typically a nocturnal pain or pain experienced at rest, of such severity that it involves the whole foot, although it may be localised in the toes or to the vicinity of an ischaemic ulcer. Rest pain may be so severe that it is not relieved even by substantial doses of opioids. Patients are typically awakened by this pain and forced to get up and do something to relieve it; this may involve rubbing and holding the foot, or walking around the room.

Any of these responses may help temporarily to relieve the pain with the help of gravity and eventually the patient learns that sleeping with the limb hanging over the side of the bed or even sleeping in a chair at night may help relieve or reduce their night-time pain. This group of patients often poses a great challenge to those involved in their care whilst awaiting revascularisation procedures to restore blood flow.

Differential diagnosis

Symptoms of pain on walking or at rest may be non-vascular in origin and patients with other forms of extremity pain are often referred to vascular surgeons under the assumption that it is circulatory in origin. For example, a painful peripheral neuritis is commonly seen in diabetics. Another extremity pain that is often mistaken for peripheral vascular pain is reflex sympathetic dystrophy (RSD); this is a syndrome of pain with motor or vasomotor instability which usually starts after a noxious event. It is not limited to the distribution of a single peripheral nerve and the patient experiences pain and hyperalgesia disproportionate to the injury with oedema and changes in skin blood flow. Like peripheral neuritis, the pain it produces is usually burning in character.

Lumbar disc disease can cause tingling, numbness and pain in the legs, which affects mobility, and spinal stenosis may cause neurogenic claudication. Similarly osteoarthritis of the hip or knee may produce pain on walking and it is important to differentiate these symptoms from those caused by arterial disease.

Leg ulcer pain

Leg ulcers are another common problem that vascular nurses are likely to encounter.

There are various types of ulcers in the lower extremity. The most common are venous or stasis ulcers, which do not typically cause excessive pain, but more a sense of discomfort. However, a significant proportion of patients with venous leg ulcers suffer moderate to severe pain (Hofman et al., 1997).

Arterial ulcers are usually accompanied by typical ischaemic rest pain. Some ulcers are of mixed aetiology, i.e. have both venous and arterial components. Other causes of leg ulcers may be vasculitic inflammatory conditions such as rheumatoid arthritis, malignancy and diabetes. Neurotrophic ulcers, which are completely painless, are often seen in patients with long-standing diabetes or peripheral neuritis.

Limb amputation

The amputation of a limb with transection of a peripheral nerve is almost invariably followed by the persistent sensation of the missing limb, which can be painful or non-painful. Furthermore, in some patients the stump can be extremely sensitive to touch (mechanical allodynia). Phantom limb and stump pain is often very intense, can be unrelenting, and may cause disruption of many aspects of life. Some patients may be intolerant of or unresponsive to many of the usual pain-relieving therapies.

The main reasons for amputation (during peacetime) are (Katz and Melzack, 1990):

- peripheral vascular disease, 60% (50% of these patients also have diabetes mellitus)
- accidents, 20%
- trauma
- tumours
- arterial thrombus
- osteomyelitis

Painless phantom limb sensations following amputation are a frequent, natural and expected consequence of amputation and usually disappear within the first year after amputation (Kao et al., 1997). In contrast, painful phantom limb and stump sensations occur in up to 80% of patients, are often difficult to treat and can be a major obstacle to successful rehabilitation (Zurmand et al., 1996). Two types of phantom limb pain usually occur: (a) burning or throbbing, and (b) ischaemic discomfort ranging from mild to excruciating (Carlen et al., 1978). It is thought that the intensity of pre-amputation pain and the severity of nociceptive injury discharge during surgery are the main factors in chronic phantom limb pain (Baron et al., 1998).

However, pre-existing underlying peripheral polyneuropathy is now proposed as a co-factor in the long-term continuation of neuropathic pain (Nikolajsen et al., 1997).

It has been suggested that ensuring good pain control before, during and after surgery will reduce the risk of chronic phantom limb pain. This has resulted in the development of pre-analgesia where epidural blockade is commenced 72 hours prior to surgery and continued for several days postoperatively. Local anaesthetic alone or in combination with opioids or clonidine can be used for epidural blockade (Baron et al., 1998). However, controversy remains about the effectiveness of these procedures (Ernst et al., 1998; Katz 1998; McQuay et al., 1998).

It is vitally important during preoperative counselling to discuss phantom limb pain and sensations with patients, reassuring them that this is usual following amputation. The type of pain an amputee experiences initially postoperatively will differ from the preoperative ischaemic pain. In some patients, such as those with painful scar tissue, puckering of the skin, inadequate closures or wound dehiscence, surgical revision of the stump may be effective.

Transcutaneous electrical nerve stimulation (TENS) has been used with some success in the treatment of phantom limb pain (Baron et al., 1998).

Psychological therapy may also be useful as stress and depression can influence the severity of phantom limb pain. Several psychological interventions are recommended such as biofeedback and relaxation therapies (Postone, 1987).

Invasive counter irritation techniques may be effective in a few patients with phantom limb pain. These techniques, such as epidural spinal cord stimulation and deep brain stimulation, are reserved for those with severe uncontrolled pain problems (Baron et al., 1998).

Neurosurgical techniques such as neurectomy, rhizotomy of dorsal root entry zone lesions, chordotomy and thalamotomy may provide short-term pain relief. However, these techniques destroy nerve fibres and patients can suffer more severe pain in the long term, so they should only be considered as a last resort in patients with severe phantom limb pain, with a short life expectancy (Baron et al., 1998).

Although complete pain relief may not always be possible, the severity of pain can be reduced, and this requires a systematic and holistic approach to the management of phantom limb pain/sensations.

Factors influencing pain

Between one-third and one-half of all surgical patients experience significant postoperative pain (Commission on the Provision of Surgical Services, 1990). Patients vary in the amount of pain they experience in relation to a specific insult and in their response to particular therapeutic approaches. These variations are partly genetic, but are also influenced by factors such as anxiety, fear, past experience of pain, and social and cultural norms for the expression of pain (Carrol, 1993).

Knowledge of the incidence and severity of pain is essential for the establishment of effective pain management programmes in patients with vascular disease.

Assessment of pain

Pain is a complex, subjective response with several quantifiable features such as intensity and duration, location, spread, aggravating and relieving factors, both at rest and during routine activities. Of prime importance in the assessment of pain is the history and examination of the patient. This should include any past experience of pain and preferences for treating and/or managing their pain. A patient's own subjective assessment of pain is the most reliable indicator of the existence and intensity of pain, and should be heeded. All members of the multidisciplinary team should be educated in the correct and consistent use of a valid pain assessment tool. Pain should be regularly measured, documented, and responded to promptly if it is to be treated effectively. Acute pain is commonly assessed using single dimension pain scales (behavioural, verbal and numerical visual analogue scale) as opposed to multidimensional pain scales, such as the McGill pain questionnaire (McGill, 1975.) In practice, verbal rating scales (VRS) tend to be simpler than visual analogue scales (VAS) for the measurement of acute pain (Melzack, 1975). Assessment tools must be reliable, accurate and easy for patients and staff to use.

Pain scoring

Patients should be asked to assess and score the severity of their pain, using a pain intensity scale (Table 6.1) both at rest, and during routine activity such as deep breathing, coughing and movement. Following pain assessment the appropriate analgesic should be selected using an analgesic ladder.

Table 6.1 Pain intensity scale

4	Worst possible/excruciating pain
3	Severe pain
2	Moderate pain
1	Mild pain
0	No pain

The World Health Organisation (WHO, 1986) has made a significant contribution in structuring a practical approach to cancer pain by devising an analgesic ladder. These principles can be applied to other acute and chronic pain problems in clinical situations. Table 6.2 (page 158) illustrates an example of an analgesic ladder.

Many of the symptoms experienced by patients with peripheral vascular disease such as phantom limb pain and sensations will need treatment with groups of drugs that are not used specifically for the relief of pain. These drugs are referred to as *adjuvant therapies* (Table 6.3, page 159), and were originally intended for the treatment of conditions other than pain. Most continue to be used in that manner, although they may also provide analgesia in specific situations. Drugs that are not classified pharmacologically as analgesics but are used alone, or in combination with narcotics to relieve pain, are known as adjuvant therapies or coanalgesics.

Assessment of analgesic efficacy

Patients with vascular disease in both hospital and community settings require regular assessments of pain levels and efficacy of

Table 6.2 Analgesic ladder (analgesic dose dependent on body weight (70 kg adult) mg/kg per day)

Pain score	Drug	Dose	Frequency	Route
0–1	Paracetamol	1 g	6 hourly (maximum dose 4 g per day or 60 mg/kg/day)	Oral/rectal Nasogastric Via jejunostomy Via stoma
1–2	Co-codamol 8/500	2 × codeine 8 mg/ paracetamol 500 mg	6-hourly	Oral/rectal Nasogastric Via jejunostomy Via stoma
2–3	Dihydrocodeine	30 mg tablets/ elixir	6-hourly up to max 4-hourly, 150–180 mg per day	Oral/via nasogastric tube IM/SC
3	NSAIDs: Diclofenac	50 mg	8-hourly, max 150 mg per day	Oral/rectal IM
4	Morphine	Dependent on pain, age, weight, condition, past use of opioids	Sevredol/ Oramorph 4-hourly MST 12-hourly MXL 24-hourly	Oral IM/SC/IV PCA Epidural

Diclofenac, or other NSAIDs, can be used for the management of moderate and severe pain in conjunction with other analgesics. Consideration should also be given to supplementing these treatments with non-pharmacological ones. For contraindications refer to the British National Formulary (BNF, 2000).
Abbreviations: MST, slow release morphine; MXL, morphine extra long; PCA, patient controlled analgesia; IM, intramuscular; IV, intravenous, SC, subcutaneous.

analgesic regimen. As pain levels alter, depending on the stage of the disease and any intervention undertaken, the need for pain relief will alter accordingly and the following action is recommended:

- Assess pain levels regularly, documenting the patient's subjective score, the analgesic requirements and effects of treatment.
- Analgesics should be prescribed on a dose/weight basis, taking

into account recommended daily dosages and contraindications.

- Step up to an analgesic on the next step of the ladder if the treatment is not effective.
- Add other drugs, such as non-steroidal anti-inflammatory drugs (NSAID) or adjuvant analgesics; as this may reduce opiate requirements.
- Review dose, frequency, and analgesic efficacy regularly.
- Patients requiring opiates may be able to reduce dosage if a simple analgesic, such as paracetamol or a NSAID is added.
- Analgesics can be stepped down as well as up if pain levels decrease.
- Patients needing opiate analgesia normally require a regular stimulant laxative; opioids can also cause nausea, which may require anti-emetics, and pruritus, which may need antihistamine treatment.
- Always try to identify the cause of nausea and/or vomiting before prescribing anti-emetic treatment.

Table 6.3 Adjuvant therapies

Anticonvulsants, e.g. phenytoin, carbamazepine, sodium valproate, gabapentin.
Antidepressants, e.g. amitriptyline.
Muscle relaxants, e.g. diazepam.
Others, e.g. caffeine, cannabinoids.

Problem	Example of drug	Dose/Route
Neuropathic pain	Amitriptyline	Orally 10–50 mg daily at night
	Phenytoin	300 mg daily
Shooting pain/numbness/tingling	Carbamazepine	Start dose 200 mg daily
	Sodium valproate	Start dose 100 mg TDS
Muscle spasm	Baclofen	5 mg TDS
	Diazepam	2–5 mg TDS
Spinal cord compression	Dexamethasone	4–24 mg daily
Sleep disturbances	Tricyclic antidepressants	(See BNF)
Anxiety	Benzodiazepines	(See BNF)
Depression	Antidepressants	(See BNF)

TDS, three times a day.
For contraindications, recommended dosages and routes of administration refer to the British National Formulary (BNF, 2000).

When prescribing or administering analgesics think:

- diagnosis
- pain levels
- documentation
- contraindications
- age/weight
- previous analgesic history
- review analgesic needs regularly

Also consider:

- analgesic – aperient – anti-emetic

Pharmacological interventions

Analgesics should be prescribed taking into account the patient's and the vascular team's assessment of pain, type and intensity. Titration of drug dosage is required to achieve the desired therapeutic effect and to maintain that effect over time. Initial administration should be on a *regular* basis.

Once an initial classification has been made, then the pharmacological treatment can be chosen from an analgesic ladder (Table 6.2). Contraindications in the medical history will influence this treatment as will previous drug history, and the patient's experiences and preferences. This treatment should then be regularly reassessed and treatment varied accordingly. Once a choice has been decided upon, careful thought should be given to the route of administration, to gain maximum compliance with treatment. The route chosen should be the least invasive that will deliver the drug of choice reliably to the patient.

Routes of administration

The routes of administration for analgesics can be considered under the following headings:

Oral

The oral route of drug delivery is the route of choice in the majority of patients, although gut absorption and general physical condition may influence the actual preparation used. A wide variety of drugs are available in dispersible, dissolvable, sublingual and liquid forms.

Drugs given by the oral route may take longer to absorb, and this should be taken into account when the dose is prescribed.

Most drugs that are available in oral preparation can also be administered via a nasogastric tube. Oral morphine; Sevredol in tablet form or Oramorph in liquid form, is an effective way to help control severe ischaemic rest pain. When the optimum dose is calculated over a 24-hour period, this can be converted to slow release morphine (MST), which lasts 12 hours, or morphine extra long (MXL), which lasts 24 hours.

Rectal

The rectal mucosa is able to absorb lipid-soluble drugs and many preparations are available in this form, although in the UK this route has remained unpopular despite its widespread use in Europe. There are many rectal NSAID preparations. Their advantage is that rectal NSAIDs are associated with roughly a 20% reduction in adverse gut effects (Cashman and McAnulty, 1995).

Parenteral

Parenteral/intravenous administration may be by bolus or continuous infusion.

Subcutaneous

In general, subcutaneous and intramuscular dose administration can be used interchangeably. Analgesic solutions should be concentrated to ensure small volumes. Infusion sites should be changed regularly dependent on appearance and patient comfort.

Intramuscular injections

This route is the most commonly used. However, absorption can be erratic with effects on speed of onset, intensity and duration of analgesia. This method necessitates repeated injections, which can be overcome by the use of an indwelling cannula such as into the deltoid muscle.

Patient controlled analgesia (PCA)

This refers to the on-demand, intermittent self-administration of analgesic drugs by a patient and is mostly used to deliver opioid analgesics, although other classes of drugs can be delivered in this way. Any opiate can be used. Traditionally the route has been intravenous but subcutaneous and epidural routes can also be used. The analgesia attained is generally good and allows for wide individual patient variation, in total dose and frequency of use. The use of background infusions is also possible, but can increase sedation and other side effects without improving analgesia. Preoperative instruction in the use of PCA is helpful. Patients express positive feelings with this technique and identified three factors: 'having better pain relief', not worrying about 'giving oneself too much drug', and not experiencing 'feeling peculiar in the head' (Chumbley et al., 1999). There are drawbacks to using PCA, such as the need for close monitoring by well-trained nurses to detect side effects of intravenous opioid administration such as respiratory depression.

Regional nerve blocks

To avoid the side effects of opioids, local anaesthetic drugs can be introduced into areas of the body no larger than the source of pain, and give extremely good analgesia. Prolonged action of the local anaesthetic is possible with insertion of catheters to the correct dermatomes, and top ups or continuous infusions of the local anaesthetic agent. Regional techniques that block pain afferents, such as extradural analgesia, intercostal and paravertebral nerve block, axillary and femoral sheath catheters and subcutaneous local anaesthetic infiltration, are useful post surgical procedures. Femoral sheath blocks are very effective following lower extremity bypass surgery to reduce pain (Rosenblatt, 1980). Lumbar sympathetic block may be indicated for pain control in severe limb ischaemia of the lower limbs. This may be performed either unilaterally or bilaterally depending on the symptoms to be treated and may be carried out using a local anaesthetic drug, for example bupivacaine (Marcain).

Surface

This may be topical or transdermal. The skin provides an impermeable barrier to most molecules but highly lipid-soluble drugs can penetrate by passive diffusion. Transdermal drug delivery permits slow but controlled release of the drug. This route is useful when the 24-hour optimum dose is calculated as a 'patch' containing opioids, usually fentanyl, which will last for 72 hours.

Inhalation

Entonox is available for inhalation via a demand only system, which means it can be delivered to a patient who actively inspires this gas via an airtight mask. A responsible trained person should supervise inhalation agents of this kind. The advantage of this route is its rapid onset and short action; the gas can be excreted without metabolism via the lungs. It is extremely useful for short, painful procedures such as wound dressing changes. Long-term use of Entonox can be associated with serious side effects, such as bone marrow depression, peripheral neuropathy and addiction.

Neural

Analgesic drugs may be delivered by direct neuraxial administration to peripheral and spinal nerves. A neurolytic agent such as phenol in glycerol injection will provide a permanent effect and may help to reduce rest pain in patients unsuitable for reconstructive surgery (Douglas Tracey and Reid, 1992).

Epidural

Opioids administered into the epidural space must pass through the dura and into the subdural space to reach the spinal cord. Some drug is lost by absorption into the systemic circulation, and some into the extradural fat. The concentration of opioid in cerebrospinal fluid (CSF) required for analgesia is very low as the dorsal horn of the spinal cord has a high concentration of opioid receptors. Local anaesthetic agents cause dilatation of blood vessels. Drugs may be administered by intermittent injection, continuous infusion or as patient controlled epidural analgesia. As with PCA, the use of epidural analgesia requires vigilant monitoring by competent nurses to detect the side effects of epidural opioid administration.

During vascular bypass surgery the combined use of general anaesthesia with intraoperative epidural analgesia is associated with increased graft blood flow and significantly lower graft occlusion rates than general anaesthesia alone (Tuman et al., 1991; Christopherson et al., 1993).

Subarachnoid

Direct injection of opioid into the CSF is associated with potent segmental analgesia. The dose is usually one-fifth of that required for epidural analgesia and onset is faster than with the epidural route. The lipid solubility of the drug is important in determining the extent and duration of analgesia.

Non-pharmacological interventions

These can be classified as cognitive behavioural approaches and physical agents. Cognitive and behavioural approaches include education and instruction, relaxation, imagery, distraction and coping mechanisms. Their purpose is to change the patient's perceptions of pain, alter behaviour patterns and help to provide a greater sense of control over pain.

Relaxation

Relaxation is freedom from mental and physical tension and stress. There are several techniques available to achieve a state of relaxation, all requiring patient participation. One or more techniques may often be combined to make a programme of relaxation therapy. Many people already practise some form of relaxation technique, which can be built on and/or combined with others. It may be achieved by various means, for example yoga, meditation, transcendental meditation. Relaxation can be used to lower anxiety and tension and encourage muscle relaxation, which has a direct bearing on pain perception, and also as distraction. Relaxation may also help with sleep, since pain is often fatiguing. It is important to realise that patients need to learn relaxation techniques.

Massage

Massage works in a similar way to relaxation and distraction, incorporating muscle relaxation. This technique can be very successful when used regularly.

Transcutaneous electrical nerve stimulation (TENS)

TENS can be used for the relief of acute and chronic pain. The mechanism by which TENS results in pain relief is not fully understood (Sindhu, 1996). TENS may act in the following ways:

- Activating nerve endings in the same way as the application of heat or cold.
- Stimulating large nerve fibres to stop the transmission of pain impulses.
- Blocking primary afferent nerve fibres.
- Stimulating the production of endorphins, the body's own naturally occurring opiate-like substances.

There are many types of devices available for the delivery of TENS which vary in size, frequency and type of amplitude. A TENS system comprises a battery-powered electronic pulse generator to which are connected two or four electrodes that are placed on the skin. TENS can be used both in hospital and at home. The positioning of the electrodes is important: they are usually placed in the area of a peripheral nerve innervating the painful site. For example, in an amputee patient experiencing phantom limb pain, electrodes can be placed over the stump and/or remaining nerves in order to stimulate the release of A-beta fibres which are thought to halt the pain impulses passing up the spinal cord to the cerebral cortex (Davis, 1993). Some amputees experience complete pain relief whilst others have little or no relief (see Chapter 11).

Acupuncture

Acupuncture is a technique developed by the ancient Chinese. During acupuncture fine needles pierce the skin at the meridian which controls the life force flow to the affected area, which may also stimulate the release of endorphins.

It should be noted that non-pharmacological interventions are intended to supplement, not replace, pharmacological techniques and may help in providing a holistic care approach to pain management in vascular patients.

Conclusion

Perfect pain relief is not always attainable in clinical practice. However, obtaining specialist advice and teaching the patient how best to cope with pain should always be the goal in caring for patients with vascular disease. Acute and/or chronic pain teams are an invaluable source of advice and practical help in assessing and treating this group of patients, and are now more readily available in both hospitals and the community.

References

Baron R, Wasner G, Lindner V (1998) Optimal treatment of phantom limb pain in the elderly. Drugs 12(5): 361–376.

British National Formulary (2000) No. 39, March. London: The Pharmaceutical Press.

Bushnell TG, Justins DM (1993) Choosing the right analgesic; a guide to selection. Drugs 46(3): 394–408.

Carlen PL, Wall PD, Nardvorna H (1978) Phantom limb and other related phenomena in recent traumatic amputations. Neurology 28: 211–217.

Carr DB, Jacox AK, Chapman CR (1992) Acute Pain Management; Operative or Medical Procedures and Trauma. Clinical Practice Guidelines No. 1. Agency for Health Care Policy and Research, US Department of Health and Human Services.

Carrol D (1993) Pain Assessment. In: Carrol D, Bowsher D (eds) Pain: Management and Nursing Care. Oxford: Butterworth Heinemann.

Cashman J, McAnulty G (1995) Nonsteroidal anti-inflammatory drugs in perisurgical pain management. Mechanisms of action and rationale for optimum use. Drugs 49: 51–70.

Christopherson R, Beattie C, Frank SM, Norris EJ, Meinert C, Gottlieb SO, Yates H, Rock P, Parker S, Perler BA, Melville Williams G (1993) Perioperative morbidity in patients randomized to epidural or general anesthesia for lower extremity vascular surgery. Anesthesiology 79: 422–434.

Chumbley GM, Hall GM, Salmon P (1999) Why do patients feel positive about patient controlled analgesia? Anaesthesia 55: 386–389.

Commission on the Provision of Surgical Services (1990) Report of the Working Party on Pain after Surgery. London: Royal College of Surgeons of England and Royal College of Anaesthetists.

Davis RW (1993) Opening up the gate control theory. Nursing Standard 7(45): 25–27.

Douglas Tracey G, Reid W (1992) Sympathectomy. In: Eastcott H (ed.) Arterial Surgery, 3rd edn. London: Churchill Livingstone.

Ernst G, Jensik G, Pfaffenzellar P (1998) Phantom limb pain. Lancet 351(Feb 21): 595–596.

Hofman D, Ryan TJ, Arnold F et al. (1997). Pain in venous leg ulcers. Journal of Wound Care 6(5): 222–224.

Kao J, Wesolowski JA, Lema MJ (1997) Phantom pain – current insights into its neuropathophysiology and therapy. Pain Digest 7(6): 333–345.

Katz J (1998) Phantom limb pain. Lancet 351(Feb 21): 595.

Katz J, Melzack R (1990). Pain 'memories' in phantom limbs: a review and clinical observations. Pain 43(3): 319–336.

McGill RG (1975) Pain management properties and scoring methods. Pain 1: 277–299.

McQuay HJ, Moore RA, Kelso E (1998) Phantom limb pain. Lancet 351(Feb 21): 595.

Melzack R (1975) The McGill pain questionnaire, major properties and scoring methods. Pain 1: 275.

Nikolajsen L, Iljaer S, Kroner E (1997) The influence of pre amputation pain on post amputation stump and phantom pain. Pain 72: 393–405.

Postone N (1987) Phantom limb pain; a review. International Journal of Psychiatric Medicine 1: 57–70.
Ready LB, Edwards WT (eds) (1992) Management of Acute Pain: A Practical Guide. Seattle: IASP Publications.
Rosenblatt RM (1980) Continuous femoral anaesthesia for lower extremity surgery. Anaesthesia and Analgesia 59: 631–632.
Rutherford RB (1995) The vascular consultation. In: Rutherford RB (ed.) Vascular Surgery, vol 1, 4th edn. Philadelphia: WB Saunders.
Sindhu F (1996) Are non-pharmacological nursing interventions for the management of pain effective? A meta-analysis. Journal of Advanced Nursing 24: 1152–1159.
Tuman KJ, McCarthy RJ, March RJ, DeLaria GA, Patel RJ, Ivankovich AD (1991) Effects of epidural anesthesia and analgesia on coagulation and outcome after major vascular surgery. Anesthesia and Analgesia 73: 696–704.
WHO (1986) Cancer Pain Relief. Geneva: World Health Organisation.
Woolf CJ (1994) A new strategy for treatment of inflammatory pain; prevention or elimination of central sensitisation. Drugs 47(Suppl 5): 1–9.
Zurmand WW, van der Zande AH, de Lange JJ (1996) Phantom pain following leg amputations; retrospective study of incidence, therapy and effect of preoperative analgesia. Nederlands Tijdschrift Geneeskdunde 140(20): 1080–1083.

Further reading

Bonica J (1990) The Management of Pain, 2nd edn. London: Lea and Febiger.
Harmer M, Rosen M, Vickers M (1995) PCA. London: Blackwell Scientific Publications
Hoskings J, Welchew E (1995) Post op Pain. London: Faber and Faber.
McCaffery M (1979) Nursing Management of the Patient with Pain, 2nd edn. St Louis: CV Mosby. Co.
Melzack R, Wall P (1985) Textbook of Pain, 2nd edn. Edinburgh: Churchill Livingstone.
Melzack R, Wall P (1988) The Challenge of Pain, 2nd edn. London: Penguin.
Orem DE (1985) Nursing Concepts of Practice. New York: McGraw Hill.
Twycross RG (1989) The Edinburgh Symposium on Pain Control and Medicine. London: Royal Society of Medical Services.

CHAPTER 7

Venous Disorders

KATHRYN VOWDEN AND PETER VOWDEN

Venous disease is common and has a significant impact on both an individual's health and the NHS, placing a major cost burden on the service. The spectrum of venous disease is vast, ranging from clinically insignificant venous flares, which may impact on a patient's body image causing great anxiety to the individual, to chronic venous hypertension and ulceration which, although not life-threatening, impacts considerably on an individual's quality of life and increases their dependence on healthcare professionals and other carers. Venous disease may also be life- and limb-threatening, conditions such as deep venous thrombosis and pulmonary embolism being a major cause of morbidity and mortality after all forms of surgery. This wide spectrum of disease and its implications are addressed in this chapter.

Nursing involvement in the patient with active or potential venous disease starts with an assessment of the patient (see Chapter 4), their general state of health and any associated medical conditions that may impact on treatment planning, and should include identification of risk factors for venous disease and possible resulting complications such as thrombosis and pulmonary embolisation. Care planning ranges from prophylaxis to general and disease-specific nursing care and this should involve other members of the multidisciplinary team to aid implementation of the most appropriate care plan for each individual. This is an active, ongoing process involving the observation and monitoring of the patient during the treatment phase, which in some cases will be during an acute illness. Risk assessment and deep vein thrombosis prophylaxis is now one of the core functions of the multidisciplinary team.

Management of the patient with venous disorders involves many teams of professionals, the roles of which cannot truly be isolated and identified as each impacts on the others. This chapter highlights the principles of specific management and allows the healthcare worker to identify and understand the actions that are taken, and the importance of recognising complications.

Some diseases of the venous system present as acute episodes, the treatment of which is largely medically led. The nurse has a pivotal role in close observation of the patient, recording the vital signs and reporting abnormalities. This will enable prompt and appropriate action to be taken which can result in the prevention of a severe life-threatening episode and reduce the incidence of later chronic complications.

Nurses are well placed to support the patient with chronic venous disease. Knowledge of the extent and position of the venous disease provided by duplex ultrasonography (see Chapter 4) can allow implementation of programmes of education, lifestyle modification and provision of compression hosiery. When medical treatment cannot be offered, nurses can also help the patient through an acute phase of their venous disease, such as treatment of ulceration in chronic venous hypertension.

Health promotion

Sometimes simple prophylactic measures can prevent the onset and progression of a disease and reduce its severity. For venous disorders this includes encouraging elevation of the limb and wearing of appropriate compression hosiery. Doing these simple things whilst also addressing general health promotion issues such as exercise and adjustments in diet will all impact on the long-term outcome for the patient with venous disease.

Where specific risk factor management is important it is highlighted in the appropriate section. General advice to prevent and modify the outcome of each venous disorder is also given.

Venous access

Gaining venous access is one of the most commonly performed invasive procedures (Vost and Longstaff, 1997). The insertion of an intravenous cannula can be life-saving. However, the choice of an inappropriate vein can destroy a patient's chance of a successful bypass graft or dialysis fistula. Venous access sites are limited and care must be taken to choose the most appropriate site for the intended infusion. Straight, soft-walled veins anchored by branching points are often the easiest to cannulate (Campbell et al., 1999). Required flow rates, solution osmolality and pH and the intended duration of the infusion, as well as patient comfort, dominant arm, vein availability and the relationship of a vein to a joint, will all influence the size and site of the vein selected. Swollen oedematous limbs or those with a functioning fistula should be avoided if at all possible. Because of the risk of line-related sepsis or the extravasation of a hypertonic or cytotoxic agent some solutions are best given via a centrally placed catheter. For long-term infusions this may be via a tunnelled line to a central vein such as the subclavian vein (Vost and Longstaff, 1997; Hamilton and Fermo, 1998).

Catheter insertion

Once the appropriate site for cannulation has been chosen the skin should be cleaned and the catheter aseptically placed within the vein. The techniques for venepuncture and catheter insertion have been reviewed by Campbell et al. (1999) and Vost and Longstaff (1997). The use of topical or subdermal local anaesthetic can reduce patient discomfort and ease catheter placement. When a suitable vein cannot be identified, ultrasound location can be helpful. Patency should be checked and the area examined for extravasation of infusion fluid before the cannula is fastened in place with tape and a transparent occlusive dressing. The advantages of specific intravenous (IV) cannula dressing types have been reviewed by Vost and Longstaff (1997). IV access sites are precious and it is therefore important that the cannula and drip tubing is well secured and that when handling the catheter site asepsis is maintained. The infusion site should be checked every 24 hours, or more frequently if the patient experiences pain, becomes pyrexial or if the catheter is dislodged or there are problems maintaining an adequate infusion rate. Department of Health guidelines suggest that the catheter be resited every 72 hours (Herbert, 1997) although if access sites are limited it may be necessary to continue infusions beyond this. In an attempt to prolong the life of a cannulation site, agents such as heparin may be added to the infusate, or a glyceryl trinitrate (GTN) patch may be placed distal to the cannula (Herbert, 1997). Some infusates are more likely to cause vein wall irritation; these include some antibiotics (vancomycin and erythromycin), amiodarone and mannitol (Clarke, 1997). Care should be taken with the dilution and infusion rates of these solutions.

Complications

Increasing discomfort or a low grade pyrexia may indicate a line complication such as sepsis or phlebitis. Some IV line complications such as air or material embolisation and thrombosis are potentially lethal. Table 7.1 outlines these and other potential complications. The nursing process relating to intravenous therapy and the avoidance of these complications has been described by several authors (Campbell and Lunn, 1997; Clarke, 1997; Vost and Longstaff, 1997). Complications are more common when lower limb veins, especially the femoral vein, are used for venous access (Vost and Longstaff, 1997). Sterile phlebitis may progress to septic thrombophlebitis and can, if not recognised, lead to septicaemia or local abscess formation. In these situations aggressive therapy with intravenous antibiotics may be necessary. The most common organisms are skin commensals including *Staphyloccocus epidermidis* and *Staphyloccocus aureus* (Vost and Longstaff, 1997). Blood cultures, especially if taken through the 'infected' line, and culture of the catheter tip will allow specific sensitivity-directed antibiotic therapy to be given.

Superficial thrombophlebitis

Phlebitis is an acute inflammation of the vein wall and most commonly results from mechanical or chemical trauma to the vein wall brought on by an IV cannula and the infusion. If unrecognised, clot may form and it may progress to thrombophlebitis (Clarke, 1997). Although it most commonly occurs at an infusion site, it may occur anywhere along the vein. It is estimated that up to 80% of patients develop phlebitis during IV therapy (Auty, 1994). This condition may also occur spontaneously either in pre-existing varicose veins or more rarely in normal superficial veins and may follow trauma to the vein (Tibbs et al., 1997). When present, the condition is acutely painful and is usually associated with pain, redness and swelling over the vein, which becomes hard and indurated. In severe examples the limb may be grossly swollen. The condition has been

Table 7.1 Intravenous therapy, complications and their prevention

Complications:
- Nerve or arterial damage during catheter placement
- Extravasation of infusate
- Pain
- Phlebitis
- Thrombophlebitis
- Infection
- Haematoma formation
- Air and material embolisation
- Equipment failure

Prevention of cannula complications by:
- Having knowledge of the underlying process
- Using an aseptic technique
- Checking the cannula site regularly (24-hourly)
- Changing giving set every 48 hours
- Resiting the cannula every 72 hours unless contraindicated
- Limiting use of cannula to the administration of fluids
- Using adequate dilutions, flow rates and large veins when giving known irritants
- Securing lines and cannulae appropriately
- Observing for early signs of the complications listed above

linked to clotting abnormalities (Hanson et al., 1998) and may be a marker of occult malignancy (thrombophlebitis migrans) (Tibbs, 1992). Although usually self-limiting, thrombophlebitis may be life-threatening and can be a cause of pulmonary embolisation if the thrombus extends to involve the saphenofemoral junction or any other major junctional site (Tibbs, 1992). It has been suggested that this condition may be associated with an increased risk of deep vein thrombosis and because of this duplex ultrasonography of the deep veins is recommended (Guex, 1996; Belcaro et al., 1999).

Management

Superficial thrombophlebitis, other than when associated with an infusion site, is rarely infected. Antibiotics do not, therefore, have a role to play in its routine treatment (Tibbs, 1992). Standard treatment regimens should include the use of a non-steroidal anti-inflammatory such as ibuprofen and support by bandage or hosiery (Herbert, 1997). Topical application of Hirudoid cream or an anti-inflammatory gel or cream may also be of benefit. Rest and elevation may help to reduce swelling and pain. Surgical drainage of a large thrombosed varix may shorten the duration of the inflammation (Tibbs et al., 1997) and may be necessary if primary or secondary bacterial infection occurs. When superficial thrombophlebitis approaches any of the major junctional sites, pulmonary embolisation becomes a significant risk and junctional ligation is recommended. When extensive superficial thrombophlebitis is present the patient should be treated with heparin. This is especially the case if other risk factors for deep vein thrombosis exist (Hanson et al., 1998).

Varicose veins and associated conditions

The prevalence of varicose veins is difficult to determine (Evans et al., 1999).Varicose veins are probably the most common condition presenting to both general and vascular surgeons. Over 50 000 patients are admitted to hospitals in the UK for treatment of varicose veins or their complications each year (Hobbs, 1991).

Risk factors

A number of predisposing risk factors for the development of primary varicose veins have been highlighted (Table 7.2). These have recently been reviewed by Burnand (1999) and have been examined in the Edinburgh Vein Study (Evans et al., 1999; Lee et al., 1999). The majority of these predisposing factors are not amenable to risk factor adjustment; however, diet, obesity, clothing, occupation and smoking habits may be. The Edinburgh group conclude that 'Based on the available epidemiological evidence, the hypothesis incriminating a fibre-deficient diet is the most consistent and would appear to offer the best prospect for any intervention aimed at reducing the prevalence of varicose veins'.

Signs and symptoms

Varicose veins are dilated, lengthened and tortuous superficial veins (Burnand, 1999) and are well illustrated in Figure 7.1. They may be simply classified into dilated venules (thread or spider veins), primary varicose veins, which are often localised and related to vein wall or valvular weakness, and secondary varicose veins, which usually follow deep vein thrombosis but which may be associated with arteriovenous shunting or congenital abnormalities such as Klippel-Trenaunay

Table 7.2 Risk factors for the development of primary varicose veins

Age	Population studies have demonstrated a rise in prevalence with increasing age (Burnand, 1999).
Gender	Most studies show a female to male ratio of between 2:1 and 4:1 (Burnand, 1999), which suggests that hormonal differences may be involved. Other studies (Evans et al., 1999) have suggested that the incidence is more equal, although women may be more likely to request cosmetic treatment.
Pregnancy	The risk of developing varicose veins during pregnancy has been investigated and found to increase with age and the number of births (Burnand, 1999).
Race	Varicose veins are uncommon in black Africans. Postmortem studies have revealed a greater number of venous valves in this group (Burnand, 1999). Others suggest that an adapted Westernised lifestyle reverses this protection and therefore is attributed to a change in diet. More studies are needed to identify the incidence of venous disease in other racial groups and their associated venous anatomy.
Height	The incidence of varicose veins increases with increasing height as this correlates with the resting venous pressure (Burnand, 1999).
Weight	Obesity is not a confirmed contributory factor but being overweight accentuates the development of varicose veins in those who are susceptible to this condition. The associated lack of exercise is suggested but not confirmed.
Diet and bowel habit	A diet that is deficient in fibre is considered a cause of varicose veins (Lee et al., 1999). Constipation, and bowel habit, has been linked with varicose veins as there is an increased pressure on the iliac veins contributing to varicosities, and straining causes increased abdominal pressure.
Increased abdominal pressure	Raised abdominal pressure as caused by sports weight lifting or playing a wind instrument or constipation and associated straining is considered to cause compression and dilatation of both the superficial and deep veins in the leg. Lee et al. (1999) suggest that squatting to defecate may provide mechanical protection for the leg veins but this is not confirmed by studies.
Clothing	Tight corsets and tight bands of clothing are said to reduce venous return (Lee et al., 1999). Flat feet, especially when associated with poor footwear and high heels (greater than 6 cm), reduce the activity of the calf muscle.
Occupation	Studies have demonstrated that those employed in standing occupations are at greater risk of varicose veins. Shop and factory workers have been studied.
Smoking	Smoking produces a decrease in fibrinolytic activity and thus would correlate with varicose veins. The few studies available seem to be conflicting (Lee et al., 1999).

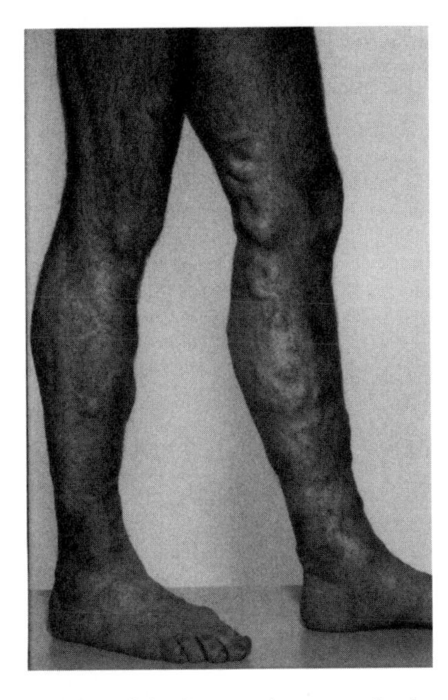

Figure 7.1 Gross varicosities of the long saphenous vein due to saphenofemoral incompetence.

syndrome (Tibbs et al., 1997). Alternative, more detailed, classification systems exist, such as the CEAP classification, which takes into account **c**linical, a**e**tiological, **a**natomical and **p**athophysiological factors (Bergan, 1999) (Table 7.3).

Symptoms attributed to primary varicose veins include aching, restless legs, feeling of swelling, heaviness, cramps, itching and tingling (Tibbs et al., 1997). The data from the Edinburgh Vein Study (Bradbury, 1999) concluded that in patients with varicose veins no particular pattern of symptoms could be used to predict future skin changes. Not all lower limb symptoms are due to varicose veins; conversely many patients with severe varicosities have experienced no symptoms. Symptoms when present are often most severe in the evening and are relieved by elevation and the use of compression hosiery.

Venous flares, particularly when situated in the gaiter area, may be associated with deep or superficial reflux, especially ankle perforator incompetence, but they may also occur in isolation. The selective use of duplex ultrasonography in these patients can be of value.

Table 7.3 CEAP classification of venous disease

Clinical	Telangiectases Prominent veins Varicose veins Oedema Skin changes Healed ulcer Active ulcer
Aetiological	Primary Secondary Primary and secondary Congenital
Anatomical	Superficial Perforating Deep
Pathophysiological	Reflux Obstruction Reflux and obstruction

Complications of superficial venous disease

Cosmetic aspects are important to the patient seeking treatment as is the fear of developing complications such as skin changes or ulceration (Hobbs, 1991). Varicose veins may be complicated by superficial thrombophlebitis, rupture and haemorrhage, and may over time be associated with skin changes due to chronic venous hypertension. These include eczema, skin pigmentation, lipodermatosclerosis, atrophie blanche and ulceration (K Vowden, 1998; Tibbs et al., 1997). Skin changes, when present, are more common in the gaiter area, particularly around the medial malleolus, but can occur anywhere in relation to varicosities of the lower limb. Duplex ultrasound studies of patients with venous ulceration suggest that up to 50% have isolated superficial reflux and thus may be suitable for superficial venous surgery, which should reduce ulcer recurrence (Grabs et al., 1996; Scriven et al., 1997; Ghauri et al., 1998).

Investigations

Inspection and clinical testing for reflux using, for example, the Brodie–Trendelenburg test can identify sites of perforator or junctional incompetence in either the long or short saphenous system. Several authors have suggested that used in isolation this is an inadequate method of assessing patients with varicose veins, indicating that hand-held continuous wave Doppler or colour flow duplex ultrasonography should be used (P Vowden, 1998b; Nicolaides, 1999; Berridge and Weston, 1999). The patient should be assessed with colour flow duplex ultrasonography when: varicosities are recurrent; if there is suspected perforator or short saphenous incompetence; if there is a previous history of a thrombotic episode such as deep vein thrombosis (DVT), pulmonary embolism (PE) or white leg of pregnancy; if there is a history of lower limb trauma or pelvic surgery.

Photoplethysmography (PPG), ambulatory venous pressure measurement, gravimetric and volumetric plethysmography and venography all provide alternative methods of assessing the patient with venous disease. The use of these investigations has been largely superseded by advances in duplex ultrasonography. The present role of these investigations has been reviewed by several authors (P Vowden, 1998; Nicolaides, 1999; Berridge and Weston, 1999). A suggested pathway for investigation of venous disease is given in Figure 7.2.

Conservative treatment, care and management

There are several elements to the care and management of a patient with varicose veins. These should include:

- A patient education programme.
- Examination and control of risk factors for venous disease.
- Advice on camouflage techniques and, where required, information on the cosmetic treatments available such as laser therapy and microsclerotherapy.

Patients also require reassurance and advice on the prevention of complications. Support hosiery is a vital element of routine care for many patients and is applicable to some individuals even after corrective surgery. Treatment by surgery is, however, the only curative option for many patients.

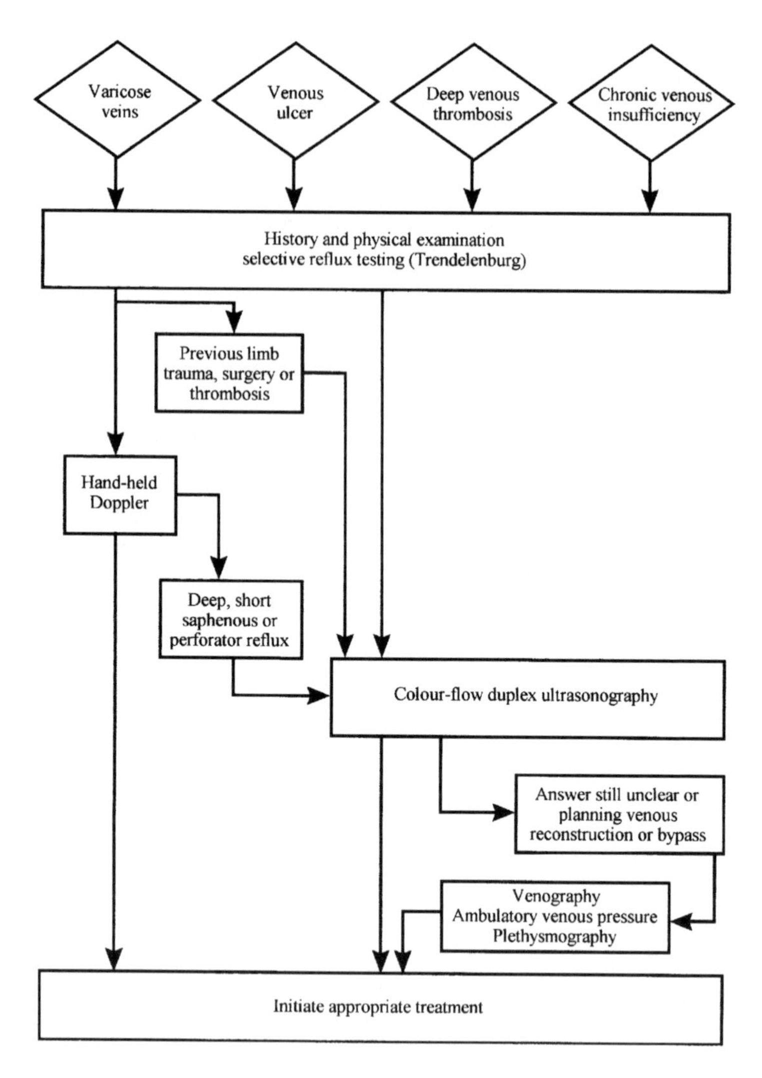

Figure 7.2 Proposed investigation pathway for patients presenting with venous disease.

Patient education and control of risk factors

Control of risk factors is important and should be instigated for all patients irrespective of other treatment intentions. Verbal information should be supported by written advice and may involve interaction with several professions allied to medicine. Advice should include information on:

- Weight control and a change in diet to include an increase in dietary fibre. This may include dietetic input.
- Exercise with correction of any abnormal gait to improve muscle pump activity and periodic lower limb elevation with the feet elevated above heart level. This may require physiotherapy input.
- Advice on footwear and foot care. This may require podiatry input.

A change in lifestyle or occupation may also be necessary for some patients to allow them to avoid complications associated with prolonged standing.

Compression

Support hosiery can relieve symptoms, conceal varicosities, prevent deterioration and may improve calf muscle pump function. To be effective compression must be graduated and provide the maximum pressure at the ankle. The level of compression needed is related to the severity of the venous disease. At present two classification systems exist, a European and a British standard. The European standard is based on the work of Stemmer (1969). The British standard is based on Department of Health classifications in the Drug Tariff. The two standards are compared in Table 7.4 which includes the suggested use of each grade of stocking.

Before introducing compression, patients should be assessed fully and significant arterial disease excluded (see Chapter 4). The Scottish surgeons study indicates the dangers of inappropriate or poorly implemented compression therapy (Callam et al., 1987). The ankle brachial pressure index should be recorded and should be repeated periodically, for example, before new garments are prescribed. A wide range of hosiery is available, each patient should be individually fitted and their suitability for the type of garment to be prescribed assessed. Exact measurements will enable correct fitting of the hosiery and encourage patient compliance with the garment. For some patients 'made-to-measure' hosiery may be required to ensure comfort and maximum use of the garment. Assessment should include not only measurements for the most appropriate size, fit and make of hosiery but also an assessment of the patient's expectations, motivation and ability to apply the garment. Their need for assistance, known allergies and the current state of the skin should be

Table 7.4 Classification of compression hosiery

European standard	Compression rating	Use	Drug Tariff equivalent
Class I (light support)	18–21 mmHg	Suitable for early varicosities including those during pregnancy	14–17 mmHg
Class II (medium support)	25–32 mmHg	Suitable for moderately severe superficial vein incompetence with varicose veins and the prevention of venous ulceration. Also used for the control of mild oedema	18–24 mmHg
Class III (strong support)	36–47 mmHg	The management of post-phlebitic venous insufficiency and prevention of ulcer recurrence in this condition. Also suitable for gross oedema	25–35 mmHg
Class IV (extra-strong support)	>50 mmHg	Used for the control of lymphoedema and congenital and acquired arteriovenous fistulae	None

recorded. Patient education allows ownership regarding self-care and maintenance of skin integrity with moisturising agents. The correct application and care of the hosiery is important to prevent complications and to extend the life of the garment.

Many of the problems that patients have to confront in relation to support hosiery can be alleviated by education and knowledgeable and creative clinical management. Elderly patients may have difficulty putting on the hosiery. Simple measures such as wearing rubber gloves to aid grip and dusting the leg with foot powder will ease application. Commercially available applicators of varied designs such as the Chinese slipper and the Valet (Medi) are available from many hosiery companies. An alternative aid to application is to wear two lower compression stockings one over the other. The compression value obtained approximates to the sum of the two stockings. A combination of above and below knee hosiery can also be used for patients with thigh problems.

Management of venous flares and telangiectasia

The appearance of minor venous abnormalities may be improved by leg make-up, laser therapy and microsclerotherapy (Tibbs et al., 1997). Laser treatment, using either argon, pulsed dye or frequency double Nd:YAG lasers or intense non-coherent pulsed light, has proved disappointing for the average patient with leg telangiectasia (very fine red or blue 'spider veins') and microsclerotherapy remains the mainstay of treatment (Quaba, 1999). Detergent solutions (sodium tetradecyl sulphate (STD), ethanolamine and polidocanol), osmotic solutions (hypertonic saline or glucose) and chemical solutions (chromated glycerine) may all be used. Generally, compression is not required and there need be no change in the patient's normal routine. Complications are uncommon but may include pigmentation, pain, oedema at the injection site, cutaneous necrosis, allergic reactions, thrombosis and development of new telangiectasia.

Management of varicose veins by sclerotherapy

Most UK surgeons with an interest in venous disease tend to favour surgery over sclerotherapy. This preference is based on the results of long-term follow-up, which suggests a higher incidence of recurrence after sclerotherapy (Belcaro et al., 1995; Tibbs et al., 1997).

Sclerotherapy is most effective when reserved for patients with local varicosities not associated with junctional incompetence and may be used for residual or small recurrent varicosities after venous surgery. The basic principles of compression sclerotherapy are that a small quantity of sclerosant is injected into a vein emptied by elevation. A compression bandage is applied to prevent blood returning to the vein. The compression holds the two vein walls together while a fibrous bonding forms between them over the next few weeks sealing the vein. Exercise is encouraged after injection to reduce the risk of thrombus extending to the deep veins. A number of sclerosants are available; most commonly varying concentrations of STD are used. Complications are rare, and similar to those following injections for venous flares. Limb ischaemia, inability to exercise, a history of allergy or previous DVT, the use of the oral contraceptive pill, pregnancy and general ill-health are all contraindications for sclerotherapy.

Management of varicose veins by surgery

Surgery addresses both the cosmetic problem of varicosities and the underlying cause. However, varicosities may recur, the incidence increasing with time. Surgery is indicated: when junctional or perforator incompetence is associated with substantial varicose veins; when a complication of superficial varicosities such as haemorrhage or ulceration occurs; when sclerotherapy is contraindicated or has been ineffective. There are three basic elements to surgery, which may be performed on a daycase basis: junctional or perforator ligation; stripping of the saphenous vein using either conventional or pin strippers; and multiple stab avulsions, which gives the best cosmetic results when phlebotomy hooks are used. Preoperatively the varicosities are mapped and marked with indelible ink with the patient standing, veins being identified both visually and by palpation. The site of perforating veins and the short saphenous junction are best located with the aid of duplex ultrasonography.

Surgical procedure

To reduce blood loss, venous surgery is usually performed with the patient's head down (Trendelenburg position) and may be performed under tourniquet. When practical, incisions are kept small in size and minimal in number and are aligned with the cleavage lines of the skin so that the most acceptable cosmetic results are obtained. Flush ligation of the saphenofemoral and/or saphenopopliteal junctions with division of all junctional branches is important and if inadequately performed early recurrence is inevitable. Stripping of the long saphenous vein to the knee or upper calf reduces recurrence and is less likely to result in damage to the saphenous nerve than more distal stripping. Phlebectomy stab incisions are usually closed with adhesive strips and larger wounds with subcuticular sutures. Local anaesthetic infiltration of groin and popliteal wounds can significantly reduce postoperative discomfort. Finally, a compression bandage is placed on the leg and this or some other form of compression is kept on the leg for 1–2 weeks.

Discharge advice

During the postoperative period the patient should be encouraged to exercise, taking frequent short walks interspersed with periods of leg elevation. Local protocols differ but in general patients should be encouraged to wear some form of support hosiery after surgery, some centres advocating the use of anti-embolism stockings for 6 weeks after surgery (Herbert, 1997). However, the evidence for the use of anti-embolism stockings in this situation is lacking. As this type of surgery is usually performed on a daycase basis, the patients should be warned that a small amount of bleeding may occur through the dressings and that bruising is common and should disappear within a few weeks.

Alternative forms of surgery exist; junctional ligation may be combined with the use of sclerosant, cryosurgery, diathermy or microwave ablation of the long saphenous vein and its varicose branches (Watts, 1972; Garde, 1994). Where major perforator incompetence is the cause of the varicose veins or ulceration there may be a role for subfascial endoscopic perforator surgery (SEPS) (Gloviczki, 1999).

The potential complications of varicose vein surgery are given in Table 7.5. The majority of complications occurring after venous surgery are minor and self-limiting. Provision of good pre- and postoperative verbal and written information will reduce the significance of these complications to the patient, and also the incidence of general practitioner consultation (Mackay et al., 1995). Of the major complications deep vein thrombosis is the most common, occurring in up to 2% of patients. Recurrent varicose veins occur in up to 20% of cases, the incidence increasing with time. Early recurrence usually results from inadequate assessment or surgery. 'New' recurrent veins may occur if a further site of junctional or perforator incompetence develops or there is recannulation or neovascularisation across a previously ligated junction (Tibbs et al., 1997). Duplex ultrasonography is essential if recurrent varicose veins are to be assessed and treated adequately.

Deep vein thrombosis

The incidence of deep vein thrombosis is difficult to estimate accurately; most figures probably underestimate the true incidence. Deep vein thrombosis is detectable in 25–35% of patients after operations

Table 7.5 Complications of varicose vein surgery

- Bruising
- Haemorrhage
- Infection
- Pain*
- Numbness*
- Superficial thrombophlebitis
- Deep vein injury
- Arterial damage
- Deep vein thrombosis
- Bandage damage

Later complications include:
- Skin discoloration
- Venous flares, especially at stab sites
- Recurrent varicose veins
- Lymphoedema
- Arteriovenous fistula formation

* These symptoms are particularly severe when they involve damage to the saphenous or sural nerves, which most commonly occurs during stripping of the long and short saphenous veins.

(Table 7.6), in 20–50% of patients after myocardial infarction or stroke, and is common after lower limb trauma (Hopkins and Wolfe, 1991b). It has been estimated that about 100 000–150 000 people in the UK have chronic leg ulceration and a further 200 000–800 000 have less severe symptoms as a direct result of deep vein thrombosis (Milne and Ruckley, 1994). In 1846 Virchow described the three components that initiate thrombosis, namely:

- changes in the coagulation mechanisms of the blood
- damage to the endothelial lining of blood vessels
- reduction in blood flow.

To these can be added a fourth, the fibrinolytic status of the patient (Hopkins and Wolfe, 1991b).

Risk assessment

The balance of these elements is altered by a number of risk factors (Table 7.7), of which immobility, particularly if prolonged, is the

Table 7.6 Incidence of thrombotic complications following general surgical procedures

Event	Incidence (%)
All DVTs	25
Clinically apparent DVTs	9
Proximal DVTs	7
All pulmonary embolic	1.6
Fatal pulmonary embolic	0.8

most important. Malignant disease, surgery, particularly if to the pelvis or lower limb, previous venous damage or DVT and a pre-existing thrombophilia may all interact to produce significantly increased risks in an individual. Risk assessment scales such as the Autar scale (Autar, 1998) now form a routine part of patient management and are specifically designed to identify high-risk individuals (Autar, 1996). The Thromboembolic Risk Factors (THRIFT) Consensus Group have reviewed these risk factors and have stratified patients into low, moderate and high risk groups and have suggested prophylaxis guidelines for each risk level (Anonymous, 1992).

Deep vein thrombosis prophylaxis

Ideally the method employed for DVT prophylaxis should be safe, effective, easy to administer or apply, inexpensive, simple to monitor, acceptable to the patient and should not interfere with other treatments or surgery (Tibbs et al., 1997; Pineo et al., 1995). There are two basic methods of DVT prophylaxis, mechanical and pharmacological; these methods may be, and often are, used in combination. Not all methods are equally applicable to individual situations as they may interact with other medical conditions and treatments or prevent access to a limb for nursing care or surgery (Milne and Ruckley, 1994; Belcaro et al., 1995). The role of post-discharge prophylaxis remains controversial but may need to be considered in high-risk patients (Agnelli, 1998).

Simple interventions such as regular physical activity and elevation of the legs without calf compression will reduce the risk of DVT. Early ambulation, which is not the same as early sitting out of bed, is a simple and effective measure, especially when combined with compression hosiery (Tibbs et al., 1997).

Table 7.7 Risk factors for deep vein thrombosis

General	Age >40 years Obesity
Vein wall abnormalities	Previous or current thrombotic episode Inflammation or infection surrounding veins • Connective tissue disorders Venous trauma Varicose veins
Stasis	Immobility • Transitory • Permanent (stroke or paralysis) Congestive heart failure Hypoperfusion states • Shock and myocardial infarction Venous compression and obstruction • Mass lesion • Calf compression
Hypercoagulability	Thrombophilia • Antithrombin III, protein S and protein C deficiency etc. Surgery, trauma, injury Pregnancy The puerperium Hyperviscosity • Polycythaemia • Thrombocythaemia Malignancy Oral contraceptive

Mechanical prophylaxis

Mechanical prophylactic measures include graduated anti-embolism elastic compression stockings, intermittent pneumatic compression (IPC) devices and electrical muscle stimulation (Hopkins and Wolfe, 1991b). Provided care is taken not to apply compression stockings to patients with significant lower limb arterial disease, elastic anti-embolism compression hosiery provides an inexpensive and safe method of DVT prophylaxis for low- and moderate-risk patients (Anonymous, 1992). Compression at the ankle is usually in the 18–23 mmHg range, falling to 14–15 mmHg at the calf; below knee anti-embolism stockings may be sufficient but further work is needed to establish whether this is in fact the case (Thomas, 1999a, 1999b, 1999c). To be effective the stocking must be of the correct size and be fitted and worn correctly. They are not a method of DVT treatment and should be used with caution in patients with microvascular disease or peripheral neuropathy in whom the risk of tissue damage and heel sores is greatest.

IPC using either a single or multichamber device is an effective method of emptying blood from areas of venous stasis within the leg and increasing the rate of blood flow. These devices have been shown to reduce the incidence of DVT. Pneumatic compression devices have been shown to exert a secondary effect by stimulating systemic fibrinolytic activity (Tibbs et al., 1997). An alternative to lower limb IPC is to use a foot impulse pump (Santori et al., 1994). Both these methods appear to offer few other advantages over anti-embolism stockings and are more expensive and less widely available but may be appropriate in some cases and have been used most extensively in orthopaedic surgery (Thomas, 1999c).

Pharmacological prophylaxis

Low-dose subcutaneous unfractionated heparin is the most widely used form of prophylactic anticoagulation and effects an overall reduction in the incidence of DVT from 25 to 8%. Similar reductions in both fatal and non-fatal pulmonary embolisation are also seen (Tibbs et al., 1997). It is less effective in major joint replacement surgery. When used as prophylaxis it should be given subcutaneously at a dose of 5000 units 2 hours preoperatively and then repeated 8- to 12-hourly. Low-molecular-weight heparins such as Fragmin and tinzaparin have been shown to be as effective and have the advantage of a longer half-life and hence a once-daily dose. Heparin prophylaxis is not recommended for patients undergoing brain, spine or eye procedures. Potential complications such as haemorrhage or heparin-induced thrombocytopenia are rare but need to be considered when this form of prophylaxis is used (Tibbs et al., 1997).

Other pharmacological methods include the use of oral anticoagulants such as warfarin, the use of antiplatelet agents and the use of dextran. The latter agent is a glucose polymer which reduces plasma viscosity and fibrin polymerisation as well as altering platelet function.

It is used widely in the prevention of thrombotic complications after hip surgery (Tibbs et al., 1997).

Diagnosis and confirmatory investigations of a possible DVT

More than half of all DVTs are clinically silent and are only detected on screening. Limb swelling, particularly when associated with calf tenderness, a positive Homan's sign (the production of calf pain during dorsiflexion of the ankle), fever and tachycardia may indicate a thrombosis. Table 7.8 lists the major signs and symptoms of a DVT. Once the clinical suspicion of thrombosis has been raised, D-dimer assay can effectively screen for a DVT in the majority of cases (Bradley et al., 2000). The patient may also be assessed by either venous duplex ultrasonography, plethysmography or venography and if the diagnosis is confirmed full anticoagulation commenced (Milne and Ruckley, 1994; Belcaro et al., 1995). Isotope scanning with iodine-125 labelled fibrinogen is useful when screening patients for DVT as it permits serial analysis over several days. This is mainly a research tool and is of little value in routine patient management. It is worth considering taking blood for a thrombophilia screen in patients with few if any risk factors for DVT before commencing treatment.

Table 7.8 Signs and symptoms of deep vein thrombosis

- Mild to severe swelling dependent upon the site and extent of the thrombosis
- Peripheral oedema
- A sensation of tension or heaviness in the leg
- Pain in the calf or along the line of thrombosis
- Positive Homan's sign or pain on movement resulting in reduced mobility
- Increased skin temperature and possibly a mild pyrexia
- Distended superficial veins

Management of the patient with a confirmed DVT

Symptomatic relief, bed rest and leg elevation are important but the mainstay of treatment for a patient with a confirmed DVT is anticoagulation. A bolus dose of unfractionated heparin is followed by a continuous heparin infusion which is continued for 5 days, the level of anticoagulation being monitored throughout this period by serial measurements of the activated partial thromboplastin time (APTT)

Table 7.9 Suggested intravenous heparin protocol (Tibbs et al. (1997) adapted from Hull et al. (1992))

1. Initial heparin bolus (80 U/kg)
2. Continuous heparin infusion (18 U/kg/h IV)
3. APTT and platelet count prior to commencing infusion
4. APTT 4 h after infusion commences
5. Repeat APTT 4–6 h after implementing any change in dosage

APTT	Change (U/h)	Additional action
<45	+240	Repeat APTT in 4–6 h
46–54	+120	Repeat APTT in 4–6 h
55–85	No change	
86–110	–120	Stop heparin for 1 h, repeat APTT 4–6 h after restarting infusion
>110	–240	Stop heparin for 1 h, repeat APTT 4–6 h after restarting infusion

6. APTT performed daily once stable

(Table 7.9). Warfarin therapy is usually commenced on day 2 of treatment following local protocols. This agent usually takes 2–3 days to reach effective levels and is monitored by the international normalised ratio (INR), which should be kept between 2 and 3 (although high ratios may be considered necessary for high-risk patients). For a primary DVT warfarin therapy is usually continued for 3 months. Increasing risk factors, previous thrombotic episodes, pulmonary embolisation or other indications for warfarin therapy may mean longer or lifelong treatment.

Recently, low-molecular-weight heparin has started to replace unfractionated heparin in the initial treatment phase of DVT and this has allowed outpatient and community management of some DVTs (Bounameaux, 1998; Buller et al., 1998). Alternative treatments include thrombolysis and surgical venous thrombectomy. Both should be considered for limb-threatening recent non-adherent thrombus, particularly if the thrombus involves the iliofemoral veins (Milne and Ruckley, 1994; Tibbs et al., 1997).

Complications of deep vein thrombosis

All patients with a suspected or confirmed DVT should be carefully monitored for potential life- or limb-threatening complications. Clearly the most significant of these is pulmonary embolisation.

Other complications include *phlegmasia alba dolens* (white leg or milk leg), where spasm and compression secondary to gross swelling compromises the arterial supply to a limb, and *phlegmasia cerulea dolens* (Szuba et al., 1998), in which the leg becomes acutely painful, massively swollen and blue-black due to almost complete venous outflow obstruction secondary to massive iliofemoral thrombosis. Both conditions may progress to moist venous gangrene and necessitate amputation (Belcaro et al., 1995). Long-term sequelae of DVTs include post-phlebitic limb, increased risk of subsequent thrombotic events and venous lower limb ulceration (Milne and Ruckley, 1994; Belcaro et al., 1995).

Upper limb thrombosis

Deep vein thrombosis may also involve the upper limb, where axillary vein thrombosis can occur producing the same symptoms of pain, swelling and dilatation of the superficial veins (in this case over the shoulder). This condition may occur as part of a thoracic outlet syndrome or may follow a prolonged period of arm use as in decorating. The basic management is the same as for lower limb thrombosis.

Pulmonary embolism

Massive pulmonary embolisation is a cause of sudden death and may occur without obvious signs of a peripheral DVT. Less massive embolisation may present with any or all of the following: pleuritic chest pain, cough, wheeze, dyspnoea, hypoxia, cyanosis, hypotension, cardiac arrhythmia, collapse, loss of consciousness, haemoptysis or pyrexia (Herbert, 1997). The major signs and symptoms of pulmonary embolisation are given in Table 7.10. Suspicion, particularly in patients known to be at high risk of DVT, is the key to prompt diagnosis.

Management

There are four main elements involved in the management of pulmonary embolisation:

1. Stabilisation and support of the cardiovascular system.
2. Confirmation of the diagnosis.

Table 7.10 Signs and symptoms of pulmonary embolisation

- Dyspnoea and occasionally wheezing
- Chest pain (can be pleuritic)
- Haemoptysis
- Altered mental state
- Tachycardia and tachypnoea
- Cyanosis
- Hypotension and hypoxia
- Pyrexia
- Rales
- Signs and symptoms of a DVT
- Elevated venous pressure
- Shock
- Pleuritic rub

3. Treatment and identification of the source of thrombotic episode.
4. Prevention of further embolisation.

The level of intervention will depend on the severity of the presenting event. Oxygen therapy should be administered, blood gases monitored and cardiac monitoring commenced. Some patients may require transfer to a high dependency or intensive care unit for more invasive monitoring and stabilisation of pulmonary and cardiac function. The diagnosis is usually confirmed by the combined results of a ventilation perfusion isotope lung scan and chest X-ray. Supporting evidence may come from blood gases, ECG (the S1, Q3, T3 pattern is pathognomonic of a large pulmonary embolus and reflects right heart strain) or pulmonary arteriography, which may be indicated in selected patients (Belcaro et al., 1995; Herbert, 1997; Tibbs et al., 1997). In the critically ill patient it is often necessary to treat presumptively without confirmatory investigations.

Treatment

As with DVT anticoagulation forms the mainstay of treatment and follows a similar regimen to that given above. Heparinisation may, however, be continued for longer with a higher APTT ratio of up to 2.5 times normal. Thrombolytic therapy, via a pulmonary artery catheter inserted at the time of arteriography, using streptokinase, tissue plasminogen activator (t-PA) or other similar agents, may be appropriate in selected patients. Surgical pulmonary thrombectomy is possible but is rarely performed (Belcaro et al., 1995; Herbert, 1997; Tibbs et al., 1997).

Once the patient's condition is stabilised the source of the embolus should be identified. This is important in a patient who has had a number of embolic episodes where prevention of further embolisation by the insertion of a vena cava filter may be indicated (Belcaro et al., 1995; Tibbs et al., 1997). *Inferior vena cava filters* are mechanical intravascular devices inserted below the renal veins under X-ray control to prevent thrombi embolising to the lungs. Permanent and temporary versions are available, temporary filters being used to protect a high risk patient during a single event such as during pregnancy. The indications for the use of an inferior vena cava filter are mainly those of recurrent embolisation despite adequate anticoagulation, but they may also be used during attempted thrombolysis, in patients with large volumes of free-floating clot or extending thrombus on anticoagulation or in patients with reduced pulmonary reserve due to pre-existing disease or embolisation.

The long-term consequences of pulmonary embolisation include adverse effects on pulmonary function and the development of chronic thromboembolic pulmonary hypertension (Tibbs et al., 1997).

Chronic venous insufficiency

The venous valvular system and physiological pumps such as those at the foot, calf and diaphragm are designed to reduce the effects of gravity on the venous system of the lower limb, allowing a fall in ambulatory venous pressure with exercise. The effectiveness of this system is diminished progressively by superficial and deep venous disease or immobility (Figure 7.3) (P Vowden, 1998). The end result is venous hypertension (Table 7.11, page 194), which itself has consequences for venous function and the skin of the lower leg.

Signs and symptoms and complications of chronic venous insufficiency

The physical signs of venous hypertension due to deep venous insufficiency or gross superficial reflux include: swelling; increased superficial collateral veins and varicosities; thickening, induration and pigmentation of the subcutaneous tissues in the gaiter area and over sites of major varicosities; varicose eczema and dermatitis; lipodermatosclerosis and atrophie blanche; ulceration or evidence of previously healed ulceration (Hopkins and Wolfe, 1991a; K Vowden, 1998). The incidence of skin changes, including lipodermatosclerosis and ulceration, increase with the duration and severity of venous insufficiency. Post-thrombotic or post-phlebitic syndrome is the commonest cause of chronic venous insufficiency and can give rise to severe disability which may impact on both social and working life (Tibbs et al., 1997; Milne and Ruckley, 1994; Belcaro et al., 1995). Within 5–10 years of a moderate to severe venous thrombosis three-quarters of patients will have developed skin changes and some symptoms of post-phlebitic limb. These symptoms will be severe in up to 40% of patients, with ulceration occurring in 4–7% of cases (Hopkins and Wolfe, 1991a).

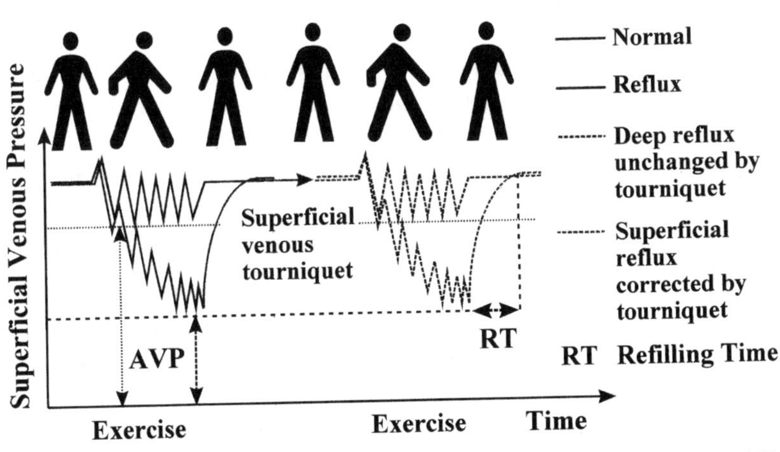

Figure 7.3 The ambulatory venous pressure (AVP), measured by inserting a needle in a vein at the ankle or in the dorsum of the foot, is defined as the lowest pressure reached during ten tiptoe exercises. It reflects the efficiency of the calf muscle pump, the degree of reflux and the level of outflow resistance. The time taken for the AVP to return to the baseline reading (the resting pressure) is the refilling time (RT). By combining the test with a superficial tourniquet, deep and superficial reflux can be assessed and the site of reflux located. The normal AVP is less than 30 mmHg and the RT longer than 18 seconds. When reflux is present, the AVP is higher and the RT shorter. With severe outflow obstruction the AVP can increase with exercise to levels above the baseline. Increasing AVP is associated with an increasing incidence of venous ulceration (Belcaro et al., 1995). Adapted from P Vowden (1998).

Table 7.11 Causes of failure of venous return leading to venous hypertension

Superficial reflux (varicose veins) overwhelming venous pump
Deep vein thrombosis causing

- Damage to intramuscular sinusoidal veins
- Deep vein obstruction (failure of recannulisation)
- Reflux through valves rendered incompetent by thrombosis
- Reflux through distended incompetent collateral veins

External venous compression, e.g. pregnancy
Congenital valvular deficiencies
Muscle inactivity due to paralysis of pain in a dependent limb

Venous ulceration

Perhaps the most significant and distressing complication of chronic venous hypertension is lower limb ulceration. Venous ulcers account for up to 70% of all lower limb ulcers (Callam et al., 1985). It is important to remember that venous ulceration may simply be due to superficial venous incompetence and that this is a correctable condition (Grabs et al., 1996; Scriven et al., 1997). Patients presenting with signs of venous hypertension do therefore require adequate investigation of both the deep and superficial venous systems. A number of theories exists as to the mechanism behind the skin changes associated with chronic venous hypertension and their progression to venous ulceration (Vowden and Vowden, 1998a). These theories, which include white cell trapping and the fibrin cuff theory, may indicate a possible future pharmacological method of controlling these conditions (Neumann, 1999). The impact of the venous hypertension on the microcirculation and the evidence for leukocyte involvement has been discussed by Coleridge Smith (1997, 1999). Chant (1999) has recently reviewed the possible biomechanics of lower limb ulceration and has shown that the forces necessary to produce capillary closure and reperfusion injury are maximal in the gaiter area, the site of most leg ulcers.

Investigations

Other than for the measurement of the ankle brachial pressure index prior to the introduction of high compression bandaging (Vowden and Vowden, 1998b), the continuous-wave handheld Doppler has little part to play in the management of a patient with possible deep vein insufficiency. Colour flow duplex ultrasonography can provide both anatomical and physiological information on both deep and superficial veins. Reflux in the popliteal vein, the gatekeeper of the calf muscle pump, appears to be one of the most important factors in the later development of chronic skin changes. Plethysmography and photoplethysmography can also provide evidence of reflux and when combined with tourniquet, can be used to identify the site of reflux. Ambulatory venous pressure measurements quantify the severity of the problem and the pattern of pressure changes can indicate the site of incompetence and reflux (Figure 7.3). Functional phlebography and ascending and descending venography can provide excellent anatomical information, including the demonstration of venous valves and their functional competence, but is invasive and may be difficult to perform. The role of these and other investigations has been reviewed by several authors (P Vowden, 1998; Tibbs et al., 1997; Belcaro et al., 1995).

Treatment

Management of the patient with chronic venous hypertension is frequently conservative but where investigations have demonstrated that surgical intervention is possible patients should be offered this form of treatment. When conservative treatment is the only option it must be lifelong. Shared care involving the patient in an individualised programme that combines risk reduction, patient education, the appropriate choice of compression hosiery and regular follow-ups, and which provides immediate and flexible access to specialised care is important if recurrent ulceration is to be kept to a minimum. Application of all these elements will reassure the patient and allow maintenance of the maximum quality of life compatible with the underlying disease.

The incidence and severity of the symptoms of chronic venous insufficiency and venous hypertension can be reduced by wearing correctly fitted high compression hosiery (European Class II or III) and this forms the mainstay of treatment. Compression bandaging using either single-layer or multilayer systems remains the mainstay of venous leg ulcer management and is covered in Chapter 8, as is the role of compression hosiery in reducing ulcer recurrence. Experimental surgery evaluating the role of venous valvular reconstruction continues, but this technique is not yet considered reliable enough to be generally applied (Tibbs et al., 1997).

Chronic venous occlusion

Following deep vein thrombosis recannulation of the vein usually occurs. Failure to do so results in chronic venous occlusion with significant lower limb swelling which increases on standing, and the development of an extensive system of venous collaterals around the obstruction. These collaterals may extend over the lower abdominal wall. Patients with severe venous occlusive disease frequently complain of a bursting pain in the leg on standing and may experience 'venous claudication' after even short periods of exercise. The pain, in contrast to that in arterial insufficiency, is frequently improved by elevation. Support hosiery may help control symptoms but needs to be used with caution as it may obstruct collateral flow and make the situation worse (Hopkins and Wolfe, 1991a). Some patients with this condition are suitable for venous bypass procedures such as the Palma cross-over procedure where the saphenous vein is swung over from the opposite side to aid venous drainage of the affected limb (Hopkins and Wolfe, 1991a; Tibbs et al., 1997).

Conclusion

This chapter has aimed to provide all healthcare professionals with an explanation of the rational basis for treatment of a patient with venous disease. The last 10 years have seen an increased understanding of the pathophysiology of venous disorders and this has allowed the introduction of scientifically based prophylaxis and treatments regimens for venous diseases. For many patients venous disease runs a chronic course punctuated by acute episodes. By empowering the patient and instituting appropriate care using members of the multidisciplinary team, the frequency of these episodes can be dramatically reduced and in this way the quality of life for the patient improved.

References

Agnelli G (1998) Postdischarge prophylaxis for venous thromboembolism among high-risk surgery patients. Vascular Medicine 3(1): 51–56.

Anonymous (1992) Risk of and prophylaxis for venous thromboembolism in hospital patients. Thromboembolic Risk Factors (THRIFT) Consensus Group. British Medical Journal 305(6853): 567–574.

Autar R (1996) Deep Vein Thrombosis: The Silent Killer. Dinton, Wiltshire: Quay Books, Mark Allen Publishing.

Autar R (1998) Calculating patients' risk of deep vein thrombosis. British Journal of Nursing 7(1): 7–12.

Auty B (1994) Free flow in IV infusion. Care of the Critically Ill 10(4): 183–187.

Belcaro G, Nicolaides AN, Veller M (1995) Venous Disorders: A Manual of Diagnosis and Treatment. London: Saunders.

Belcaro G, Nicolaides AN, Errichi BM, Cesarone MR, De Sanctis MT, Incandela L, Venniker R (1999) Superficial thrombophlebitis of the legs: a randomized, controlled, follow-up study. Angiology 50(7): 523–529.

Bergan JJ (1999) How should venous disease be classified? In: Ruckley CV, Fowkes FGR, Bradbury AW (eds) Venous Disease: Epidemiology, Management and Delivery of Care, pp 73–79. London: Springer-Verlag.

Berridge DC, Weston MJ (1999) Should every patient with chronic venous disease have a duplex scan? In: Ruckley CV, Fowkes FGR, Bradbury AW (eds) Venous Disease: Epidemiology, Management and Delivery of Care, pp 203–211. London: Springer-Verlag.

Bounameaux H (1998) Unfractionated versus low-molecular-weight heparin in the treatment of venous thromboembolism. Vascular Medicine 3(1): 41–46.

Bradbury AW (1999) Venous symptoms and signs and the results of duplex ultrasound: Do they agree? In: Ruckley CV Fowkes FGR, Bradbury AW (eds) Venous Disease: Epidemiology, Management and Delivery of Care, pp 98–114. London: Springer-Verlag.

Bradley M, Bladon J, Barker H (2000) D-dimer assay for deep vein thrombosis: its role with colour Doppler sonography. Clinical Radiology 55(7): 525–527.

Buller HR, Kraaijenhagen RA, Koopman MMW (1998) Early discharge strategies following venous thrombosis. Vascular Medicine 3(1): 47–50.

Burnand K (1999) What makes veins varicose? In: Ruckley CV, Fowkes FGR, Bradbury AW (eds) Venous Disease: Epidemiology, Management and Delivery of Care, pp 42–50. London: Springer-Verlag.

Callam MJ, Ruckley CV, Harper DR, Dale JJ (1985) Chronic ulceration of the leg: extent of the problem and provision of care. British Medical Journal 290(6485): 1855–1856.

Callam MJ, Ruckley CV, Dale JJ, Harper DR (1987) Hazards of compression treatment of the leg: an estimate from Scottish surgeons. British Medical Journal 295(6610): 1382.

Campbell H, Carrington M, Limber C (1999) A practical guide to venepuncture and management of complications. British Journal of Nursing 8(7): 426–431.

Campbell T, Lunn D (1997) Intravenous therapy: current practice and nursing concerns. British Journal of Nursing 6(21): 1218–1228.

Chant A (1999) The biomechanics of leg ulceration. Annals of the Royal College of Surgeons of England 81(2): 80–85.

Clarke A (1997) The nursing management of intravenous drug therapy. British Journal of Nursing 6(4): 201–206.

Coleridge Smith PD (1997) The microcirculation in venous hypertension. Vascular Medicine 2(3): 203–213.
Coleridge Smith PD (1999) How does a leg ulcerate? In: Ruckley CV, Fowkes FGR, Bradbury AW (eds) Venous Disease: Epidemiology, Management and Delivery of Care, pp 51–70. London: Springer-Verlag.
Evans CJ, Lee AJ, Ruckley CV, Fowkes FGR (1999) How common is venous disease in the general population? In: Ruckley CV, Fowkes FGR, Bradbury AW (eds) Venous Disease: Epidemiology, Management and Delivery of Care, pp 3–14. London: Springer-Verlag.
Garde C (1994) Cryosurgery of varicose veins. Journal of Dermatological Surgery and Oncology 20(1): 56–58.
Ghauri ASK, Nyamekye I, Grabs AJ, Farndon JR, Whyman MR, Poskitt KR (1998) Influence of a specialised leg ulcer service and venous surgery on the outcome of venous leg ulcers. European Journal of Vascular and Endovascular Surgery 16(3): 238–244.
Gloviczki P (1999) Subfascial endoscopic perforator vein surgery: indications and results. Vascular Medicine 4(3): 173–180.
Grabs AJ, Wakely MC, Nyamekye I, Ghauri AS, Poskitt KR (1996) Colour duplex ultrasonography in the rational management of chronic venous leg ulcers. British Journal of Surgery 83(10): 1380–1382.
Guex JJ (1996) Thrombotic complications of varicose veins. A literature review of the role of superficial venous thrombosis. Dermatological Surgery 22(4): 378–382.
Hamilton H, Fermo K (1998) Assessment of patients requiring IV therapy via a central venous route. British Journal of Nursing 7(8): 451–460.
Hanson JN, Ascher E, DePippo P, Lorensen E, Scheinman M, Yorkovich W, Hingorani A (1998) Saphenous vein thrombophlebitis (SVT): a deceptively benign disease. Journal of Vascular Surgery 27(4): 677–680.
Herbert LM (1997) Caring for the Vascular Patient. New York: Churchill Livingstone.
Hobbs JT (1991) Varicose veins. British Medical Journal 303: 707–710.
Hopkins NFG, Wolfe JHN (1991a) Deep venous insufficiency and occlusion. British Medical Journal 304: 107–110.
Hopkins NFG, Wolfe JHN (1991b) Thrombosis and pulmonary embolism. British Medical Journal 303: 1260–1262.
Hull RD, Raskob GE, Rosenbloom D, Lemaire J, Pineo GF, Baylis B, Ginsberg JS, Panju AA, Brill-Edwards P, Brant R (1992) Optimal therapeutic level of heparin therapy in patients with venous thrombosis. Archives of Internal Medicine 152(8): 1589–1595.
Lee AJ, Evans CJ, Ruckley CV, Fowkes FGR (1999) Does lifestyle really affect venous disease? In: Ruckley CV, Fowkes FGR, Bradbury AW (eds) Venous Disease: Epidemiology, Management and Delivery of Care, pp 32–41. London: Springer-Verlag.
Mackay DC, Summerton DJ, Walker AJ (1995) The early morbidity of varicose vein surgery. Journal of the Royal Navy Medical Service 81(1): 42–46.
Milne AA, Ruckley CV (1994) Venous insufficiency following deep vein thrombosis. Vascular Medicine Review 5(3): 241–248.
Neumann HAM (1999) Medical treatment for venous diseases. In: Ruckley CV, Fowkes FGR, Bradbury AW (eds) Venous Disease: Epidemiology Management and Delivery of Care, pp 153–160. London: Springer-Verlag.

Nicolaides A (1999) How do we select the appropriate tests of venous function? In: Ruckley CV, Fowkes FGR, Bradbury AW (eds) Venous Disease: Epidemiology Management and Delivery of Care, pp 80–88. London: Springer-Verlag.

Pineo GF, Hull RD, Raskob G (1995) Prevention of venous thrombosis in general surgery and orthopaedics. Vascular Medicine Review 6: 185–192.

Quaba A (1999) Telangiectasia: Is treatment worthwhile and who should pay? In: Ruckley CV, Fowkes FGR, Bradbury AW (eds) Venous Disease: Epidemiology, Management and Delivery of Care, pp 161–173. London: Springer-Verlag.

Santori FS, Vitullo A, Stopponi M, Snatori N, Ghera S (1994) Prophylaxis against deep vein thrombosis in total hip replacement. Journal of Bone and Joint Surgery 76B(4): 579–583.

Scriven JM, Hartshorne T, Bell PR, Naylor AR, London NJ (1997) Single-visit venous ulcer assessment clinic: the first year. British Journal of Surgery 84(3): 334–336.

Stemmer R (1969) Ambulatory-elasto-compressive treatment of the lower extremities particularly with elastic stockings. Kassenarzt 9: 1–8.

Szuba A, Cooke JP, Rockson SG (1998) Images in vascular medicine: Plegmasia coerulea dolens – venous gangrene. Vascular Medicine 3(1): 29–31.

Thomas S (1999a) Graduated compression and the prevention of deep vein thrombosis (Part 1). Journal of Wound Care 8(1): 41–43.

Thomas S (1999b) Graduated compression and the prevention of deep vein thrombosis (Part 2). Journal of Wound Care 8(2): 93–95.

Thomas S (1999c) Graduated compression and the prevention of deep vein thrombosis (Part 3). Journal of Wound Care 8(3): 133–139.

Tibbs D J (1992) Varicose Veins and Related Disorders. Oxford: Butterworth-Heinemann.

Tibbs DJ, Sabiston DC, Davies MG, Mortimer PS, Scurr JH (1997) Varicose Veins, Venous Disorders, and Lymphatic Problems in the Lower Limb. Oxford: Oxford University Press.

Vost J, Longstaff V (1997) Infection control and related issues in intravascular therapy. British Journal of Nursing 6(15): 846–857.

Vowden K (1998) Lipodermatosclerosis and atrophie blanche. Journal of Wound Care 7(9): 441–443.

Vowden K, Vowden P (1998a) Anatomy, physiology and venous ulceration. In: The Philosophy of Compression Therapy, pp 1–5. London: EMAP Healthcare.

Vowden K, Vowden P (1998b) Venous leg ulcers Part 2: assessment. Professional Nurse 13(9): 633–638.

Vowden P (1998b) The investigation of venous disease. Journal of Wound Care 7(3): 143–147.

Watts GT (1972) Endovenous diathermy destruction of internal saphenous. British Medical Journal 4(831): 53.

CHAPTER 8

Leg Ulcers

CHRISTINE MOFFATT

The last decade has seen a considerable change in the profile of leg ulceration as a healthcare problem. Many factors have contributed to this, not least the development of effective treatment modalities. In addition, it is now recognised that leg ulceration affects the multidisciplinary team. New models of care delivery have promoted this concept, with the nurse often playing a pivotal role (Moffatt et al., 1992). While many patients will receive all their care in a community setting, the important link to vascular surgeons and dermatologists helps to ensure the patient receives the most appropriate care, wherever they are being treated.

The epidemiology of leg ulceration is still poorly defined. However, it is thought to affect between 1 and 2% of the adult population in the United Kingdom (Callam et al., 1985; Cornwall et al., 1986). This translates into a population of 80 000–100 000 patients with an open ulcer at any one time. In addition, there is likely to be half a million patients with a healed ulcer that will recur at some time. The figure may in fact be much larger. Studies in Sweden have found the problem to be twice as large (Nelzen et al., 1991). While this may be partially explained by the different methodologies used, these studies identified a large number of patients who were not known to professionals but were treating their own ulcer. The Riverside leg ulcer project found that 25% of the patients within this study of over 500 patients were not known to professionals before a system of community clinics was established (Moffatt et al., 1992). Delay in patients presenting to professionals may result in them developing large intractable ulceration that is more difficult to heal.

The last decade has also shown the considerable amount of suffering associated with leg ulceration. Patients with leg ulcers have a considerable reduction in their quality of life and ability to function socially (Franks et al., 1994).

For treatment of these patients to reach full potential it is vital that practitioners understand how to assess and treat patients using research-based practice. National clinical guidelines now exist to guide the nursing management of patients with venous ulceration (RCN Institute, 1998). These guidelines are based on a systematic review of the literature (Cullum, 1994).

Causes of leg ulceration

There are many causes of leg ulceration. These range from a simple traumatic ulcer to ulceration resulting from complex autoimmune diseases. Understanding the aetiology of the patient's ulcer is one of the primary goals. It is the basis upon which subsequent plans for treatment are made. In Western populations over 70% of patients have venous disease as the predominant factor causing their leg ulceration (Browse and Burnand, 1982). The second major cause of ulceration is peripheral vascular disease. Cornwall found that over 50% of patients over the age of 80 with a leg ulcer had concomitant arterial disease (Cornwall et al., 1986). In considering the aetiology of leg ulceration it is very important to remember that we are treating an increasingly elderly population where peripheral vascular disease may become the dominant factor. Approximately 20% of patients will suffer with both venous and arterial disease. Table 8.1 shows other causes of leg ulceration seen in clinical practice.

Venous ulceration

Venous ulceration occurs on the lower third of the leg (Figure 8.1, page 204). The commonest site is the medial malleoli followed by the lateral malleoli. Ulceration may occur insidiously but is often precipitated by minimal trauma. Venous ulcers are usually shallow with evidence of granulation in the wound bed. The size of the ulcer is dependent on many factors including the length of time the patient has had the ulcer and the appropriateness of the wound management strategies that have been used. A sudden increase in size is often linked to acute infection or uncontrolled oedema.

Table 8.1 More unusual causes of leg ulcers

Malignant ulcers	
Squamous cell carcinomas	Can be seen as a primary carcinoma or with an ulcer that undergoes malignant change (Marjolin's ulcer).
Basal cell carcinomas	Usually found on the face but may occur on the leg. Lesion usually presents as a scab which, when knocked, bleeds profusely.
Melanomas	Currently on the increase, probably because of exposure to ultra-violet sunlight. These tumours metastasise rapidly. Ulceration of the lesion is indicative of an advanced stage of malignancy.
Kaposi's sarcoma, lymphangiosarcoma and bone tumour	Seen often in patients with HIV infection. The lesions can mimic the presentation of a melanoma or of a venous ulcer.
Blood disorders	
Sickle cell disease	Small, perforating ulcers on the lower limb frequently follow a sickle cell crisis. Frequently wrongly described as arterial in origin, they develop because of thrombosis occurring in the veins after sickling. Treatment is therefore compression therapy.
Thalassaemia	Small painful ulcers, most commonly in teenagers and young adults.
Polycythaemia	Seen in older people usually occurring as typical ulcers on the foot.
Macroglobulinaemias	Rare blood disorders in which ulceration presents as one of many symptoms. Ulceration occurs because of damage in the microcirculation after the accumulation of large protein molecules.
Infection	
Tuberculosis	Currently on the increase. Skin ulceration may present alone but often with chest involvement. The ulcer base is usually grey-pink with irregular, bluish, friable edges.
Syphilis	Rare cause of ulceration today but still occurs occasionally. Often presenting in the tertiary stage of the disease with accompanying osteomyelitis. Tends to occur high on the calf or outer aspect of the lower leg (Walzman et al., 1986).
Leprosy	Progressive destruction of digits and ulceration with associated neuropathy, ulcers usually occur on plantar surface.
Fungal infection	Occurs in tropical areas associated with malnutrition, poor hygiene and poverty.

Table 8.1 (contd)

Metabolic disorders	
Pyoderma gangrenosum	Often accompanies systemic disorders such as ulcerative colitis, Crohn's disease, rheumatoid arthritis or myeloma.
Pretibial myxoedema	Rare type of ulceration occurring in patients with myxoedema.
Necrobiosis lipodica	Occurs predominantly in patients with diabetes mellitus. Pigmented areas with ulceration in the gaiter region involving secondary infection of the dermis which becomes progressively necrotic.
Lymphoedema	(i) Primary lymphoedema caused by congenital absence of lymphatic vessels, rarely presenting with ulceration (ii) Secondary lymphoedema accompanying venous disease (iii) Parasitic elephantiasis caused by filariasis causing lymphatic destruction.
Iatrogenic	e.g. Compression-induced ulceration when there is arterial insufficiency or overnight bandaging over a bony prominence when compression is indicated.
Self-inflicted ulceration	Deliberate attempts to create or sustain ulceration Possible indicators include: – Ulceration in unusual sites – No other pathology – Immediate improvement when limb is immobilised and protected from damage. Evidence of tampering with dressings or bandages is not in itself evidence of self-inflicted injury.

Reprinted from Morison M, Moffatt C, Bridel-Nixon J, Bale S, Peripheral vascular disease. In: Nursing Management of Chronic Wounds, p 192, 1997 by permission of the publisher, Mosby.

In order to understand the clinical signs and symptoms associated with venous ulceration it is important to review the anatomy and physiology of the vascular system found in Chapter 1.

The common pathway to venous ulceration is the development of high venous ambulatory pressures. This is frequently called chronic venous hypertension. A number of factors contribute to this. Damage to the valves within the veins allows the blood to flow

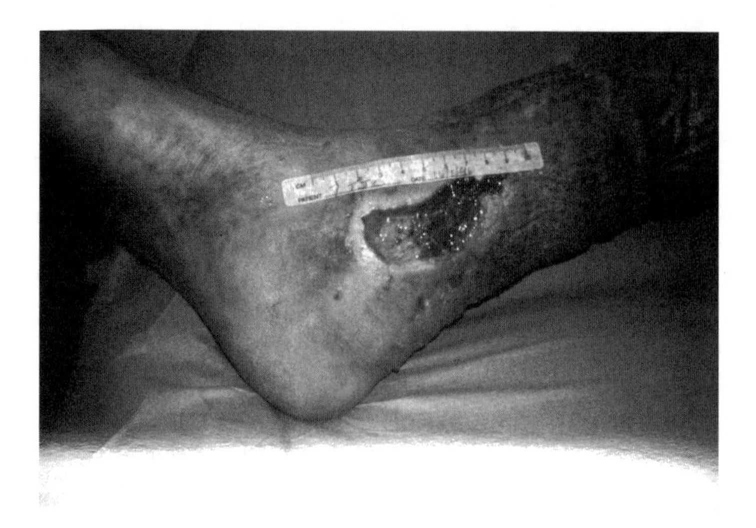

Figure 8.1. Classic skin changes in a patient with a venous ulcer; see Plate 3.

backwards down the vein. The reflux of blood results in high pressure in the dermal capillary bed and damage to the microcirculation. These factors predispose the patient to the development of leg ulceration. The situation may be compounded in patients with reduced mobility who have poor calf pump function.

The damage to the microcirculation results in a number of skin changes. There is much debate as to the exact mechanism that leads to ulceration in these patients. A number of key theories have emerged which are fiercely debated. However, it is likely that these mechanisms are working together. The most significant theory is the white cell entrapment theory which describes the inflammatory effects of neutrophil activation in ulcer formation (Browse and Burnand, 1982; Coleridge-Smith et al., 1988; Chant, 1990; Higley et al., 1995).

Clinical signs associated with venous ulceration

Chronic venous hypertension results in a number of typical changes to the skin of the lower leg.

Staining

The skin of patients with venous ulceration looks dry, scaly and discoloured. These changes result from leakage of substances from the damaged microcirculation. The brown colour is caused by leakage of red blood cells into the interstitial spaces which deposit their haem content. The degree of staining varies between patients but may extend throughout the gaiter region in patients with severe disease.

Lipodermatosclerosis

Lipodermatosclerosis is the term used to describe the hard, woody, indurated feeling of the lower leg in these patients (Browse and Burnand, 1982). This is caused by the laying down of fibrous tissue in the gaiter region. Patients may develop an inverted champagne bottle shape leg over time due to the progressive scarring and loss of subcutaneous tissue. This is usually a chronic, progressive problem but may be seen as an acute symptom in patients following a deep vein thrombosis. Patients with these skin changes show progressive thinning of the dermis which makes them extremely vulnerable to trauma.

Varicose veins

Varicose veins are a common accompaniment to venous ulceration. Although varicose veins affect between 10 and 20% of the adult population, only 3% of patients with varicose veins actually go on to develop a venous ulcer (Callam et al., 1985). Patients may complain of having varicose veins for many years or have developed secondary varicose veins following a deep vein thrombosis.

Ankle flare

This is distension of the tiny venules over the medial aspect of the foot. It is seen frequently in patients with venous ulceration, particularly in the presence of perforating vein incompetence.

Varicose eczema

Patients with venous ulceration suffer with a number of dermatological problems. Varicose eczema is by far the commonest. It is caused by the extravasation of irritating proteolytic enzymes and other metabolic waste products within the dermis. Patients may develop secondary infection due to scratching. *Staphylococcus aureus* infection is the commonest infective organism in this situation. Contact dermatitis is also a serious problem, which may affect between 50 and 80% of patients (Cameron, 1995). The patient becomes sensitised to the wound care products used to treat the ulcer. Contact dermatitis is frequently missed in patients who have gone on to develop a total body eczematous reaction due to the lymphocytic hypersensitivity.

Atrophie blanche

Atrophie blanche is the term used to describe white areas of scar tissue on the lower legs of these patients. Debate exists as to why these areas form (Moffatt and Harper, 1997). Atrophie blanche is seen in a number of other skin conditions including autoimmune conditions such as systemic lupus erythematosus and a wide range of vasculitic conditions. Ulceration occurring in these areas is often exquisitely painful, which suggests that the local blood supply to the area is reduced. Histology of these lesions frequently shows micro-occlusions, which supports the concept of a localised area of infarction.

Symptoms of venous ulceration

Patients with venous disease frequently complain of aching heavy legs, particularly at the end of the day. It is only in recent years that we have begun to appreciate the degree of pain associated with venous ulceration. Research has shown that up to 80% of patients with venous ulceration experience pain, with 20% describing it as unremitting (Franks et al., 1994).

Arterial ulceration

Arterial ulceration is due to a lack of adequate blood supply to ensure tissue perfusion. Atherosclerosis is the commonest cause of arterial ulceration. Cornwall et al. (1986) and Callam et al. (1985) suggest that approximately 20% of patients with ulceration have peripheral vascular disease. In the leg, the common sites for disease are the lower superficial femoral artery (60%) and the aortic vessels (30%). However 7% of patients have disease in a number of different sites (Orr and McAvoy, 1987). Other causes of arterial ulceration include trauma that interrupts blood flow, vasospastic disorders such as Raynaud's disease and cold injuries such as frostbite. A number of risk factors have been identified as important predictors of peripheral vascular disease (see Chapters 2 and 3). By far the most important factors are smoking and diabetes (Rose, 1991). In addition, male sex, hypertension and hyperlipidaemia have also been identified in this patient group. It is important to remember that it is the combination of risk factors working together that appears to have the most devastating effect.

Patients may also develop an arterial ulcer following an acute event such as an arterial embolism or following a severe injury that disrupts blood flow. The site of occlusion is different for thrombotic and embolic conditions. In an arterial embolism the site of occlusion depends on the relative size of the embolus and arterial conduit, whereas in a thrombosis the site of occlusion is determined by the underlying site of atherosclerotic plaque. These embolic events may have more severe effects than in a patient who has progressive atherosclerosis and has developed collateral circulation to compensate for the occluded vessels. Patients may also present with microemboli which lodge in the distal microcirculation causing small localised areas of cyanosis and gangrene. The general circulation of the foot may not be disordered. However, progressive accumulation of these microemboli may lead to major occlusion and microcirculatory failure eventually in the absence of a major emboli. Patients with aortic aneurysm are at risk of developing these microemboli.

The severity of the symptoms experienced by these patients varies greatly depending on the degree of blockage and the site of occlusion. Patient who spend their time resting may not experience symptoms despite 70% of the blood vessel being occluded. Patients will often have 90% occlusion before they experience rest pain. The European Working Group on Critical Leg Ischaemia has defined critical ischaemia as 'Persistently recurring rest pain requiring regular analgesia for more than 2 weeks with an ankle systolic pressure <50 mmHg or toe systolic pressure <30 mmHg or ulceration or gangrene of the foot or toes.'(European Working Group on Critical Leg Ischaemia, 1992).

Clinical signs associated with arterial ulceration

Skin condition

The skin of the patient's lower limbs is cold, atrophic and shiny. Pedal pulses are absent or diminished. Dependent oedema is a common feature as patients cannot elevate the limbs without increasing their pain. Consequently they sit with the limb dependent most of the time. Patients may show considerable loss of subcutaneous tissues due to ischaemia and wasting of the calf muscle due to disuse. Nail deformities and fungal infections are found frequently in these patients.

Poor tissue perfusion

Poor localised tissue perfusion is seen when there is a delay of colour returning to the toenail when localised pressure is applied. A delay of greater than 3 seconds is considered significant. It is often not possible to find a Doppler signal in these patients' limbs. Occasionally a weak signal may be found if the limb is held in a dependent position. The signal will disappear as the limb is elevated. When dropping the severely ischaemic leg over the side of the bed after a period of elevation, the veins refill very slowly, often taking up to 90 seconds. After a further few minutes reactive hyperaemia occurs, the ischaemic metabolites causing maximum vasodilatation. The bright red colour slowly subsides to leave a dusky blue colour on dependency. The limb turns pale on elevation and in very severe cases venous guttering occurs, where the vein is not only empty and collapsed, but depressed by the effect of gravity applying a negative pressure along the lumen of the vessel.

Ulceration and gangrene

Ulceration and gangrene develop when tissue perfusion cannot meet the metabolic demands of the tissues. Ulceration occurs on any site including the medial malleoli, but is frequently seen on the dorsum of the foot and the lateral aspect of the leg (Figure 8.2). The site occurs distal to the occluded vessels. The base of the ulcer usually contains grey slough. Tissue, bone, tendon and ligament are quickly exposed if the vascularity of the base is insufficient to support the growth of granulation tissue. Gangrene of the toes occurs as distal perfusion reduces. Patients with diabetes and peripheral vascular disease frequently have ulceration and gangrene of the toes (Japp and Tooke, 1994). This is because the disease frequently affects the distal vessels particularly in these patients (Caputo et al., 1994). In addition, patients with diabetes are likely to have disease affecting the microcirculation. Infection may cause rampant gangrene to develop in these patients due to the synergistic effect of polymicrobial infection and a failing microcirculation.

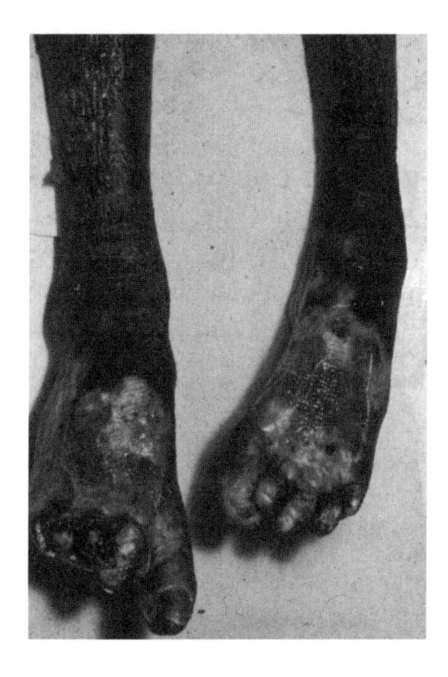

Figure 8.2 Ulceration due to severe peripheral vascular disease; see Plate 4.

Symptoms of arterial ulceration

Patients with arterial disease develop progressive symptoms beginning with intermittent claudication, and ending in the critically ischaemic limb with rest pain.

Intermittent claudication: this is a cramp-like pain in the calf, thigh or buttocks in response to exercise. Rapid relief is gained on resting. The position of the claudication is linked to the site of occlusion (see Chapter 9).

Nocturnal pain: patients complain of neuritic type pain in the middle of the night which is relieved by hanging the leg out of bed.

Pain develops due to a drop in blood pressure causing reduced peripheral circulation in the middle of the night.

Rest pain: nocturnal pain and rest pain may occur simultaneously. The patient complains of intractable pain in the foot, particularly the toes and heel. Patients frequently sleep upright in a chair with their legs in the dependent position to gain relief.

Patients with a large acute embolus may present with a much more dramatic clinical picture. Pain is extreme and accompanied by pallor and complete absence of pedal pulses. This progresses rapidly to paraesthesia and paralysis within hours (see Chapter 10).

Assessment issues

The most important priority in the assessment of patients with leg ulceration is to identify the underlying aetiology. It is also important that the patient has a thorough medical assessment to identify other medical conditions that may delay healing. Assessment requires an understanding of how the ulcer is impacting on the patient's life and that of their family. Bringing together all these aspects will provide the holistic assessment that will allow for effective care planning (Moffatt, 1998).

Identifying the underlying aetiology

In order to identify the underlying aetiology it is important to make a differential diagnosis to determine whether the patient has a venous ulcer, an arterial ulcer or a combination of both. The priorities of management will be based on the arterial status of the patient's leg.

Rarer aetiologies must also be identified, although their assessment and management lie outside the scope of this chapter. The clinical signs and symptoms already described are a useful guide in determining whether the patient has a venous or arterial ulcer. However, it is necessary to have more objective assessment of the patient's arterial circulation using Doppler ultrasound to record an ankle to brachial pressure index (ABPI). The rationale and procedure can be found in Chapter 4. It is now recommended that all leg ulcer patients have this recorded and that reassessment of the patient's circulation occurs frequently. The current clinical guidelines recommend re-Dopplering every 3 months in patients with an ulcer, and 6-monthly for healed ulcer patients (RCN Institute, 1998).

Research has shown the importance of using the correct procedure and of not simply relying on manual palpation of pedal pulses to predict arterial disease (Moffatt and O'Hare, 1995). Analysis of the wave form of the Doppler signal is also useful, particularly in patients with calcified vessels, where the ABPI reading does not reflect the arterial status of the patient.

An ABPI can be performed on almost every patient with a leg ulcer, except if the ulceration is circumferential and involves all pedal pulse sites. The ulcer can be covered with a piece of cling film or a sterile dressing towel.

An ABPI measurement will not provide information about the site of arterial disease. Toe pressures may be required in patients with extensive calcification, particularly diabetics. If a patient has a reduced ABPI below 0.8 a referral to a vascular unit is advised. Particular care should be taken if there is a significant difference between the ankle systolic readings of the different vessels as this may indicate there is occlusive disease of an individual vessel. Further investigations using Duplex ultrasonography are needed to identify the site and severity of disease. It is very important when considering the findings from investigations to consider the patient's previous medical history and how their symptoms present.

Leg ulcer history

It is important to identify the immediate cause of the patient's ulcer (which is often trauma). Patients frequently report several episodes of ulceration and there may be evidence of a family history of ulceration. A number of risk factors have been found to predict delayed healing in venous ulcer patients; these include ulcers of long duration and large size. Patients with reduced general mobility as well as reduced ankle function take longer to heal, probably due to the effect on overall venous function (Franks et al., 1995). Approximately 40% of patients with venous ulceration will have experienced a deep vein thrombosis. (Stacey et al., 1991). Many patients will be unaware of this and it is useful to ask questions about serious illnesses, operations or leg injuries which may have led to a 'silent' deep vein thrombosis.

Patients should be questioned about the presence of varicose veins and any treatment they may have received. It is also useful to find out about the patient's lifestyle or occupation. Patients whose occupation requires long periods standing are at greater risk of developing varicose veins and potentially venous ulceration (Burkitt, 1972).

Patients with arterial ulceration may have evidence of other cardiovascular disease. Callam et al. (1987) found that a history of stroke, angina, myocardial infarction and transient ischaemic attacks were all associated with peripheral vascular disease.

General medical history

Leg ulcer patients frequently suffer with other medical conditions. Patients with lower leg oedema may be treated for a potential leg ulcer when in fact the problem is cardiac in origin. Other medical causes for oedema may be related to renal failure or liver disease. Leg ulcers in patients with heart disease or respiratory failure will often fail to heal due to inadequate oxygen profusion. It is important to identify the medication the patient is receiving. Drugs such as immunosuppressants and cytotoxic therapy have a detrimental effect on wound healing. Patients may also be taking vasoactive drugs such as Oxpentifylline, Paroven or aspirin. Patients with a history of thrombosis may be being treated with anticoagulant therapy.

Mobility status

Limited mobility occurs in over 50% of patients with leg ulceration and may be due to many causes such as osteoarthritis (Franks et al., 1995). Ulceration may lead to secondary immobility. Patients with leg ulceration are reluctant to move and keep their ankle in a fixed position. Reduced ankle function has a direct effect on venous return (Alexander, 1972) (Figure 8.3). Assessment of the patient's mobility and the appropriateness of footwear is needed before commencing a bandaging regime. Foot deformities such as hallux valgus and equinus deformity are found frequently in these patients.

Limb assessment

It is important to note any alterations in sensation within the patient's limb. This is found in over 80% of patients with diabetic foot ulceration but also occurs in patients with conditions such as rheumatoid arthritis, alcoholic neuropathy or following nerve entrapment (Fernando et al., 1991). Micro-filaments are a particularly useful tool in guiding assessment of neuropathy. Neuropathy assessment should

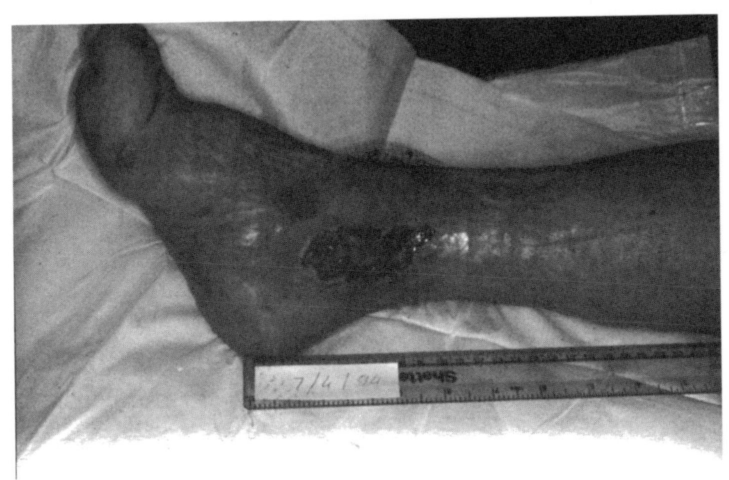

Figure 8.3 Foot deformity leading to reduced healing in a venous ulcer patient; see Plate 5.

aim to identify changes in patients' appreciation of painful stimuli and hot and cold. Changes in gait and proprioception should be noted. Foot deformities are an inevitable precursor to the development of diabetic neuropathic ulceration due to the combined effects of sensory and motor neuropathy. Identifying reduced sensation is vitally important if compression bandaging is to be used. Patients with reduced sensation will not know if the bandage is too tight. The size and shape of the patient's limb should be recorded. The ankle should be measured using a tape measure. This is necessary for all patients receiving compression therapy. Bandages are designed to apply the correct pressure to a given ankle range. Many patients with venous disease present with deformed limb shape. Manifestations include the inverted champagne limb. Bandages applied to this shape limb frequently slip, leading to oedematous bands above the bandage and the danger of the bandage acting as a tourniquet. Many patients lose their calf muscle over time and the limb becomes thin and wasted. These patients are at risk of excessive bandage pressure being applied to the bony tibial crest. Pressure damage may easily occur. All vulnerable pressure points should be assessed in these patients.

Skin and wound assessment

Assessment of the patient's skin and wound should be undertaken every time the patient is treated. Changes in the skin and wounds of patients with arterial disease can be rapid. All areas of the skin should be assessed including the nail beds, which are prone to infection in patients with peripheral arterial disease. The toe webs should be inspected for signs of fungal infection, which provides a portal of entry to pathogenic organisms, including bacteria, fungi and viruses. Poor compression bandaging may lead to an accumulation of oedema in the forefoot and toes. Over a prolonged period of time secondary lymphoedematous changes develop.

Contact dermatitis can be a major clinical problem in patients with venous ulceration (Cameron, 1995). The combined effects of the loss of barrier function and the occlusive environment beneath dressings create an ideal environment for a contact allergy to develop. Contact dermatitis is often mistaken for cellulitis. Figure 8.4 shows the line of demarcation seen in patients with contact allergy. Sensitisation may occur over a long time of exposure to the allergen. The patient presents with an erythematous, oedematous limb and complains of intense irritation (Figure 8.4). The reaction may involve the entire surface of the skin, causing a generalised eczema.

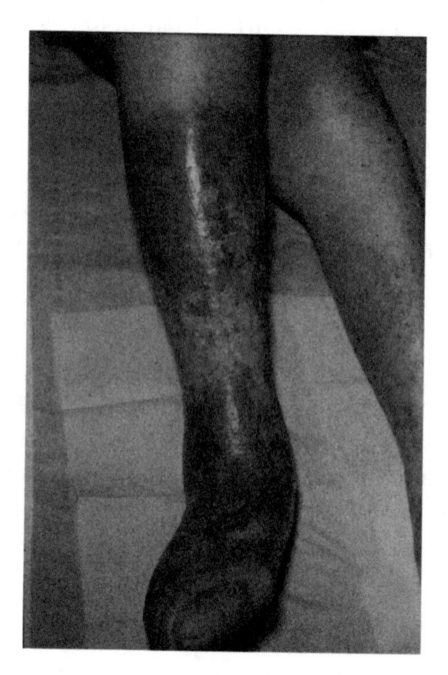

Figure 8.4 Acute parabens-induced contact dermatitis; see Plate 6.

The wound should be assessed and measured regularly – a number of methods exist including simple tracing on to acetate sheets (see Chapter 14). Photography is also useful and may be a great encouragement to patients who can see the progress they are making. A structured format is useful in the assessment process. It is important to evaluate the stage of wound healing as this will determine the wound care regime to be used. Routine wound swabbing is not recommended as all leg ulcers are heavily colonised with bacteria (Gilchrist, 1996). Wound swabs should be taken when clinical signs of cellulitis are present. More reliable assessment of infection may be obtained from tissue sampling. Wound swabs may lead to an over-prediction of colonising organisms and may fail to identify deep invasive anaerobic bacteria, which may be catastrophic in an ischaemic limb. The most noticeable clinical change is the increase of pain, accompanied by erythema, oedema and increased exudate. Patients with severe peripheral vascular disease are at great risk of catastrophic infection which may lead to amputation and possibly death. Many patients with severe peripheral vascular disease may be given prophylactic antibiotics.

However, practitioners should be warned that not all very elderly patients develop clear clinical signs of infection, such as cellulitis and pyrexia. Patients taking corticosteroids may show no signs of impending severe infection within the wound but may proceed to severe septicaemia.

Pain assessment

Pain assessment and management is an important issue for all patients with leg ulceration. Chapter 6 explores these issues in more depth. Relatively little is known concerning management of venous ulcer pain. However, compression bandaging has been shown to reduce pain as a consequence of ulcer healing (Franks et al., 1994). Understanding the patient's perception of their pain is important if patients are to comply with their treatment regimes.

Other investigations

In addition to the Doppler investigations, a number of other investigations provide useful information. Tests such as a BM stix should be performed routinely on all patients with leg ulceration to detect undiagnosed diabetes, which is associated with peripheral vascular disease. Recording of HbA1 (glycosylated haemoglobin) may be a more reliable guide of diabetic status over previous weeks. Blood tests for rheumatoid and antinuclear factor may indicate that the patient has a potential autoimmune disorder. A full blood count should be taken on all patients. This will identify patients with anaemia, who may have delayed healing, as well as helping to ensure that other metabolic problems are identified. Patients with myxoedema or thyrotoxicosis will benefit from thyroid function tests. Tissue biopsy is used if malignant changes are suspected. Chronic non-healing wounds may undergo malignant change. The commonest lesion to develop is a squamous cell carcinoma (Figure 8.5). Patch testing for allergens (e.g. antibiotics) within wound care products is very useful in patients who present with chronic varicose eczema (Cameron, 1995). Wound swabs should be used in cases of cellulitis to determine the nature and sensitivity of the organism and to ensure that the correct antibiotic is prescribed. The presence of osteomyelitis may be detected on X-ray or by magnetic resonance imaging (MRI).

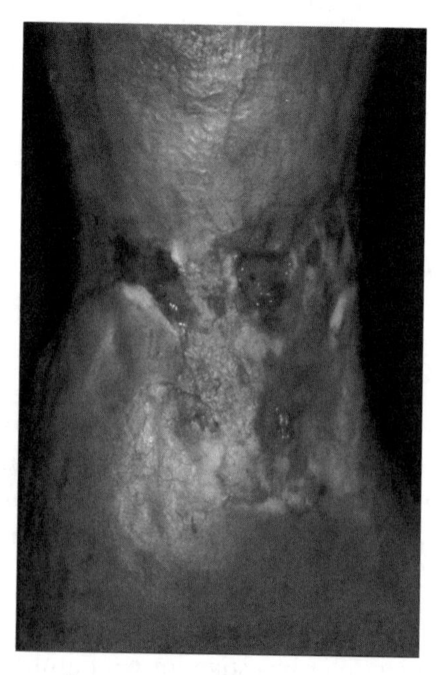

Figure 8.5 Development of a squamous cell carcinoma (Marjolin's ulcer) in an existing venous ulcer; see Plate 7.

Psychosocial assessment

Successful treatment of leg ulceration requires the cooperation of the patient and, where possible, the involvement of the carer or family. Research undertaken in the last decade has highlighted the impact that leg ulceration has on a patient's quality of life (Lindholm et al., 1993). Assessment requires the practitioner to understand the issues that are important to the patient. Many leg ulcer patients become socially isolated because they withdraw from society due to the smell and pain associated with ulceration. Assessment of the patient should aim to identify whether they are depressed or anxious over their condition. The practitioner must assess the patient's understanding of their condition and what their expectations are concerning treatment. Patients with peripheral vascular disease may need to be persuaded to change their lifestyle (see Chapter 3). Practitioners must be aware of punitive regimes that fail to take account of patients' needs while attempting to encourage patients to reduce their risk factors, such as smoking.

Treatment priorities

A careful assessment will have identified the underlying aetiology of the patient's leg ulcer. Should practitioners be in doubt about the findings from the assessment such as the Doppler readings, the patient should be referred for a specialist opinion. The National Clinical Guidelines stress the importance of working as a team in order to ensure the best care is delivered to patients (RCN Institute, 1998). Every patient with an arterial ulcer should be assessed and monitored by a vascular department.

Irrespective of the type of ulcer, a number of priorities are common to all patients:

1. To correct the underlying problem that is causing the ulceration, e.g. revascularisation, reducing venous hypertension through compression therapy.
2. To manage the wound using appropriate wound management strategies that optimise the environment for healing.
3. To prevent any avoidable complications that may inhibit healing such as infection and contact dermatitis.

4. To improve the wider factors that impact on healing such as the medical status of the patient, their nutritional status, mobility etc.
5. To provide psychological support to the patient and family during the treatment process, taking account at all times of the patient's perspective on treatment.
6. To ensure the multidisciplinary team work effectively to maximise the chances of ulcer healing.
7. To prevent a recurrence of ulceration through providing appropriate strategies and patient education.

The above principles apply to all patients irrespective of the underlying aetiology.

Wound management issues

Wound cleansing

Historically, a wide range of solutions have been used to cleanse wounds. While it is now generally accepted that powerful antiseptics such as the hypochlorites damage tissue, little research is available to guide practice in this area (Cullum, 1994). Current best practice recommends simple wound cleansing techniques such as cleansing the wound with warm isotonic normal saline or immersing the limb in a bucket of warm water with an emollient added. This leaves the patient feeling 'clean' and removes much of the odour associated with the exudate. The use of the emollient will hydrate the skin, thus helping to maintain its barrier function. Many patients with leg ulceration describe this procedure as the most therapeutic part of treatment. Patients may opt to shower prior to the dressing changes (Moffatt and Harper, 1997).

Patients with critical ischaemia should never have the limb immersed in very warm water. The sudden rise in temperature will increase the metabolic rate within the limb. Because of the ischaemia further oxygen cannot be supplied to the area and this may exacerbate the ischaemia. Patients with areas of gangrene on the foot and toes should keep the area dry as moisture may increase the risk of superseding infection.

Skin care

The skin has an important barrier function. Any break in the skin may lead to infection, particularly in the patient with peripheral vascular disease. Emollient creams can be applied to the limb at each dressing change. Paraffin-based mixes such as 50% white soft paraffin and 50% liquid paraffin are particularly useful if patients have dry flaky skin or complain of irritation due to bandaging. Products containing lanolin should be avoided as this is one of the most potent sensitisers in leg ulcer patients. Homeopathic creams may also cause contact allergy. When applying cream it is important to apply it in a downward direction to avoid folliculitis developing due to the clogged hair follicles. The area between the toes should be checked regularly for signs of fungal infection. If this occurs treatment with antifungal agents may be required for several months.

Many skin care problems in these patients are caused by poor wound care practice. Inappropriate choice of wound dressings may lead to maceration as well as contact dermatitis. Control of exudate is an important priority, particularly in patients with large venous ulcers.

Patients with peripheral vascular disease are particularly at risk of developing pressure ulcers (see Chapter 5). The heel is a very vulnerable area where the local blood supply is often poor. All patients should be assessed regularly for pressure ulcer risk and appropriate pressure-relieving devices used. Heels may be protected from pressure by simple foam gutters in which the patient rests the leg with the heel off the surface of the bed. Patients should be protected from trauma to the skin at all times. Patient education should include advice on regular podiatry and avoiding self-care removal of calluses. Adhesive tapes that cause irritation or may strip the outer layer of the epidermis on removal should be avoided where possible.

Wound infection

Leg ulcers are chronic wounds and are colonised with many different sorts of bacteria. Colonisation refers to the presence of potentially pathogenic organisms within an ulcer without signs of clinical infection (Gilchrist, 1994). A colonised wound does not require the same treatment as an infected wound. Evidence of clinical infection is required before systemic antibiotics are given to patients with venous ulceration. Patients with severe peripheral vascular disease or diabetic foot ulceration may require long-term antibiotic therapy because of the risk of infection leading to gangrene and loss of limb. Patients with diabetic foot ulceration are particularly prone to developing polymicrobial infection involving several organisms (Caputo et al., 1994). Antibiotic cover must ensure that Gram-negative, Gram-positive and anaerobes are treated. Patients may continue antibiotics until the ulcer is nearly healed. When prescribing antibiotics it is essential that a wound swab is taken to ensure the correct antibiotic is prescribed. Many of the pathogens, such as haemolytic streptococcus, are developing resistance to the main antibiotics groups. One of the many difficulties these patients have is that because perfusion to the limb is poor, adequate levels of antibiotic do not reach the tissues. Even patients with venous ulceration may require 10 to 14 days of antibiotics rather than the traditional 5-day course.

Many chronic leg ulcers are colonised with *methicillin-resistant Staphylococcus aureus*. While this rarely causes a clinical problem to the patient's wound it does, however, pose an important infection control issue. Treatment of leg ulcer patients requires rigorous adherence to infection control procedures. Aprons should be worn at all times and changed between patients. Gloves should be worn for all procedures. Vinyl gloves are preferable to latex as patients with rubber allergy may develop severe contact dermatitis following treatment. Adherence to strict hand washing procedures is vital, particularly in wounds that are producing copious exudate. All equipment such as buckets and scissors should be washed with detergent, rinsed with clean water and dried between each patient. A plastic bin liner should also be inserted into the bucket and changed between patients. In a clinic situation it is vital that the room is cleaned well after use. Patients with methicillin-resistant Staphylococcus aureus should not be brought to a clinic unless this is unavoidable and should be seen at the end of a clinic session. Instructions should be given to the cleaning staff that a patient with methicillin-resistant Staphylococcus aureus has been treated in the clinical area. Any inpatients with methicillin-resistant Staphylococcus aureus should be treated according to the local infection control procedures and liaison with the infection control nurse is essential (Hosein, 1996).

Wound debridement

It is generally agreed that wounds containing large amounts of necrotic, possibly infected, tissue should be debrided owing to the risk of overriding infection (Leaper, 1995). There are a number of methods used to debride necrotic wounds. However, there is little research in this area and no conclusive evidence as to which method is most effective. In patients with peripheral vascular disease the most important factor is to be aware of the significance of the underlying ischaemia in the patient's limb. Debridement of these necrotic wounds can lead to exposure of deeper structures such as tendons, with the risk of secondary infection greatly increased. Infection in an already compromised foot can lead to amputation. Surgical debridement should be undertaken by a vascular surgeon in these patients. Patients with diabetes may develop small patches of gangrene on isolated areas of the toes and foot due to failing microcirculation and infection. Individual digits may autodebride when the infection is under control. The toes become dry and mummified and eventually fall off leaving a clean site, which can then heal by secondary intention. Venous ulceration is often covered with a superficial layer of slough, particularly in the early stages of the ulcer developing. Radical debridement in these patients is rarely required as the wound develops granulation tissue when effective compression is applied. This is because the correct wound environment for healing has now been achieved.

There is increasing interest in biotechniques of debridement using sterile maggots (Bale and Jones, 1997). Maggots have been known to be effective debriders over the centuries and saved many limbs from amputation in the First World War. The maggots remove all necrotic tissue and also produce enzymes which may have a stimulatory effect on wound healing. Patients must be adequately prepared for this treatment as some may find the concept alarming.

The final method of debridement involves creating a moist environment that rehydrates the slough, which then separates from the wound. A number of different dressing types are used for this. These include hydrogels, hydrocolloids, alginates, polysaccharide pastes and enzymatic products (Morison et al., 1997). When the slough has softened it is often possible to remove the slough mechanically with scissors and fine-toothed forceps. It is important to remember when debriding these wounds that unless the underlying vascular problem has been corrected the slough will quickly reform.

A number of other methods have been used to debride wounds over the decades. Hypochlorites such as eusol were used regularly in these wounds despite evidence of their toxicity and inactivation in wounds (Gilchrist, 1996). However, much of the research in this area is limited to laboratory experiments, and virtually no research has been carried out on patients with wounds due to peripheral vascular disease. Saline-soaked gauze, which is packed in the wound and allowed to dry, is still used in some parts of the world. When it is then removed from the wound both necrotic and healthy tissue is debrided. This is an inhumane method of treatment which is likely to cause extreme pain to the patient as well as damage to healthy tissue.

Wound dressings

A wide range of wound dressings are available to treat patients with chronic wounds. There is often inadequate research into many of these products, and it is not possible to state that one type of dressing speeds healing over another (Cullum, 1994). The concept of creating a moist wound environment at the wound interface is now broadly accepted (Winter, 1962). A number of classifications have been written which attempt to describe the properties of an ideal dressing. Chapter 14 gives an in-depth discussion on the types of wound dressings and their use in patients with peripheral vascular disease.

Management of venous ulceration

The primary aim of management in the patient with venous ulceration is to reverse the effects of venous hypertension by the use of high compression therapy (Moffatt and Harper, 1997). As already described, venous ulceration occurs because of reverse flow of blood in the leg veins. This causes a rise in pressure in the superficial venous system and the microcirculation. High compression therapy applies an external pressure which counteracts this pressure, improves the overall venous function and reduces the inflammatory processes occurring in the damaged microcirculation. Importantly, the external pressure forces oedema from the interstitial spaces into the venous circulation and lymphatics.

High compression therapy

A systematic review of the literature on compression bandaging has shown that high compression bandaging is more effective than lower levels of compression in ulcer healing (Fletcher et al., 1997). In the United Kingdom high compression systems aim to apply a pressure at the ankle of 35 to 40 mmHg. It is important to ensure the patient has an adequate arterial supply before application. An ABPI should be recorded on all patients. High compression is recommended for all patients with an ABPI greater than 0.8 (Table 8.2).

Table 8.2 Criteria for using compression therapy

ABPI Doppler findings	Suitable bandage systems	Comments
ABPI >0.8	High compression: Single layer high compression bandaging (applied over padding layer), e.g. Setopress, Surepress, Tensopress. Multilayer high compression bandaging, e.g. Charing Cross 4 layer, Profore, Ultra 4. Short stretch bandaging (applied over padding layer), e.g. Comprilan, Rosidal K, Elastocrepe.	Care should be taken in patients with ABPI readings >0.8 who have concurrent diabetes mellitus and rheumatoid arthritis.
ABPI 0.6–0.8	Reduced compression: Short stretch bandages (applied over padding), e.g. (low resting pressure) Comprilan, Rosidal K, Elastocrepe. Reduced multilayer systems, e.g. (pressure approx. 17 mmHg) Velband, Crepe, Elset or Velband, Crepe, Coban (pressure approx. 23 mmHg) Profore Lite.	Practitioners must take account of the patient's arterial symptoms when applying compression. This group of patients already have established arterial disease. Regular assessment is essential.
ABPI <0.5	High compression must *not* be applied.	Refer for vascular opinion. Compression only to be applied under *strict* vascular supervision.

High compression can be applied using different methods of bandaging:

Elastic compression systems (long stretch)

- Single layer high compression bandages, e.g. Setopress, Surepress, Tensopress.
- Multilayer bandage regimes, e.g. Original Charing Cross 4 layer bandage, Profore, Ultra four.

The bandages described above all contain elastomers which ensure that the pressure the bandage applies is maintained until the bandage is removed.

Inelastic bandaging systems (short stretch)

- Single layer short stretch bandages, e.g. Comprilan, Rosidal K.
- Multilayer short stretch regimes, e.g. padding and Comprilan.

Short stretch bandages do not contain elastic but are made entirely of natural fibres such as cotton. These bandages apply a rigid support to the calf. Unlike elastic bandages these bandages apply lower levels of pressure when the patient is at rest. However, when exercising the calf muscle the pressure rises beneath the bandage due to the rigidity of the bandage. Short stretch bandaging may be particularly useful in very active patients because of the high working pressure. These types of bandages are used extensively in mainland Europe and there is growing interest in their use in the United Kingdom.

High compression can also be applied using hosiery. This can be very useful for patients with small, low exudating ulcers who wish to care for their own ulcers. Hosiery is used extensively in the prevention of venous ulcer recurrence.

Intermittent pneumatic compression

Intermittent pneumatic compression is the application of cycles of controlled pressure to a limb using compressed air. The patient applies an inflatable garment which inflates cyclically. The amount and frequency of compression can be modified. Intermittent pneumatic compression has been shown to improve the venous return and is particularly useful in patients with chronic oedema, where it has been shown to enhance the healing rates (Coleridge-Smith et al., 1990). Intermittent pneumatic compression can be used on the top of existing compression bandaging in venous ulcer patients. However, this should never be undertaken in patients with a degree of arterial disease as the combined pressure of the bandage and the pump may be sufficient to interrupt arterial inflow. Intermittent compression has also been used successfully in the treatment of patients with lymphoedema, sports injuries and following deep vein thrombosis. In a patient with deep vein thrombosis it is essential to undertake a Duplex scan to identify the site and adherence of the clot to ensure that the patient is not at risk of a pulmonary embolism.

Application issues in applying high compression bandaging

The application of high compression requires an understanding of the scientific principles behind its use, as well as skill in its correct application. Effective compression bandaging has revolutionised the outlook for patients with venous ulceration who frequently failed to heal for months and years.

Regardless of the choice of bandage, it is essential to identify any changes in the limb conformity prior to bandaging. Figure 8.6 describes the issues that should be considered when applying a bandage in a spiral or a figure of eight technique. There is increasing recognition of the need to apply a protective padding layer prior to application of any compression bandage. All of the multilayer systems have incorporated this into their design (Moffatt et al., 1992). The Profore high compression system has four layers as follows:

- Layer 1: orthopaedic wool which absorbs exudate and protects limb.
- Layer 2: cotton crepe which adds absorbency and preserves elastic energy.
- Layer 3: Litepress which applies compression (17 mmHg at the ankle in a figure of eight).
- Layer 4: Coplus which applies compression (23 mmHg) and keeps bandage system in place.

Multilayer systems such as this are designed to accommodate different sizes and shapes of limbs. The compression is applied in layers using weaker elastic bandages. This overcomes the problem of applying excessive pressure, which can happen when using the single

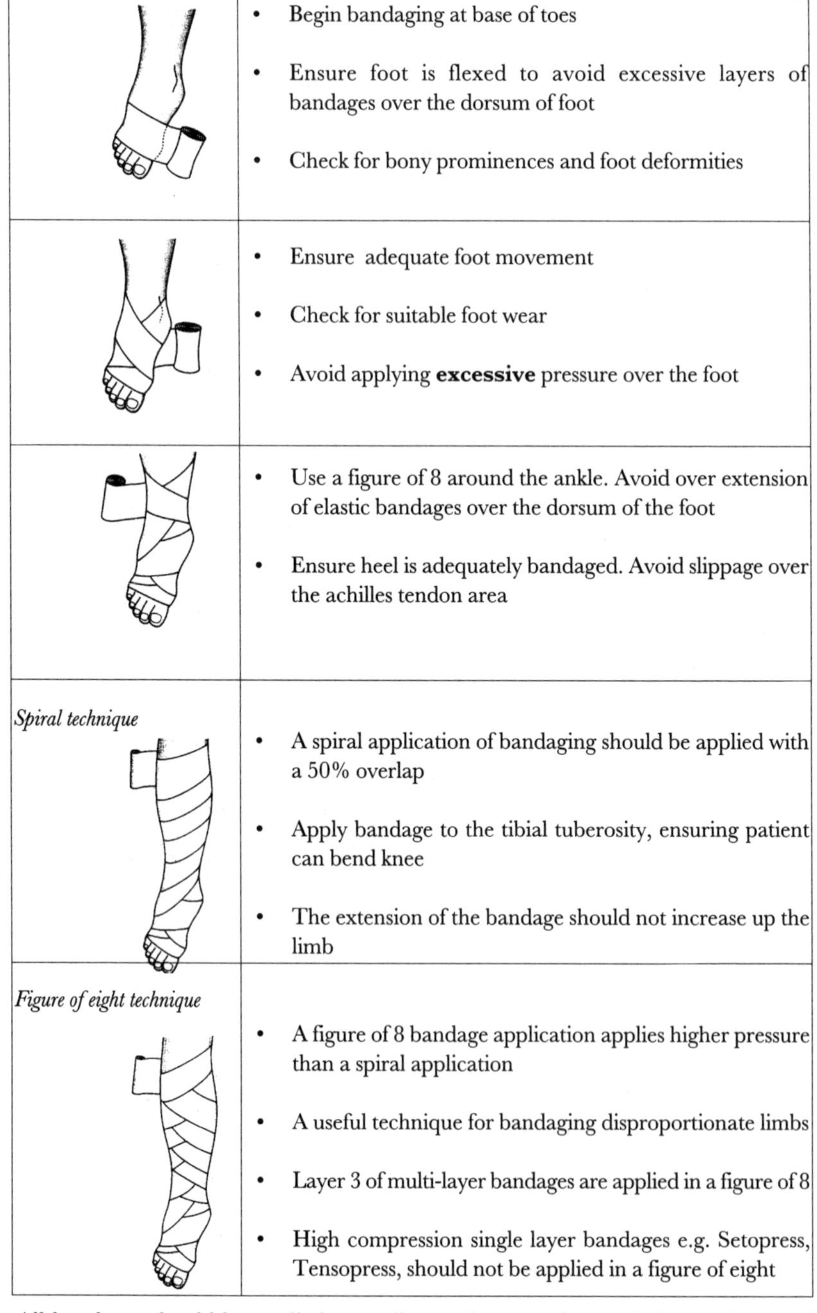

	• Begin bandaging at base of toes • Ensure foot is flexed to avoid excessive layers of bandages over the dorsum of foot • Check for bony prominences and foot deformities
	• Ensure adequate foot movement • Check for suitable foot wear • Avoid applying **excessive** pressure over the foot
	• Use a figure of 8 around the ankle. Avoid over extension of elastic bandages over the dorsum of the foot • Ensure heel is adequately bandaged. Avoid slippage over the achilles tendon area
Spiral technique	• A spiral application of bandaging should be applied with a 50% overlap • Apply bandage to the tibial tuberosity, ensuring patient can bend knee • The extension of the bandage should not increase up the limb
Figure of eight technique	• A figure of 8 bandage application applies higher pressure than a spiral application • A useful technique for bandaging disproportionate limbs • Layer 3 of multi-layer bandages are applied in a figure of 8 • High compression single layer bandages e.g. Setopress, Tensopress, should not be applied in a figure of eight

All bandages should be applied according to the manufacturer's instructions and following appropriate training.

Figure 8.6 Application of compression bandages.

layer elastic bandages. Some of the single layer bandages have incorporated bandage symbols which show the practitioner how far to extend the bandage (Figure 8.7). Patients who have oedematous toes may benefit from the application of a narrow toe bandage applied to each individual digit. This technique has been extensively used in the field of lymphoedema. Modifications have been made to the four-layer bandage systems to ensure the correct pressure is applied to all limbs

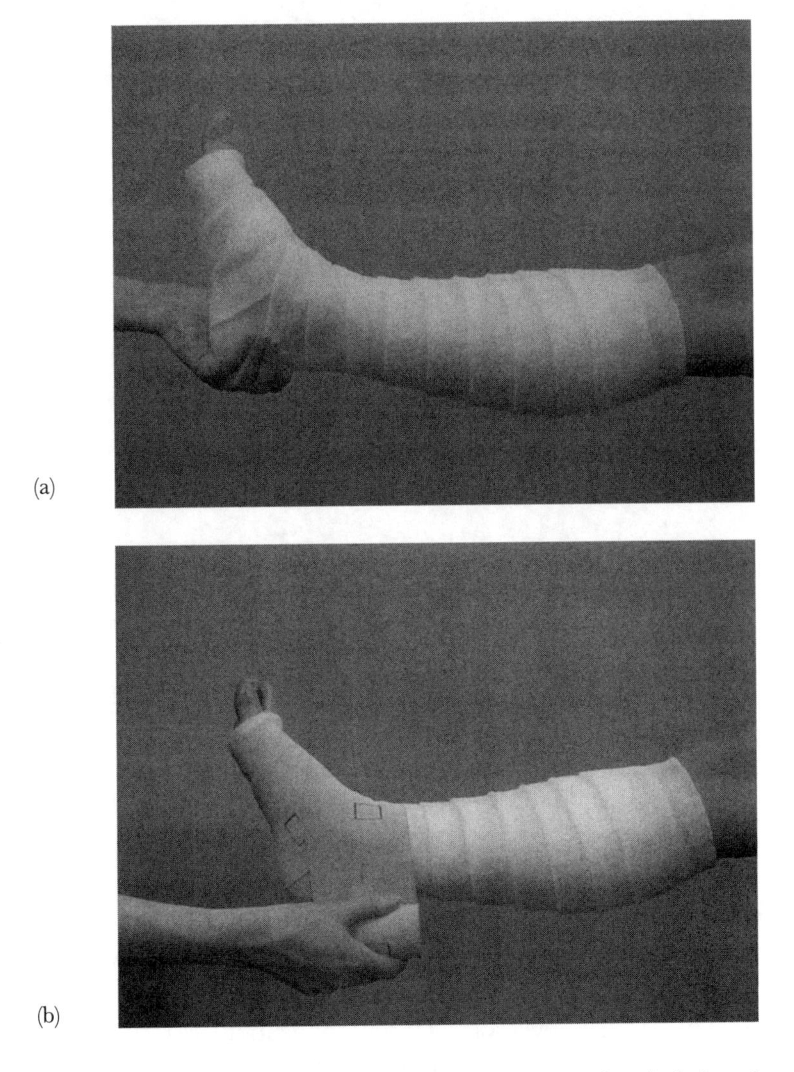

(a)

(b)

Figure 8.7(a–d) Application of (Setopress) a high compression single layer bandage over orthopaedic padding.

(contd)

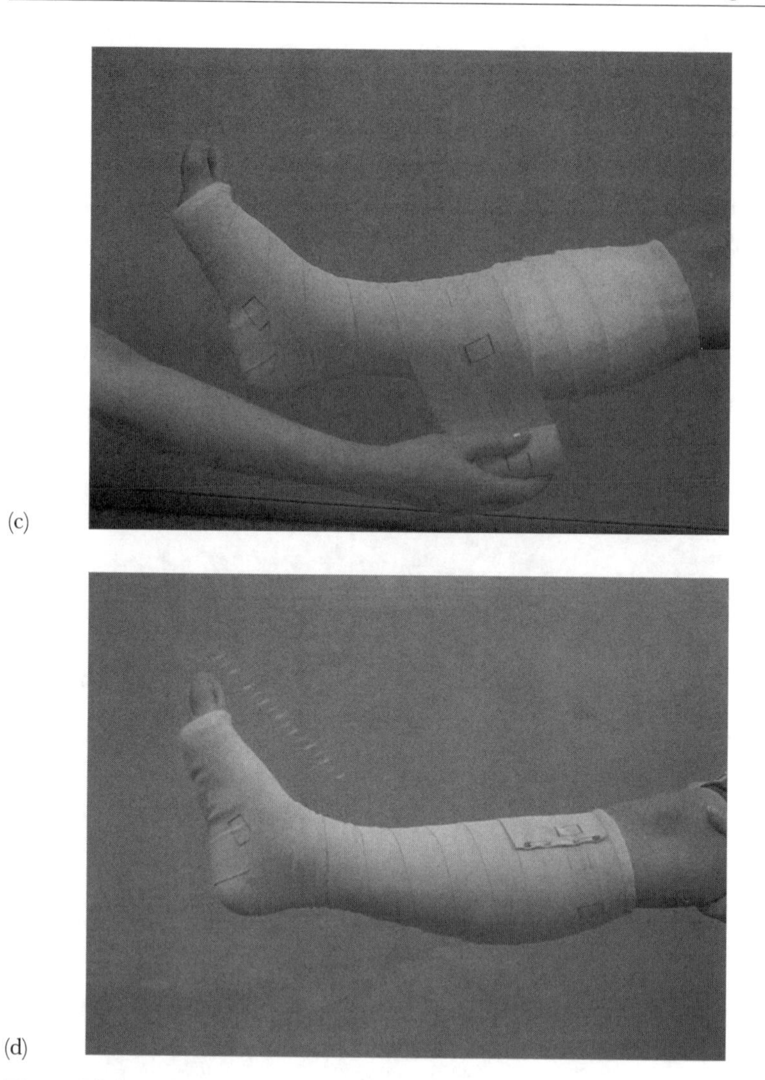

(c)

(d)

Figure 8.7 (contd).

irrespective of the size of the ankle. Table 8.3 shows the modifications to the original four-layer bandage system and the new Profore system. Note that the ankle circumference measurement informs the practitioner of the required regime. Thin limbs, with an ankle circumference of less than 20 cm, are at risk of excessive pressure resulting in skin damage. This is easily overcome by the application of a little extra padding. Large, oedematous limbs frequently do not receive a therapeutic level of compression. A more powerful compression bandage is

Table 8.3 Modifications to four-layer bandaging according to limb size and shape to ensure 35–40 mmHg pressure is applied to all limbs. Patient's ankle circumference is measured in centimetres. If oedema is present the limb should be regularly measured.

Ankle circumference	Bandage combinations
Less than 18 cm	2 orthopaedic wool layers (extra padding protects thin limbs) 1 cotton crepe 1 elastic (e.g. Elset, Litepress) 1 cohesive (e.g. Coban, Coplus)
18–25 cm	1 orthopaedic wool layer 1 cotton crepe 1 elastic (e.g. Elset, Litepress) 1 cohesive (e.g. Coban, Coplus)
25–30 cm	1 orthopaedic wool layer 1 high compression bandage (e.g. Setopress, Surepress, Tensopress) 1 cohesive (e.g. Coban, Coplus)
Greater than 30 cm	2 orthopaedic wool to cover larger limb 1 elastic (e.g. Elset, Litepress) 1 high compression bandage (e.g. Setopress, Surepress, Tensopress) 1 cohesive (e.g. Coban, Coplus) Few patients will have ankle circumference of this size

substituted. Using this simple method it is possible to ensure that all patients have the correct level of pressure to achieve ulcer healing.

Skin problems in venous ulcer patients

Patients with venous ulceration suffer from a number of skin conditions ranging from flaky skin to acute contact dermatitis. All patients require the wound cleansing and skin care regimes already outlined. Patients with severe intractable varicose eczema may require a short course of topical steroids to control the situation. Steroids should always be applied sparingly according to the instructions. Steroids must never be applied to a wound as this will inhibit the inflammatory response. The strength of steroid may be reduced over time and increasing amounts of emollients substituted. Steroids should not be stopped suddenly as this may cause a rebound reaction in which the skin appears worse than before treatment (Cameron, 1995). Practitioners should be aware that when steroids are applied beneath occlusive dressings or bandages, this has a depot effect increasing the potency and absorbency of the steroids (Varghese et al., 1986). Long-term use of steroids should be avoided as this will lead to dermal thinning which makes the skin more vulnerable to trauma. Contact dermatitis occurs due to an allergic response to an allergen. Common leg ulcer allergens include preservatives such as parabens, wool fats, antibiotics and rubber (Cameron, 1995). A patient with an acute contact allergy may require topical steroids initially. The allergen should first be washed from the leg with warm water. All possible allergens contained within dressings or bandages should be removed and the patient's leg covered with an inert dressing and cotton liner prior to bandaging. Occasionally a patient may present with a total body eczematous reaction. All patients with contact allergy should be patch tested in order to identify what they are allergic to. Patients can then be educated about what to avoid in the future. Although steroids are often the first line treatment in these patients, occasionally patients may actually become sensitised to the steroids themselves, particularly if they have used excessive amounts of hydrocortisone (Dooms-Goosens et al., 1986).

Skin grafting of venous ulceration

A number of skin grafting techniques are used in the management of patients with large venous ulcers. Traditional meshed grafting techniques are used for patients admitted to hospital. Frequently these patients will undergo vein surgery during the admission if the primary cause of the ulceration is due to varicose veins. Increasingly, nurses are using the technique of pinch grafting, which involves taking tiny pinches of full thickness skin from an anaesthetised area of skin on the thigh (Figure 8.8) and applying them to a granulating ulcer bed (Poskitt et al., 1987). Many of these patients are grafted in an outpatient or community setting and do not require admission to hospital.

Hospitalised patients receiving *meshed grafts* will frequently be on bed rest following the procedure for a number of days, preferably with the foot elevated. It is vital that compression bandaging is applied to the patient's limb before they are allowed to mobilise. The major cause of graft failure in this group is the lack of understanding that the underlying venous hypertension that led to the ulcer remains. If oedema or a haematoma develops the graft will fail, as

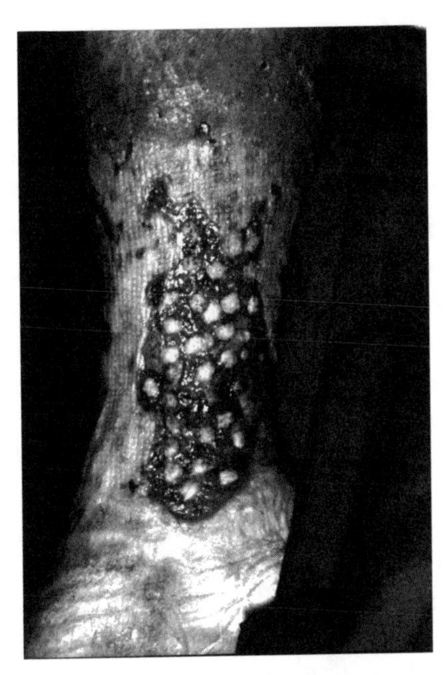

Figure 8.8 Pinch grafts applied to a venous ulcer; see Plate 8.

the newly established vascular structure will be damaged. All patients undergoing skin grafting should be screened for bacteria in the wound before a graft is applied. In particular, haemolytic streptococci and pseudomonas have a devastating effect on graft take. Patients will often be given prophylactic antibiotics in order to avoid the problem. Every effort must be made to avoid damage to the graft during dressing changes. A truly non-adherent dressing should be used. Dressings such as Mepitel, which has a non-adherent contact layer that can be left on the wound over several dressing changes, are far superior to the traditional tulle dressings which dry out and adhere and inhibit healing due to the meshed structure. The pain associated with the donor sites can be helped greatly by the use of occlusive type dressings such as foams, semipermeable film dressings and hydrocolloids.

Health promotion issues in venous ulceration

It is vital to encourage these patients to participate in their treatment programme and to realise that there are many things they can do themselves to aid healing. Research has highlighted that many of these patients are passive and do not necessarily want to become actively involved in their care, preferring to rely on the professional (Cullum and Roe, 1995). Patients need to understand the importance of exercise and, if they are able, to walk several miles a day. They should understand why they should avoid standing for long periods or keeping the limb in a dependent position. Even very immobile patients can be encouraged to spend time each afternoon lying on the bed or a settee. The patient needs to understand that their legs must be above the level of their heart to be therapeutic. The end of the patient's bed can easily be raised on blocks or a suitcase placed under the mattress. Some patients are purchasing recliner chairs which are also useful. Immobility is frequently coupled with obesity in this patient group. Referral to a dietician may provide the necessary impetus to lose weight. However, many of these patients have other health care problems that make these recommendations impossible. The practitioner must always remain realistic in their expectations of patients, while maintaining an optimistic outlook to the patient.

Management of patients with mixed aetiology ulceration

Many patients with leg ulceration have more than one aetiology contributing to non-healing. It is beyond the scope of this chapter to discuss all the possible combinations of problems. Of particular mention are the complex problems of patients with diabetic foot ulceration which are often due to peripheral neuropathy and peripheral vascular disease.

Many patients with venous ulceration also have arterial disease of the lower limb. The priority in managing these patients is always to determine the degree of ischaemia. Patients with a mild degree of ischaemia may tolerate reduced levels of compression. While more research is required to determine the effectiveness of the different regimes some recommendations can be made for practitioners based on the National Clinical Guidelines (RCN Institute, 1998).

The findings from the ABPI readings have been used successfully to guide practitioners concerning the level of compression to apply (Table 8.2). However, it is vital that the patient's symptoms and signs are taken into account. Some patients with fairly minimal levels of compression find the pain intolerable, while others with severe disease may manage well.

Patients with an ABPI of 0.7 or 0.6 may tolerate compression of around 20 mmHg. This can be applied in a number of ways. Multi-layer systems can be used by simply removing either the third or fourth layer. Paste bandaging with a cotton elastocrepe is also often used. Patients who find high compression elastic systems painful may find short stretch regimes better due to the low pressure beneath the bandage when at rest. The skin and wound management issues in this group do not differ from those already highlighted. However, the most important factor to remember in these patients is the need for constant assessment. These patients already have established arterial disease which may progress rapidly. The patient should be re-Dopplered regularly, particularly if the patient notices an acute change in symptoms. Patients should be advised to remove the bandage if they get an acute exacerbation of pain or change in sensation and to get immediate medical advice. Any patient with an ABPI lower than 0.5 should not have compression unless under the regular supervision of a vascular team.

Patients with conditions such as rheumatoid disease or diabetes may also have microvascular disease which cannot be identified on routine Doppler assessment. In these patients compression should be used with caution, as tight compression may exacerbate an already failing microcirculation leading to tissue necrosis.

Management of arterial ulceration

The priority of management in patients with ulceration due to ischaemia is to improve blood flow and increase tissue perfusion. A limb with critical ischaemia is unlikely to heal even with the most effective wound care strategies.

Skin care issues are very important to these patients who are at risk of infection and for whom minor trauma may result in gangrene.

There has been considerable debate concerning the use of occlusive type dressings in these wounds (Thompson and Smith, 1994). While the research suggests that occlusion does not increase the risk of infection in other wounds, it is not clear what the effects are on a wound with a greatly diminished blood supply where it is impossible to create an optimum environment for healing, due to lack of oxygen to the area. The concept of moist wound healing relies on the ability to create the best environment to allow healing. Occlusion of ischaemic wounds may lead to overriding levels of pathogens accumulating and clinical infection developing. However, whether this does actually occur is poorly understood. Because of the nature of these wounds it is essential that they are assessed regularly as change can occur rapidly. Occlusive dressings should not be used to debride gangrenous areas unless under vascular supervision.

These patients require considerable psychological support as many will face major surgery or amputation. The practitioner's role may often be palliative, and control of symptoms becomes the main priority. Patients with ischaemic pain need adequate control of their pain, which can be difficult. Opiates are often required in high doses. Chapter 6 discusses the issues of pain management in more detail.

Control of risk factors and advice on lifestyle change can be a major challenge. Attempting to get the patient to stop smoking can be a difficult task. Patients frequently do not believe that cessation will help their condition and for many the effect is questionable if they have smoked heavily for decades. Patients may also report tangible relief of symptoms when smoking, particularly reduced levels of anxiety. For some patients there is a sense that there is little else left in life except smoking. However, every attempt should be made to encourage the patient and enlist the family's help. Advice on diet and reduction of cholesterol levels may be needed. Control of the patient's blood pressure and other medical conditions should be aimed for, as these impact on wound healing.

Prevention of leg ulcer recurrence

The epidemiological information on recurrence is sparse. The Lothian and Forth Valley study found that two-thirds of patients had experienced two or more episodes of recurrence and that 21% had experienced more than six (Callam et al., 1985). Until recently very little work had been done to identify which patients with leg ulceration were most at risk of recurrence. A community study found that a history of deep vein thrombosis and a previously large ulcer increased the risk of the patient's ulcer returning (Moffatt and Dorman, 1995). These two factors are likely to indicate that these patients had more severe underlying venous disease. Patients with arterial ulceration may heal after vascular intervention but any change in the patient's vascular status will lead to a recurrence of the problem.

Even though evidence is sparse most practitioners would agree that the most effective tool in preventing venous ulcer recurrence is the use of graduated compression hosiery. The research suggests that the higher the level of compression the patient can have, the lower the recurrence rate (Harper et al., 1995). However, the compliance rate is likely to fall the greater the compression level applied. Elderly patients or their carers must be educated not only in the method of application but just as importantly in understanding the importance of continuing with the treatment even though the ulcer has apparently healed.

The management of patients with leg ulceration is both challenging and rewarding. Practitioners must attempt to stay abreast of the developments occurring within the field of tissue viability. For management to be effective it is important to understand the underlying aetiology of the patient's ulcer. Assessment requires a holistic approach that never loses sight of the patient and family in the quest for healing.

References

Alexander CJ (1972) Chair sitting and varicose veins. Lancet i: 822–823.

Bale S (1997) Wound dressings. In: Morison M, Moffatt CJ, Bridel Nixon J, Bale S. Nursing Management of Chronic Wounds, 2nd edn, pp 103–118. London: Mosby.

Bale S, Jones V (1997) Wound Care Nursing. A Patient Centred Approach. London: Baillière Tindall.

Browse NL, Burnand KG (1982) The causes of venous ulceration. Lancet ii: 243–245.

Burkitt DF (1972) Varicose veins, deep vein thrombosis and haemorrhoids: epidemiology and aetiology. British Medical Journal ii: 556-561.

Callam MJ, Ruckley CV, Harper DR, Dale JJ (1985) Chronic ulceration of the leg: extent of the problem and provision of care. British Medical Journal 290: 1855–1856.

Callam MJ, Harper DR, Dale JJ, Ruckley CV (1987) Chronic ulcer of the leg: a clinical history. British Medical Journal 294: 1389–1391.

Cameron J (1995) The importance of contact dermatitis in the management of leg ulcers. Journal of Tissue Viability 5(2): 52–55.

Caputo GM, Cavanagh PR, Ulbrecht JS, Gibbons GW, Karchmer PR (1994) Assessment and management of foot disease in patients with diabetes. New England Journal of Medicine 331(13): 854–860.

Chant AD (1990) Tissue pressure, posture and venous ulceration. Lancet 336: 1051–1501.

Cohen JI, Prystowski JH (1992) Treatment of ulcerated HIV-associated Kaposi's sarcoma with combination chemotherapy. Wounds 4: 208-214.
Coleridge-Smith PD, Thomas P, Scurr JH, Dormandy JA (1988) Causes of venous ulceration – a new hypothesis. British Medical Journal 296: 1726–1727.
Coleridge-Smith P, Sarin S, Hasty J, Scurr JH (1990) Sequential gradient pneumatic compression enhances venous ulcer healing: a randomised trial. Surgery 108: 871-875.
Cornwall J, Dore CJ, Lewis JP (1986) Leg ulcers: epidemiology and aetiology. British Journal of Surgery 73: 603–696.
Cullum N (1994) The nursing management of leg ulcers in the community: a critical review of research. Department of Health. London: HMSO.
Cullum N, Roe B (1995) Leg Ulcers: Nursing Management: A Research Based Guide. London: Scutari.
Dooms-Goosens A, Verschaeve H, Degreef H, van Berendoncks J (1986) Contact allergy to hydrocortisone and tixocortal pivalate: problems in the detection of corticosteroid sensitivity. Contact Dermatitis 14: 94–102.
European Working Group on Critical Leg Ischaemias (1992) Consensus Document on Chronic Critical Leg Ischaemia European Journal of Vascular Surgery 6 (Suppl A): 1–14.
Fernando DJS, Hutchinson A, Veves A, Gokal R, Boulton AJM (1991) Risk factors for non ischaemic foot ulceration in diabetic nephropathy. Diabetic Medicine 8(3): 223–225.
Fletcher A, Cullum N, Sheldon TA (1997) A systematic review of compression treatment for venous leg ulcers. British Medical Journal 315: 576–580.
Franks PJ, Moffatt CJ, Connolly M, Bosanquet N, Oldroyd M, Greenhalgh RM, McCollum CN (1994) Community leg ulcer clinics: effects on quality of life. Phlebology 9: 83–86.
Franks PJ, Moffatt CJ, Oldroyd M, Bosanquet N, Connolly M, Greenhalgh RM, McCollum CN (1995) Factors associated with healing leg ulceration using high compression. Age and Ageing 24: 407–410.
Gilchrist B (1994) Treating bacterial wound infection. Nursing Times 90(5): 56–58.
Gilchrist B (1996) Wound infection 1. Sampling bacterial flora: a review of the literature. Journal of Wound Care 5(8): 386–388.
Harper DR, Nelson EA, Gibson B, Prescott RJ, Ruckley CV (1995) A prospective randomised trial of Class 2 and Class 3 elastic compression in the prevention of venous ulceration. Phlebology '95, Negus et al (eds) Phlebology Suppl 1: 872–873.
Higley HP, Ksander GA, Gerhardt CO, Falanga V (1985) Extravasation of macromolecules and possible trapping of transferring growth factor in venous ulceration. British Journal of Dermatology 132: 79–85.
Hosein IK (1996) Wound infection 2. MRSA. Journal of Wound Care 5(8): 386–388.
Japp AJ, Tooke JE (1994) Is microvascular disease important in the diabetic foot? In: Boulton AJM, Connor H, Cavanagh PR (eds) The Foot in Diabetes, 2nd edn. Chichester: Wiley.
Leaper D (1995) The management of venous ulcers – the medical and surgical options. Journal of Wound Care 4(10): 477–481.
Lindholm C, Bjellrup M, Christenson O, Zederfelt B (1993) Quality of life in leg ulcer patients. An assessment according to the Nottingham Health Profile. Acta Dermato Venerologica (Stockh) 73: 440–445.

Moffatt CJ (1998) Issues in the assessment of leg ulceration. Journal of Wound Care 7(19): 469–473.
Moffatt CJ, Dorman MC (1995) Recurrence of leg ulcers within a community leg ulcer service. Journal of Wound Care 4(2): 57–61.
Moffatt CJ, O'Hare L (1995) Ankle pulses are not sufficient to detect impaired arterial circulation in patients with leg ulcers. Journal of Wound Care 4(3): 134–138.
Moffatt CJ, Harper P (1997) Access to Clinical Education Leg Ulcers. New York: Churchill Livingstone.
Moffatt CJ, Franks PJ, Oldroyd M, Bosanquet N, Brown P, Greenhalgh RM, McCollum CN (1992) Community clinics for leg ulcers and impact on healing. British Medical Journal 305: 1389–1392.
Morison M, Moffatt CJ, Bridel Nixon J, Bale S (1997) Nursing Management of Chronic Wounds, 2nd edn. London: Mosby.
Nelzen O, Bergvist D, Lindehagen A, Hallbrook T (1991) Chronic leg ulcers: an underestimated problem in primary health care among elderly patients. Journal of Epidemiology and Community Health 45: 184–187.
Orr MM, McAvoy BR (1987) The ischaemic leg. In: Fry J, Berry HE (eds) Surgical Problems in Clinical Practice, pp 123–135. London: Edward Arnold.
Poskitt KR, Lloyd Davies ERV, James A, Walton J, McCollum CN (1987) Pinch grafting or porcine dermis in venous ulcers: a randomised clinical trial. British Medical Journal 294: 674–676.
RCN Institute (1998) Clinical Practice Guidelines: The Management of Patients with Venous Leg Ulcers. London: RCN Institute.
Rose G (1991) Epidemiology of atherosclerosis. British Medical Journal 303: 1537–1539.
Stacey MC, Burnand KG, Lea Thomas M, Pattison M (1991) Influence of phlebographic abnormalities on the natural history of venous ulceration. British Journal of Surgery 78(7): 868–877.
Thomas S (1990) Functions of a wound dressing. In: Wound Management and Dressings. London: The Pharmaceutical Press.
Thompson PD, Smith DJ (1994) What is infection? American Journal of Surgery 167 (1A) (Suppl: Symposium: wound infection and occlusion – separating fact from fiction: 7S–11S).
Varghese MC, Baun AK, Carter DM, Caldwell D (1986) Local environment of chronic wounds under synthetic dressings. Archives of Dermatology 122: 52–57.
Walzman M, Wade AAH, Drake SM, Thomas AMC (1986) Rest pain and leg ulceration due to syphilitic osteomyelitis of the tibia. British Medical Journal 293: 804–805.
Winter GD (1962) Formation of the scab and the rate of epithelialisation of superficial wounds in the skin of the domestic pig. Nature 193: 293–294.

CHAPTER 9

Chronic Ischaemia

SHELAGH MURRAY

Management of patients with *chronic ischaemia* is a challenging area of care which requires a collaborative approach between nurses, doctors, and other healthcare professionals. The word 'ischaemia' comes from the Greek 'ischein haima' which means to suppress blood. This chapter focuses on nursing care, support, and management of patients with chronic ischaemia, which is caused by peripheral arterial occlusion due to atherosclerosis, diabetic vascular disease, vasculitis and vasospastic conditions. Limb-threatening ischaemia is discussed in Chapter 10.

Studies have revealed significant major arterial stenosis in 15% of men and 5% of women (Mitchell and Schwartz, 1965). Atherosclerosis, the underlying cause of peripheral arterial occlusive disease (PAOD), is insidious, often producing no symptoms for many years (Fowkes, 1996). The major arteries in the lower limbs, most frequently the superficial femoral artery, are most commonly affected (Figure 9.1).

Atherosclerosis is known to be a significant cause of morbidity and mortality in patients with peripheral arterial occlusive disease due to the co-incidence of coronary artery, cerebrovascular, and renal disease (Fowkes et al., 1991; Missouris et al., 1994). Coronary artery and cerebrovascular disease is primarily responsible for more than 30% of deaths in patients with peripheral arterial occlusive disease (Kallero, 1981; Greenhalgh et al., 1988), whereas limb disease can cause chronic disability and lifestyle handicap which can significantly affect a patient's quality of life.

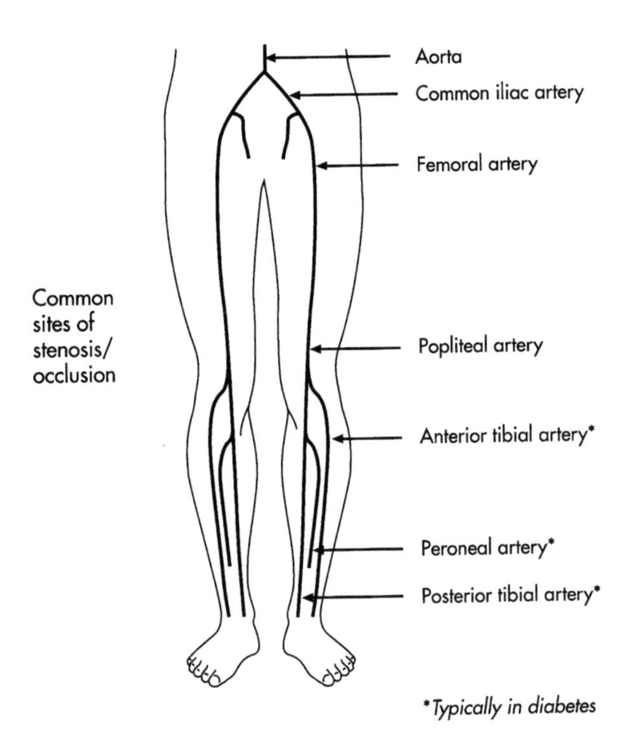

Figure 9.1 Location of atherosclerotic disease in the lower limbs.

Peripheral vascular disease is often linked to a certain lifestyle where modifying risk factors such as smoking, lack of exercise, and hypertension, may help to improve a patient's general health. Hyperglycaemia due to poorly controlled diabetes, or an unhealthy high fat diet causing obesity, may predispose to atherosclerosis. Non-modifiable factors include age, gender and hereditary conditions.

A patient with chronic ischaemia who is experiencing early symptoms of mild or moderate intermittent claudication may be able to cope with the disability for many years by making a few lifestyle changes. Studies have demonstrated an association between sedentary lifestyles and increased risk of claudication (Housley et al., 1993). Intervention will need considering if a patient becomes so severely handicapped that claudication results in a significant deterioration in quality of life. If an acute on chronic situation occurs resulting in signs of critical limb ischaemia (CLI) such as rest pain, ulceration or gangrene, then reconstructive bypass surgery may be indicated.

Intermittent claudication

Intermittent claudication is the equivalent to cardiac angina pectoris in the extremities, where there is a deficiency of the blood flow to the limb muscles during exercise. The term 'claudication' comes from the Latin 'claudicare', meaning 'lame' or 'limping' and was associated with the Emperor Claudius who walked with a limp. Intermittent claudication is the commonest symptom of vascular disease and is classified as the second stage of *Fontaine's classification* of signs and symptoms of peripheral arterial occlusive disease (Table 9.1).

Patients complain of aching, cramping, or tiredness of the leg muscles that is brought about by exercise and relieved by resting for a few minutes. Depending on the level of disease, the patient may experience pain in the lower back, buttocks, thigh, calf or foot. Calf claudication is most common and occurs when the superficial femoral artery is diseased. In aortoiliac disease, the patient is more likely to have lower back, hip, buttock or thigh claudication and may also complain of impotence.

Patients usually experience a gradual onset of symptoms with claudication beginning in one leg, which gradually worsens over a period of months or years. As the iliac or femoral arteries become more narrowed, the patient may notice a sudden deterioration in their pain-free walking distance, which worsens further when walking up hills or stairs. Many patients will find improvement in their symptoms over the following months as the collateral vessels develop and symptoms can sometimes completely disappear (Housley, 1992).

The extremity of the affected limb may be pale, with cyanosis and dependent rubor, and may feel cooler than the other limb. Depending on location of the disease, the femoral, popliteal, and pedal pulses may be reduced or absent on palpation. Aortic, iliac or femoral bruits may be present in aortoiliac disease.

Table 9.1 Fontaine's classification of peripheral arterial occlusive disease

Stage 1	Asymptomatic
Stage 2	Intermittent claudication
Stage 3	Rest pain
Stage 4	Development of ulceration and/or gangrene

Patients with intermittent claudication usually have no symptoms at rest although they may eventually experience increased frequency of night cramps as the disease worsens (Coffman, 1996). Development of pain at rest would indicate more severe disease when the blood supply to the limb is compromised to an extent that the skin's nutritional requirements are not being met. Rest pain occurs in the foot at night, or when the patient is resting in a chair, and may be relieved by keeping the foot down or hanging the foot over the edge of the bed.

Assessment of the patient with intermittent claudication

It is important to establish at the initial baseline and follow-up assessments how far the patient is able to walk before claudicating, as a decrease in distance usually indicates progression of the disease. However, patients are often unable to accurately report their pain-free walking distance and whilst objective measures using a fixed-speed treadmill are used, as discussed in Chapter 4, patients can often walk substantially further at their own speed using a corridor walking test (Watson et al., 1997). Many centres find treadmill testing impractical and although there appear to be variations in assessment of walking distance, Watson et al. (1997) suggest that assessment of the patient's lifestyle handicap rather than their walking disability, is fundamental to their management and treatment.

Other investigations also discussed in Chapter 4 should include a baseline Doppler assessment of the ankle brachial pressure index (ABPI). Depending on the severity of arterial occlusion there may be a significant reduction in ABPI to less than 0.8. A change in the pressure index of greater than 0.15 indicates improvement or deterioration of the vascular disease (Coffman, 1996). In some patients, the ABPI at rest may be normal; therefore a pre- and post-exercise pressure should be performed to demonstrate an abnormality (Chapter 4). Colour flow duplex scan or more invasive investigations may be indicated in patients with more severe claudication or lifestyle handicap.

Hip or lumbar spine X-rays may be required to distinguish vascular from non-vascular causes of leg pain such as arthritis of the hips and knees, or compression or ischaemia of the lower spinal cord during exercise.

Conservative management of the claudicant patient

Conservative treatment should be the primary treatment for intermittent claudication (Whyman et al., 1996). Patients with mild to moderate symptoms are generally treated conservatively. However, variations in initial management remain substantial within the UK (Whyman, 1998). Although bypass surgery is successful in up to 90% of claudicant patients (De Vries and Hunink, 1997), it is not without risk as the graft may become infected, or blocked by thrombus, putting the patient in a limb-threatening situation which would probably never have occurred without surgery. In addition, the coexistence of cardiac and cerebrovascular disease in many claudicant patients increases the risk of perioperative morbidity and mortality. Reconstructive surgery is therefore more commonly reserved for patients who develop critical leg ischaemia whose lesions are not amenable to less invasive radiological intervention.

The majority of claudicant patients will require only outpatient care and many can be discharged safely from the vascular clinic if their condition is stable. Those with more severe disease will need to be seen in the vascular outpatient clinics every 3–6 months to assess progression of their condition. Some vascular centres have developed nurse-led conservative management clinics for claudicant patients which provide ongoing monitoring of their condition, as well as improved continuity of care (Murray, 1997). Patients will also be seen by general practice nurses for annual health checks.

The main goal of conservative management in claudicant patients should focus on intensive control of cardiovascular risk factors where possible, and relief of symptoms and resultant disability, thus returning the patient to normal functional status. For many patients this will involve addressing lifestyle issues and changing lifetime habits. Nurses in both community and acute settings need to develop a therapeutic relationship to help patients adjust. The natural history of intermittent claudication has shown that significant deterioration in symptoms occurs in 25–35% of patients over 3–5 years with 1–2% of patients requiring amputation (Bloor, 1961; Dormandy and Murray, 1991; Dormandy et al., 1999). Many claudicant patients will express their fears of limb loss and will need reassurance that only a small proportion of claudicants will develop critical leg ischaemia or undergo amputation

(Housley, 1992; Coffman, 1996). The nurse can address this problem by promoting discussion, openness, and understanding which will help the patient to verbalise any fears and anxieties. Assessing patients' understanding of their condition and explaining the disease process to them will help to accommodate patient participation in their management plan.

Conservative nursing management will involve prioritising and setting realistic goals, and developing an action plan which should provide the catalyst to encourage patients to make change. Patients may benefit by keeping a record card of their personal goals, recording their walking distance achievements, as well as other agreed targets in smoking cessation, or weight reduction. Patients will be more motivated to continue their exercise programme and not to resume smoking, when they feel the positive effect on their overall fitness and self-image. An outline for a conservative nursing management programme for patients with intermittent claudication can be seen in Table 9.2. The reader should refer to Chapter 3 for details of risk factors and health promotion strategies.

Table 9.2 Conservative nursing management programme for patients with intermittent claudication

Assess the patient's understanding of their condition and its treatment – provide verbal and written information to allow patient to make informed choices

Help develop a therapeutic relationship by:

- allowing the patient to express their fears/anxieties by promoting openness, discussion, and understanding.
- allowing the patient greater control and choices in decision making.

Agree realistic goals for reduction of identified risk factors as follows:

Smoking
Educate patient on the effects of nicotine and carbon monoxide.
Give advice on use of nicotine patches, sprays or chewing gum.
Refer to smoking cessation support group.

Hyperlipidaemia
Provide information on reducing dietary fat intake and refer to dietician if necessary.
Advise patient on advisable alcohol intake to prevent elevated triglyceride levels.
Refer patient to general practitioner for lipid lowering drugs if required.

(contd)

Table 9.2 (contd)

Diabetes mellitus
Discuss the importance of good glycaemic control and refer to dietician and diabetic specialist nurse if necessary.
Ensure footwear is appropriate and give foot care advice to both diabetic and non-diabetic claudicants stressing importance of avoiding trauma. Refer patient to hospital or community chiropodist if required.

Hypertension
Refer patient to general practitioner, or blood pressure clinic if required.
Educate patient regarding medication compliance and stress reduction.

Obesity
Give dietary advice advising patient that weight loss may help to increase pain-free walking distance and refer to dietician if required.

Antiplatelet therapy
Discuss the importance of taking aspirin or other antiplatelet therapy to reduce the risk of coronary or cerebrovascular events.

Exercise programme
Refer patient to a supervised hospital, or home-based exercise programme as appropriate.
Educate patient regarding the benefits of undertaking regular walking exercise 5 times per week, or indoor exercise during bad weather, e.g. using an exercise bike or treadmill.
Advise the patient to walk more slowly which may help increase their pain-free distance and to rest at onset of intolerable pain, continuing when it subsides.

Avoiding extreme temperatures
Inform patient that pain may be worse in cold weather and to wear warm clothing.
Discourage the use of hot water bottles and sitting too close to fires or radiators.
Discourage the patient from bathing in hot baths and from soaking feet in water for long periods.

Claudicant exercise programme

Exercise therapy in intermittent claudication is widely recognised as an effective treatment alternative to invasive intervention for many patients (Regensteiner and Hiatt, 1994). Larsen and Lassen (1966) revealed a three-fold increase in walking distances over a one-year period in their controlled study, and Ericsson et al. (1970) found exercise groups were able to double their walking distance, with more recent trials continuing to support this evidence (Hiatt et al., 1990, Regensteiner et al., 1997a). Exercise is not only beneficial in helping to

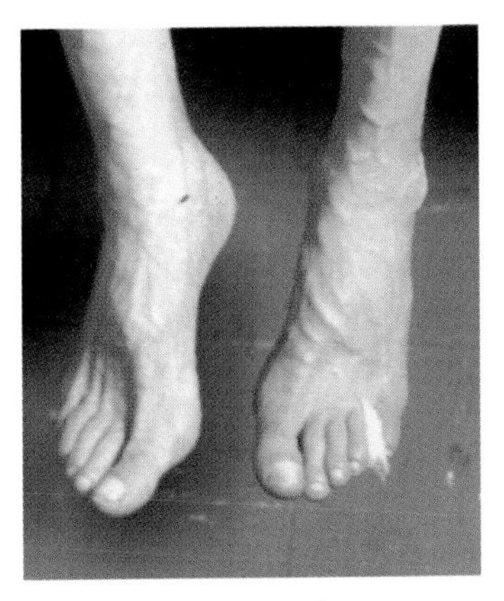

Plate 1 Dependent rubor.

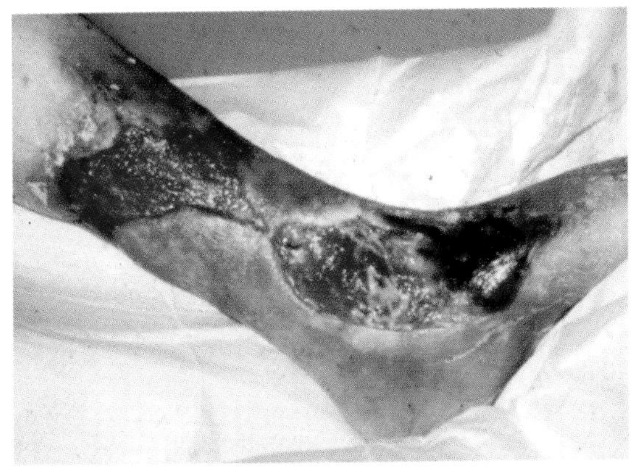

Plate 2 Pressure ulceration caused by compression bandaging. (Courtesy of M Bliss.).

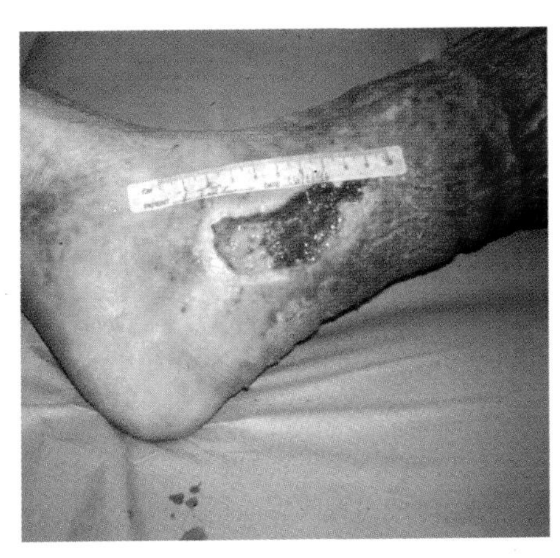

Plate 3 Classic skin changes in a patient with a venous ulcer.

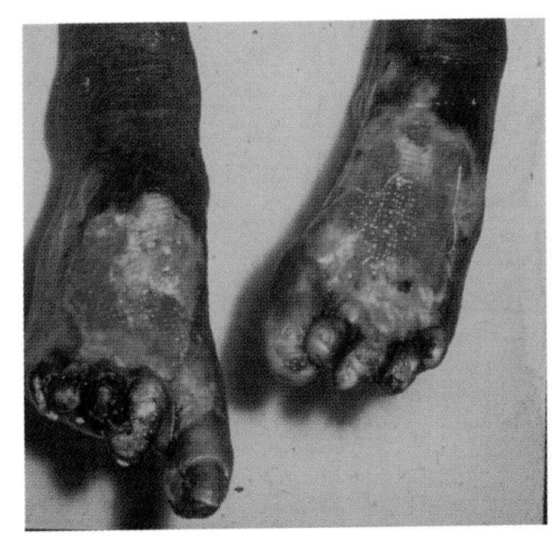

Plate 4 Ulceration due to severe peripheral vascular disease.

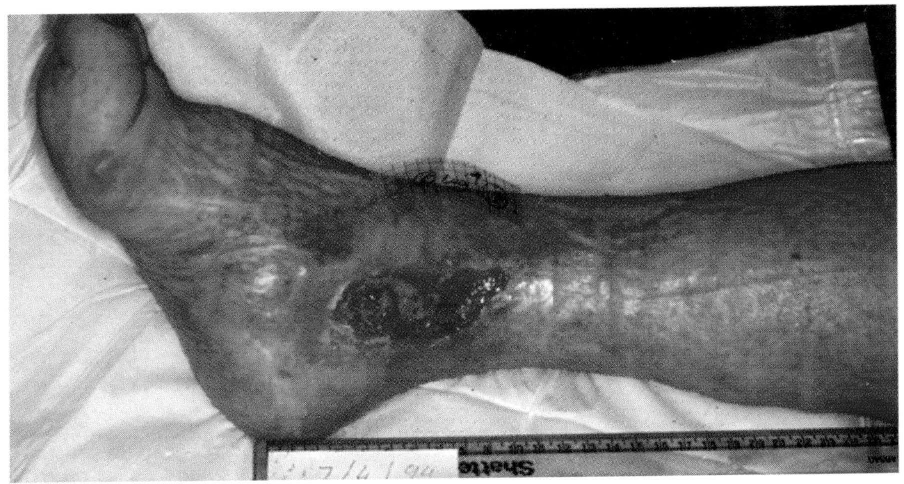

Plate 5 Foot deformity leading to reduced healing in a venous ulcer patient.

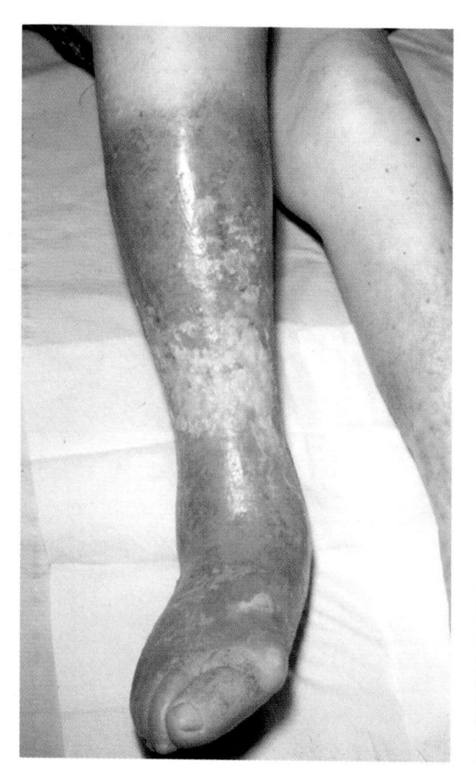

Plate 6 Acute parabens-induced contact dermatitis.

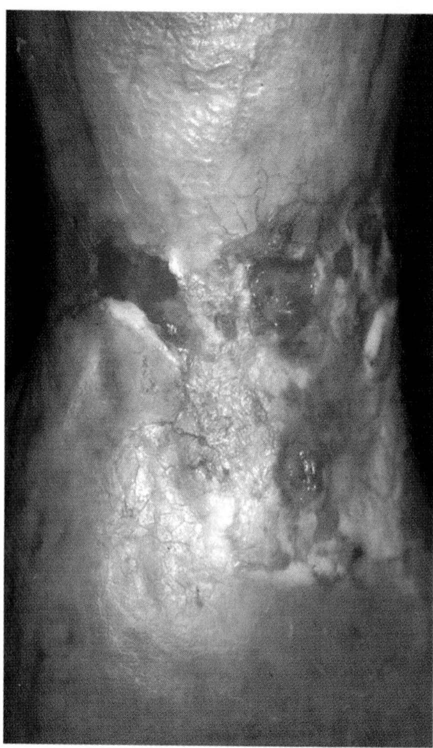

Plate 7 Development of a squamous cell carcinoma (Marjolin's ulcer) in an existing venous ulcer.

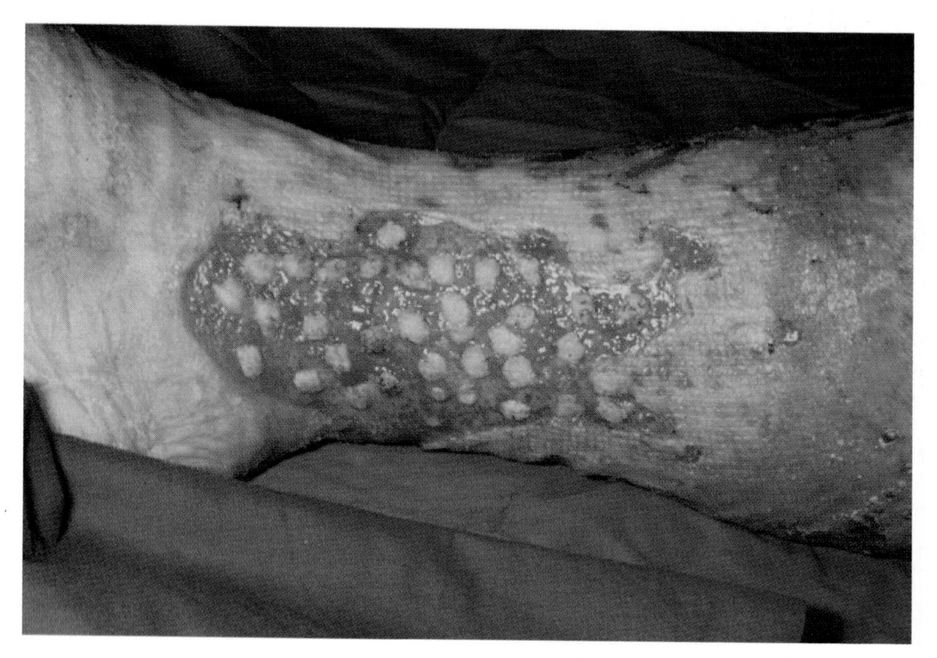

Plate 8 Pinch grafts applied to a venous ulcer.

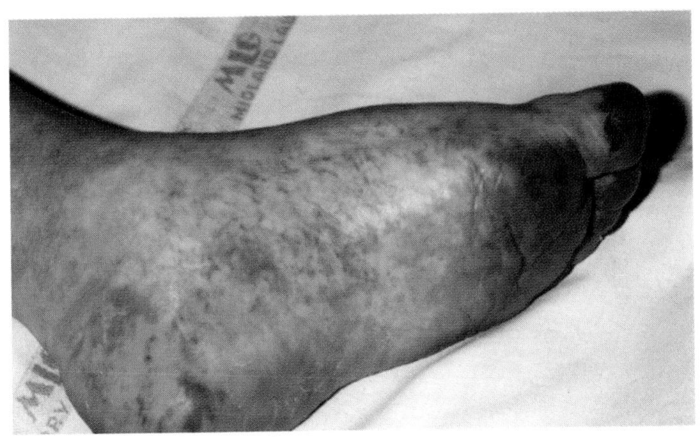

Plate 9 Chronic ischaemia, left foot.

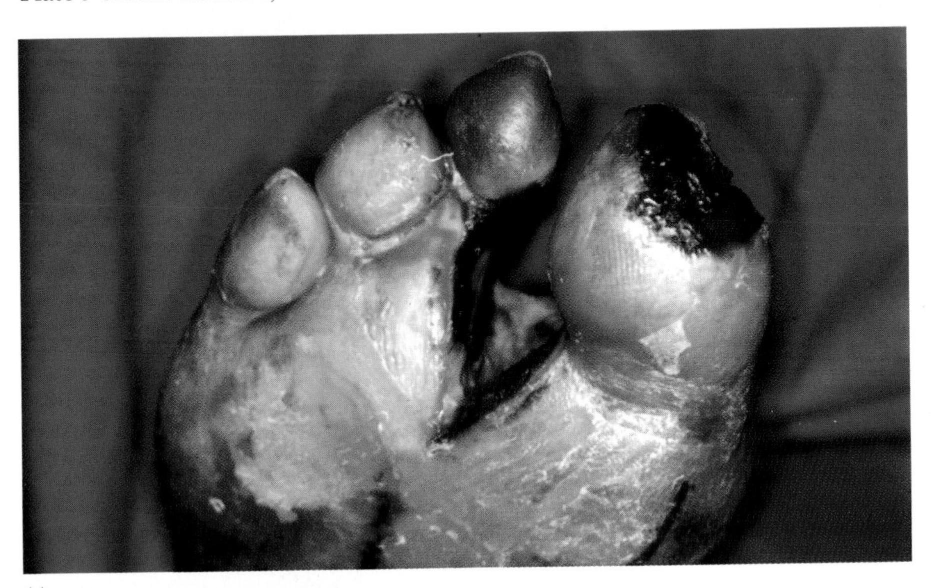

(a)

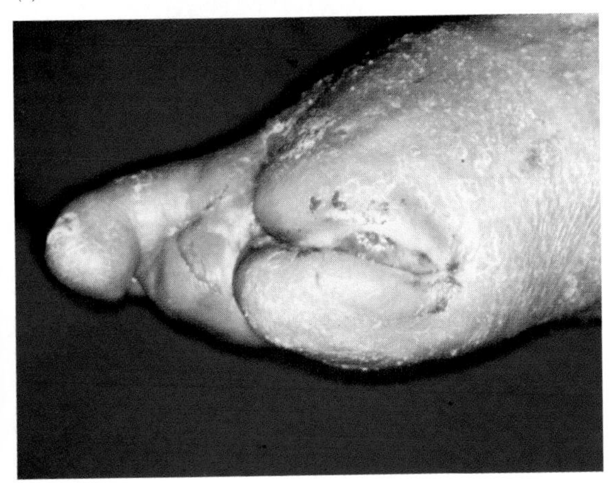

(b)

Plate 10 (a) Foot prior to distal venous arterialisation. (b) Healing foot following distal venous arterialisation. Courtesy of Mr R.S. Taylor, St George's Hospital, London.

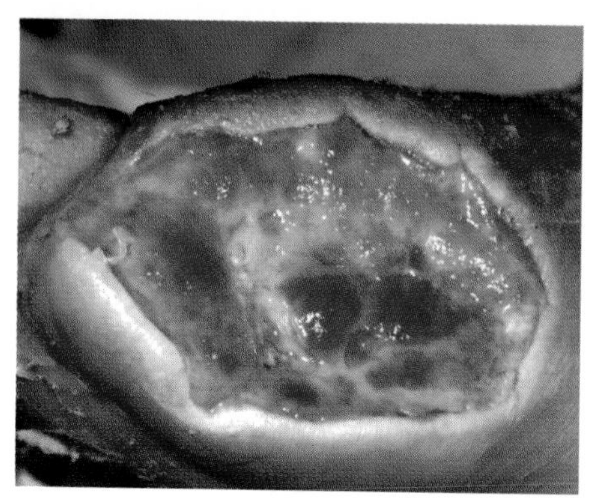

Plate 11 Slough and fibrin in a wound.

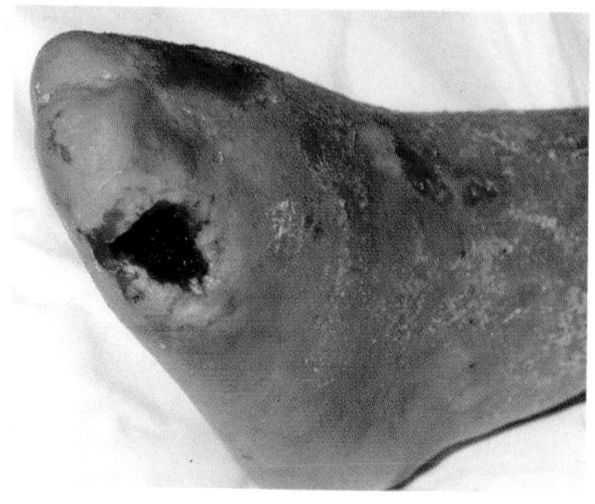

Plate 12 Haematoma in the base of a wound.

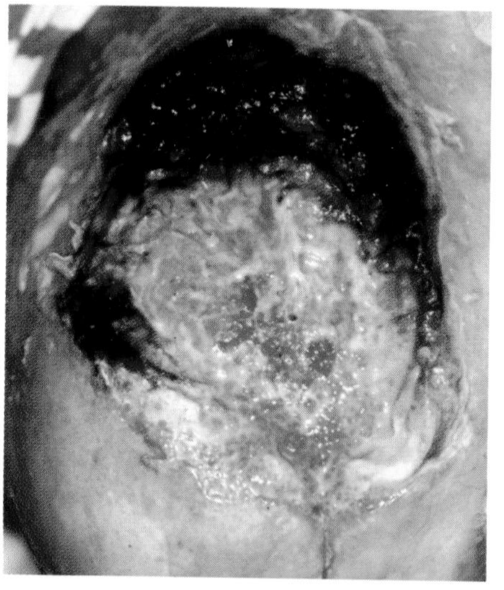

Plate 13 Necrotic tissue in stump wound to which larvae are to be applied.

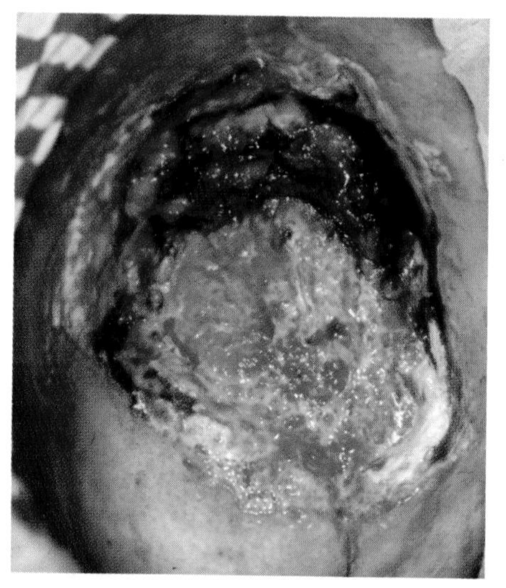

Plate 14 Necrotic tissue in stump wound reduced following application of larvae.

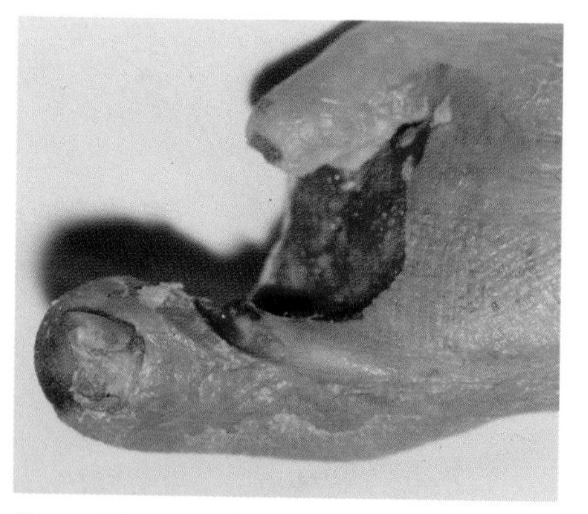

Plate 15 Amputation stump wound with fragile surrounding tissue.

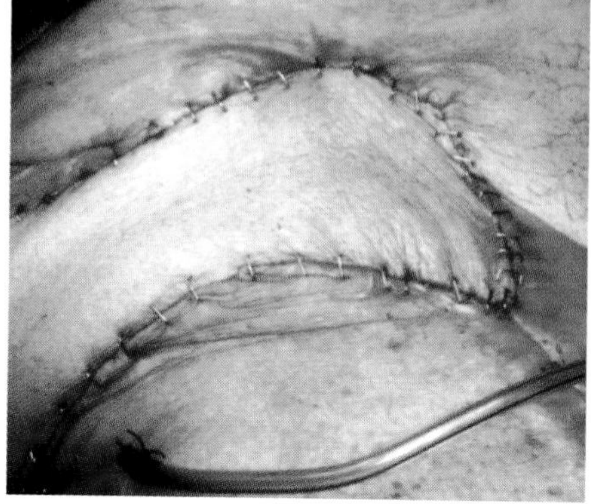

Plate 16 Myocutaneous flap to reconstruct a groin wound post-bypass.

develop collateral blood vessels (Figure 9.2), thereby reducing muscle pain, but will also help improve patients' general wellbeing and self-esteem, and allows them to return to a more active lifestyle.

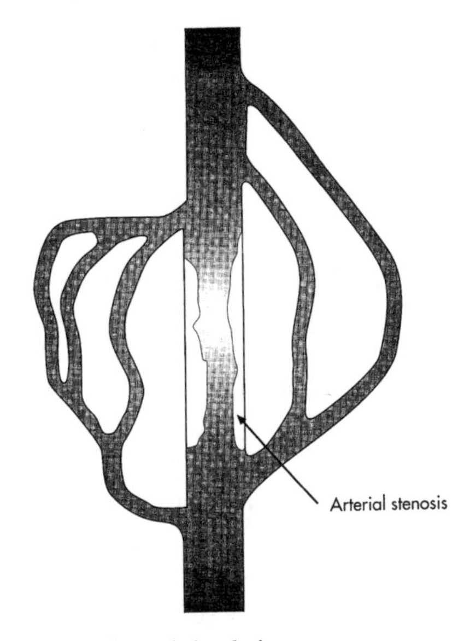

Figure 9.2 Development of collateral circulation.

Patients whose walking pain interferes with their work or daily activities should be considered for exercise programmes. It is not recommended to include patients with rest pain, or ischaemic ulceration. Patients with cardiopulmonary disease will need careful screening as patients with uncontrolled hypertension, symptoms of heart failure, or arrhythmias, will need stabilising before commencing an exercise programme. Many patients will also have coexisting diabetes or angina, although this should not exclude them from exercising unless their angina is unstable.

Depending on resources available in vascular centres, exercise programmes can be either unsupervised home-based programmes, or supervised hospital-based structured programmes (Patterson et al., 1997; Regensteiner et al., 1997b). Objective pre- and post-exercise programme treadmill tests can be performed to measure patients' walking distance and to assess progress, or patients can be asked to record their progress on a record card. The practitioner should be aware that although treadmill testing is useful in assessing progress following exercise programmes, it may bear little relation to a patient's subjective estimate of their normal walking routine as many report walking further on a treadmill. Providing handrail support during treadmill assessment of claudication distance can increase pain-free walking distance, thus reducing the reliability of the test (Gardner et al., 1991). Differences in a patient's walking speed, nature of terrain, surrounding temperature, footwear and psychological factors may also contribute to the inaccuracy of treadmill claudication (Watson et al., 1997).

Home-based programmes typically involve patients being taught simple warm-up exercises followed by dynamic calf exercises involving heel raising, step-ups, and sit-ups, as shown in Figure 9.3. Patients are advised to undertake each exercise for as long as they can tolerate the leg pain, rest until the pain disappears, and then commence the next exercise. They are encouraged to undertake these exercises at least five times weekly for 30–60 minutes, as well as other forms of exercise tailored to the patient's capabilities and fitness. With unsupervised programmes it is important to follow up the patients regularly to provide encouragement and support for them to continue exercising. Many types of exercise can be undertaken but this should be in the upright position such as walking, running, stair climbing, cycling or dancing (Coffman, 1996). Although any of these exercises will improve a patient's aerobic capacity, treadmill walking is more effective in improving exercise performance and pain-free distances in claudicants (Hiatt et al., 1994).

Supervised hospital-based exercise programmes are known to provide superior increased walking ability (Patterson et al., 1997) but require greater resources and may be inconvenient for patients who work, or need to travel long distances, to attend two to three times weekly. The positive benefits of this type of programme are that patients with intermittent claudication may be socially isolated and will undoubtedly benefit from building supportive relationships with other claudicant patients. Programmes can include general physical reconditioning, dynamic calf exercises, and treadmill training, which can be accompanied by music. The programme ideally should incorporate a multidisciplinary approach involving informal health promotion and basic anatomy sessions from specialist nurses, smoking cessation counsellors, dieticians, physiotherapists, chiropodists and stress counsellors. Hospital-based programmes vary in duration from 6 to 12 weeks and patients need to understand that the sessions are only the building blocks to the goal of undertaking regular exercise at home.

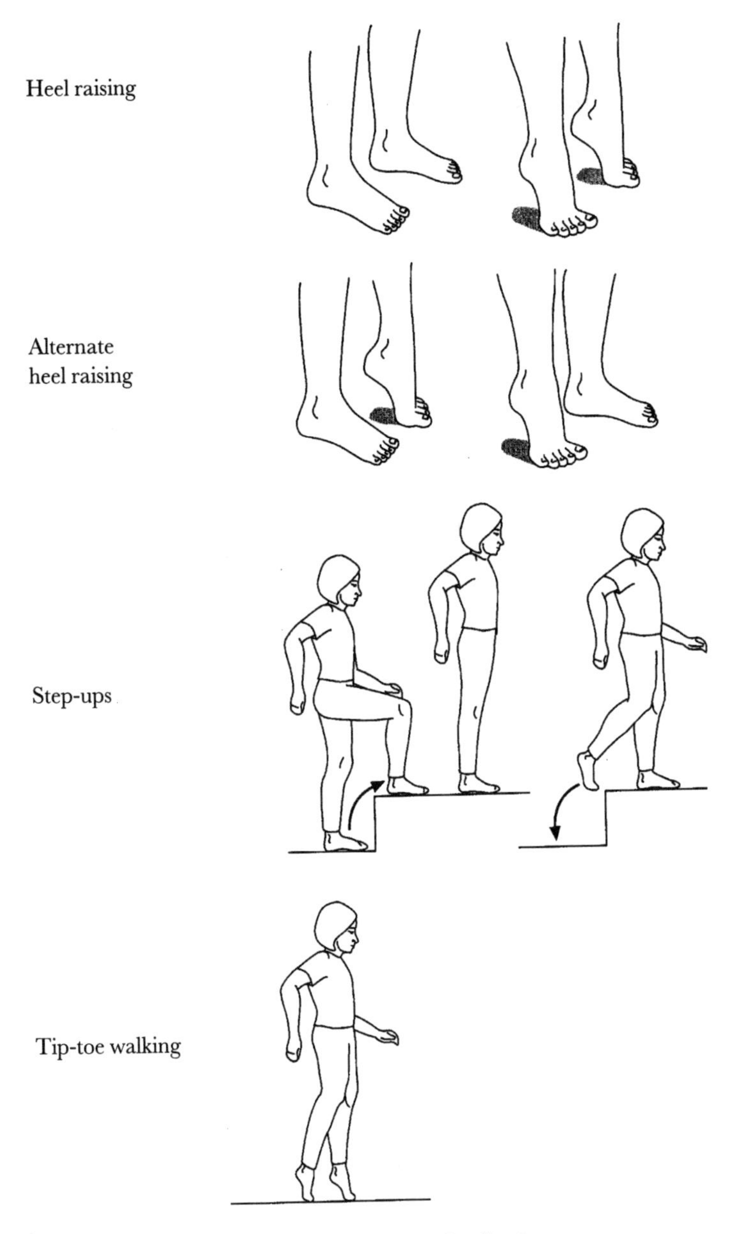

Figure 9.3 Dynamic calf exercises for intermittent claudication.

With regular exercise, patients should experience an increase in their pain-free and maximum walking distance after 3 months (Coffman, 1996).

Drug therapy for claudication

Drug therapy in patients with intermittent claudication may be given to improve walking distance or slow down the progression of atherosclerotic lesions. A number of drugs have been studied to assist in treating claudicants such as vasodilators, calcium channel blockers, prostaglandins and their analogues, anticoagulants, and antiplatelet drugs.

Vasodilators have been used in the treatment of intermittent claudication with little success. The distal arterial bed is dependent on collateral vessels which offer a high resistance to blood flow. During exercise, the distal blood pressure is further reduced and blood flow may stop completely due to muscle contraction of the small arteries. No vasodilators have so far been developed that have the ability to dilate collateral vessels (Coffman, 1996). Naftidrofuryl has a vasodilatory effect and has been shown to be of some benefit in patients who claudicate at more than 150 metres (Lehert et al., 1990). Oxpentifylline, which increases blood flow by lowering blood viscosity, has been shown to increase treadmill walking distance. However, patients did not report any subjective improvement in their walking ability (Porter et al., 1982).

Antiplatelet drugs are commonly used in patients with peripheral arterial disease. Although they have little effect on pain-free walking distance, they appear to reduce the risk of coronary or cerebrovascular events (Antiplatelet Triallists Collaboration, 1994). Low-dose aspirin is the drug of choice although dipyridamole can be used as an alternative if the patient is unable to tolerate aspirin, or has a history of peptic ulceration. Plavix is a new antiplatelet drug which has been shown to be slightly superior to aspirin (Caprie Steering Committee, 1996).

Prostaglandin (PGE1), which has a potent vasodilatory effect and inhibits platelet aggregation, has been used intravenously for critical leg ischaemia. However, an effective oral substitute has not been developed. Recent preliminary studies of a chemically modified PGE1 using daily bolus injections found significant improvements in the maximum walking distance of patients with intermittent claudication (Belch et al., 1997).

Lipid lowering drugs, such as simvastatin, are often prescribed for patients with intermittent claudication to reduce hyperlipidaemia, which is a major risk factor for peripheral arterial disease. Claudicant patients who have raised lipid levels are at high risk of myocardial infarction and should therefore be prescribed lipid lowering agents (Fowkes, 1996). Although there is an association with stabilisation or regression of femoral artery disease, lipid lowering drugs have no effect on pain-free walking distance (Duffield et al., 1983).

Percutaneous transluminal angioplasty (PTA)

Further investigation and treatment is required for patients with intermittent claudication when their symptoms severely limit their lifestyle, or ability to work, or if signs of critical leg ischaemia such as rest pain and/or ulceration occur.

There are now several percutaneous endovascular interventional techniques available in the treatment of peripheral arterial occlusion. Percutaneous transluminal angioplasty (PTA) is the most commonly practised procedure and the first choice of treatment for patients severely handicapped by claudication (Belli and Buckenham, 1996). Dotter and Judkins (1964) first described dilatation of arterial stenosis, although it was not until 1974, when Gruntzig reported the use of a double lumen balloon catheter, that the technique became widely adopted as a less invasive treatment. Angioplasty has a greater success rate in short, localised stenosis in patients with good run-off vessels in the calf than in those with longer diseased segments and poor run-off (Belli and Buckenham, 1996). However, the use of angioplasty in intermittent claudication remains controversial (Coffman, 1991; Creasy and Fletcher, 1991), with long-term outcomes similar to patients undertaking exercise programmes only (Perkins et al., 1995). Indications for undertaking angioplasty in claudicants can be seen in Table 9.3.

Technique for angioplasty

Balloon dilatation of the artery is performed under local anaesthetic. Access into the artery can be from a variety of sites; the common femoral artery via a groin puncture is the usual site of entry. Other sites of access include the popliteal, axillary and brachial arteries. A guidewire is inserted into the arterial lumen and passed across the stenosis/occlusion. A balloon catheter is then passed over the wire with the balloon placed across the diseased segment (Figure 9.4). The balloon is inflated with the dilute contrast for several seconds at varying

Table 9.3 Indications for lower limb angioplasty

Patients with intermittent claudication at 200 metres or less, or claudication that limits lifestyle, which has not improved on conservative therapy
Rest pain
Ulceration or gangrene
Blue toe syndrome
A significant stenosis threatening the patency of a bypass graft

Source: Belli and Buckenham (1996).

pressures depending upon the site of the lesion. An angioplasty can be performed when the diagnostic arteriogram is performed if a skilled radiologist is present. Laser-assisted angioplasty techniques using laser probes have been developed during the last decade which enable long occlusions to be crossed. However, long length angioplasties have a high re-occlusion rate and this technique has largely been abandoned (Belli et al., 1992). The long-term success rate of angioplasty depends on the length and position of the stenosis, operator experience, catheter

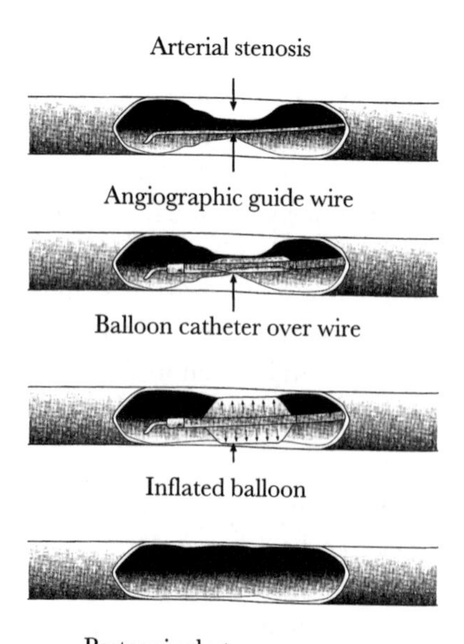

Figure 9.4 Percutaneous angioplasty of arterial stenosis.

technology and patient compliance with a healthy lifestyle. Johnston et al. (1987), reported 5-year patency rates of 60–70% for iliac vessel disease, and 40–70% for femoral lesions.

Intraluminal stents

Expandable intraluminal stents, which are usually made from a meshed metal material, can also be sited in the vessel lumen at the angioplasty site. Stents help maintain vessel patency by acting as a scaffold to prevent the artery from collapsing (Figure 9.5). Stents are usually reserved to treat complications of angioplasty, recurrent disease, and occlusions where stenting will prevent embolisation of the distal vessels (Belli, 1996). There is some evidence that patency rates are improved in the iliac arteries if stents are inserted at the initial angioplasty (Vorwerk et al., 1995).

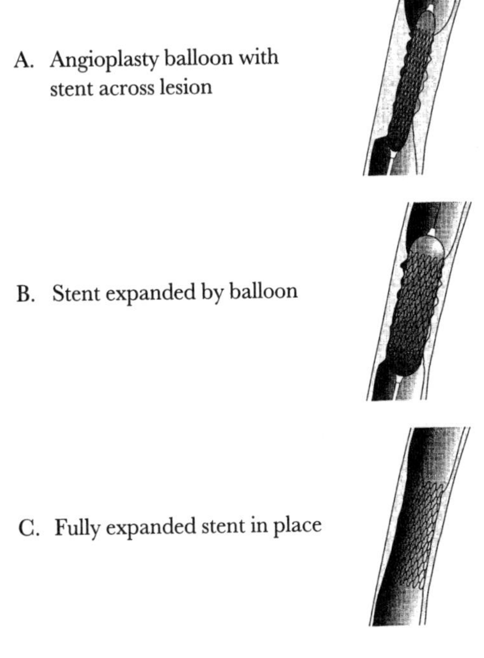

Figure 9.5 Balloon expandable mesh stent.

Complications following angioplasty

Despite advances in radiological technique, complications will inevitably arise. These may occur at the puncture, or angioplasty sites, either during or following the procedure and may include the following:

- haematoma formation and haemorrhage
- thrombosis or occlusion
- distal vessel embolisation
- perforation or rupture of the vessel wall
- false aneurysm
- cerebrovascular accident
- infection at the puncture site
- renal failure due to contrast medium
- arteriovenous fistula

Patient preparation for angioplasty

- Nursing care and preparation is similar to that provided prior to angiography as discussed in Chapter 4, except that the patient will need to fast for 2–3 hours prior to the procedure as emergency surgery may be required should complications arise.
- During angioplasty and stent insertion, the patient will be required to lie still for a long period of time and will require pressure-relieving aids to prevent skin breakdown, especially to the heels.
- Due to the increased risk of complications, the patient should be cannulated prior to the procedure with a large intravenous cannula (e.g. 16 or 17G Venflon).
- Prophylactic intravenous antibiotic cover will be required for patients who have artificial bypass grafts or stents in situ, or those undergoing stent insertion.
- Patients with, or at risk of, renal impairment will require intravenous fluids for 12–24 hours to maintain hydration, commencing prior to the procedure.

Care following angioplasty

- Nursing care is similar to that following angiography as described in Chapter 4. However, there is an increased risk of complications arising and the patient will require careful monitoring.

- Signs of haemorrhage, haematoma formation, or thrombosis, should be reported immediately.
- Limb perfusion should be monitored hourly and pedal pulses located using a handheld Doppler. Pressure relief for heels will be required during the bedrest period.
- Aspirin antiplatelet therapy should be prescribed unless contraindicated.
- Health promotion advice should be reinforced before the patient is discharged and the patient should be referred to smoking cessation groups if required. Exercise should be encouraged to help develop collateral circulation. Diabetics must ensure their diabetes is kept well controlled.

Atherectomy

Atherectomy is another endovascular procedure performed using a catheter-mounted device which rotates and cuts away atheroma from the vessel wall (Figure 9.6). A positioning balloon helps to push the cutting device against the atheroma and the cutter then shaves off the atheromatous plaque widening the vessel lumen. Particles of removed plaque are collected in a chamber to prevent migrating particles causing further occlusions. As only small lesions can be treated at present, atherectomy is most useful for treating anastomotic lesions in stenosed bypass grafts.

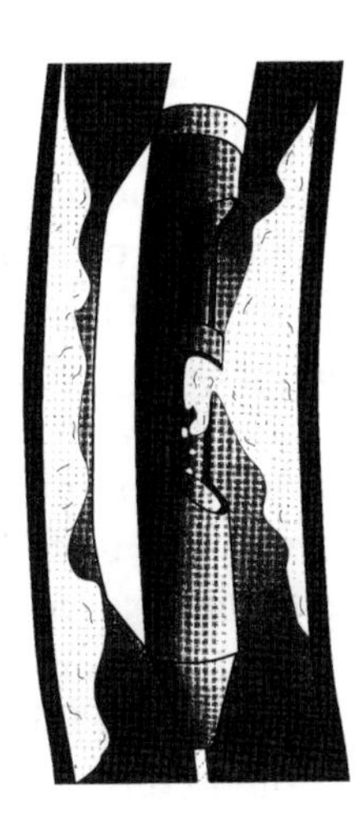

Figure 9.6 Atherectomy cutting device removing atheroma from artery wall.

Diabetic peripheral vascular disease

Vascular disease is a leading cause of morbidity and mortality in diabetics due to the extensive and more rapid progression of atherosclerosis than in non-diabetics (Jaap and Tooke, 1996). More than one-fifth of diabetics will die within 2 years of being diagnosed with peripheral vascular disease, which is five times the rate of non-diabetics, and amputation rates in diabetics are estimated to be 15 times higher (Most and Sinnock, 1983; Coffman, 1986).

Diabetics can be affected at a younger age, and may develop signs of critical leg ischaemia such as rest pain or ulceration, without ever having experienced earlier symptoms of intermittent claudication. It is still unclear whether this is due to coexisting peripheral neuropathy, or to the location of the diseased vessels, which tends to differ in patients with diabetes mellitus from non-diabetics with peripheral vascular disease (Coffman, 1996). As seen in Figure 9.1, there is known to be more involvement of the tibial and peroneal arteries between the knees and ankles in diabetics, than of the larger aortic and iliac vessels. However, diabetics and non-diabetics have similar involvement of the femoral vessels in the thigh (Conrad, 1967).

Care of the patient with diabetic peripheral vascular disease

Conservative management and care of the diabetic patient presenting with early signs and symptoms of intermittent claudication is similar to the non-diabetic patient, as discussed earlier in this chapter. Lifestyle issues and health promotion as discussed in Chapter 3, particularly in relation to control of diabetes and foot care, need to be addressed in order to prevent the onset of foot complications. These occur due to a combination of ischaemia and neuropathy, which frequently predispose to infection and tissue necrosis. Smoking must be strongly discouraged as this will further accelerate atherosclerosis in diabetics.

The introduction of specialist community and hospital based diabetic foot clinics may prevent up to 50% of diabetic foot ulcers (Edmonds et al., 1986). A collaborative approach to care of the diabetic patient with chronic ischaemia requires the combined skills of a number of healthcare professionals (Figure 9.7).

Nursing management should consider other factors thought to identify diabetics as being at high risk of developing foot complications,

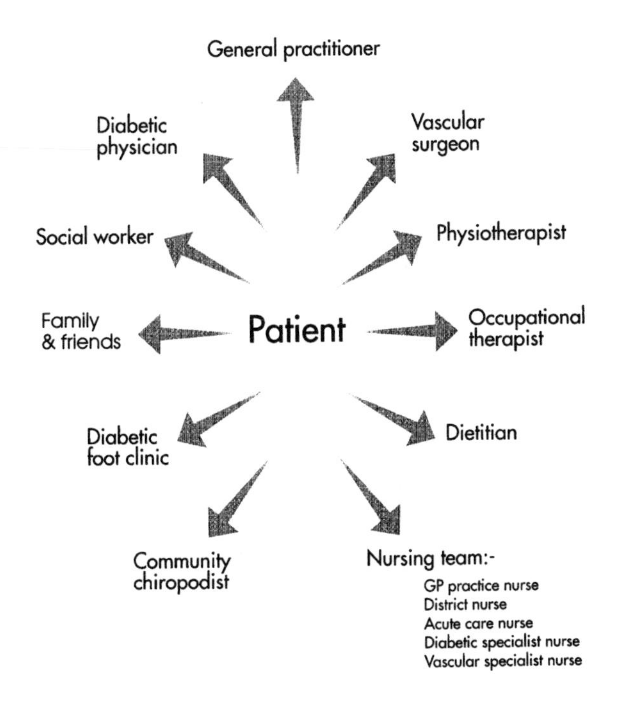

Figure 9.7 Services and support available to the diabetic patient with chronic ischaemia.

such as social isolation, low socio-economic status, and poor eyesight. An elderly diabetic patient presenting with peripheral vascular disease may be unable to comply with foot care advice, such as daily foot inspections, due to poor eyesight and joint mobility; therefore involving a family member or carer in education may be more appropriate.

The need for intervention in diabetics is the same as in non-diabetic patients with peripheral vascular disease. Radiological or surgical intervention would be considered in severe claudication or the onset of critical leg ischaemia. However, the extent and distal location of large vessel disease may render the diabetic patient unsuitable for angioplasty or reconstructive bypass surgery (Jaap and Tooke, 1996).

Vasculitis

The term *vasculitis* is defined as an inflammation of the blood vessel walls commonly associated with occlusive and necrotic conditions and can apply to various conditions already discussed in Chapter 2.

Buerger's disease (thromboangiitis obliterans)

Buerger's disease is a chronic inflammatory condition affecting the small and medium-sized arteries of the arms and legs which may often result in ulceration and gangrene. The inflammatory process also affects the nearby veins, resulting in superficial thrombophlebitis (Buerger, 1908).

Horton (1938) considered the disease to be almost exclusively confined to the 20–40-year-old male smoker. Although there is still a male predominance, the incidence of Buerger's disease in women has increased as more women smoke (Lie, 1987).

The exact cause is unknown, although there is a clear link with cigarette smoking as approximately 95% of patients suffering from Buerger's disease are heavy smokers (Hill, 1974; Mills et al., 1987). Current opinion considers Buerger's to be a distinct peripheral vascular disease and not a variant of atherosclerosis (Fiessinger, 1996).

Clinical presentation and diagnosis

The commonest symptoms of Buerger's disease are cyanosis, coldness and paraesthesia of the limbs. The patient may experience severe localised foot claudication and a squeezing pain on the sole of the foot which rapidly progresses to severe ischaemic rest pain, ulceration, gangrene and tissue loss. Ischaemic symptoms clearly manifest themselves in the distal region of the upper and lower limbs and digital ulceration and gangrene may be present. A patient may present with symptoms involving two or more limbs. Examination will reveal cold and hypersensitive fingers and toes with reactive hyperaemia when the limb is in the dependent position. This may also be accompanied by inflamed, raised lesions in upper and lower limbs if superficial thrombophlebitis is present.

Establishing an early diagnosis is vital to the patient's future although confirmation is often complex (Table 9.4).

Table 9.4 Diagnostic criteria for Buerger's disease

Mostly male
Age of onset <50 years
History of heavy smoking
Frequent upper limb involvement
Frequent thrombophlebitis migrans
Absence of popliteal entrapment syndrome and classical risk factors for atherosclerosis
Angiography – normal proximal arteries with abrupt distal occlusions only and 'corkscrew' collaterals distally

European Consensus Document on Critical Limb Ischaemia (1989).

Investigations

The aim of investigations is to first exclude other causes of ischaemia such as popliteal entrapment syndrome, emboli, collagen disease, diabetes and hypercoagulability. Investigations may include the following:

- Blood screening for full blood count, platelets, erythrocyte sedimentation rate (ESR), glucose, rheumatoid factor, serum complement, and antinuclear factor (ANF).
- Angiography – this will often confirm the classic pattern of 'corkscrewing' and multiple abrupt occlusions of the distal collateral vessels (Figure 9.8).
- Allen test – this determines the patency of the radial and ulnar arteries.
- Ankle systolic pressures – these may often be normal if the occlusions are below the popliteal arteries.
- Toe systolic pressures – these are more reliable in confirming the existence of critical leg ischaemia.
- Biopsy of superficial thrombophlebitic lesion.

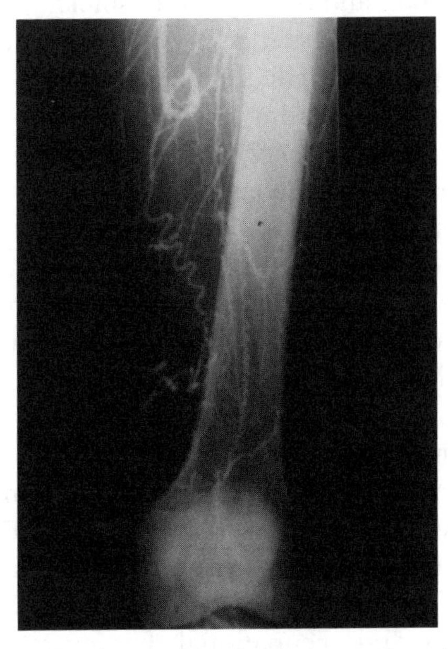

Figure 9.8 Angiogram showing classic corkscrew-type collateral vessels in a patient with Buerger's disease. (Courtesy of Professor J.A. Dormandy, St George's Hospital, London.)

Nursing care and conservative management

The progressive course of Buerger's disease is characterised by acute exacerbations and long remission periods. Central to all nursing care is the emphasis on the whole patient, not just the symptoms of the disease. Buerger's disease will also have an adverse effect on the patient's family, particularly when the patient is young and suddenly faced with major lifestyle changes and possible limb loss. Gibson and Kenrick (1998) found that vascular patients experienced a feeling of powerlessness from the direct effects of their disease; therefore nurses need to develop a therapeutic relationship with the patient and their family by acknowledging the distress they are suffering, and assisting them to draw upon positive coping mechanisms. In both acute and community settings, the patient and their relatives will require a great deal of psychological and practical support, as well as education regarding the management of their condition.

The following are important aspects of management and care:

- Stopping smoking is the primary feature of conservative management as cessation and resumption of smoking relates to disease remission and exacerbation, respectively, and is a major factor in determining prognosis (Hill, 1974; Mills et al., 1987). Despite the devastating and mutilating consequences of the disease, the patient may experience great difficulty in quitting and will require expert and continuous counselling and access to smoking cessation support networks.
- Walking exercise should be encouraged during remission periods.
- Any ulcerated gangrenous lesions will need to be managed as discussed in Chapter 7. Antibiotics will be required if there are any clinical signs of cellulitis or ulcer infection.
- Assessment of pressure areas and prevention of sores is essential as discussed in Chapter 5.
- Limbs should be kept warm and protected from trauma as this will help prevent onset of exacerbations (Hill, 1974).
- Pain should be assessed, monitored and evaluated regularly, as discussed in Chapter 8.
- Physiotherapy and occupational therapy referrals should be made at an appropriate stage as patients may require mobility

help improve their quality of life.

assessment, and advice on home alterations, and aids which will help improve their quality of life.

- A social services referral should be made for advice regarding disability, mobility and attendance allowances, or rehousing if required. A young patient in employment will also need advice and support from their employer regarding returning to work or job retraining programmes, to allow them a feeling of self-worth and wellbeing which will help raise their self-esteem.

Drugs

Various medical treatments including steroids, vasodilators, and anticoagulation have been tried with little success in the treatment of Buerger's disease (Fiessinger, 1990). Some preliminary results with prostaglandin therapy are more promising in patients with Buerger's disease than in those with atherosclerosis, and further research is currently being undertaken (Fiessinger and Schaffer, 1990; Dormandy, 1991).

Surgical intervention for Buerger's disease

Surgical sympathectomy may provide short-term pain relief and promote ulcer healing but carries no long-term benefit in preventing amputation (Lau and Cheng, 1997). Controversy still remains as to benefits of bypass surgery in patients with Buerger's disease compared to those performed in patients with atherosclerosis. Graft patency rates are poor as the disease mainly involves the small distal vessels (European Consensus Document on Critical Limb Ischaemia, 1989; Sasajima et al., 1997). Some patients with Buerger's disease will face the possibility of upper or lower limb loss. McPherson et al. (1963) reported a 12.5% incidence of major limb loss over a 10-year period following diagnosis, which is supported in more recent studies (Ohta and Shionoya, 1988; Fiessinger, 1990).

Vasospasm

Acrocyanosis

Acrocyanosis is a vasospastic condition of the small vessels which is difficult to distinguish from Raynaud's phenomenon and is characterised by symmetrical, cold, cyanosed hands and feet with mottled blue/red skin discoloration. Unlike Raynaud's, it is differentiated by the lack of blanching, and is a *constant cyanotic condition.*

Livedo reticularis

This vasospastic condition is characterised by *reddish-blue mottling* of the skin of the lower extremity, which is exacerbated by exposure to cold. It may also be present in the lower limbs and apart from cosmetic appearance the condition causes little disability.

Raynaud's disease or phenomenon

Raynaud's disease or phenomenon is the most frequently encountered vasospastic disorder. The condition was first identified by Maurice Raynaud in 1862 (Raynaud, 1888). The term *Raynaud's disease* has historically been used to imply a benign condition without any evident cause, whilst *Raynaud's phenomenon* may be seen in association with a variety of conditions including atherosclerosis, thoracic outlet syndrome, connective tissue disorders, and vasculitic conditions. Vasospasm may also be induced by hypothyroidism, or drug induced through excessive use of ergot for migraine relief, or from oral contraceptives. In young patients the condition may spontaneously disappear.

The condition can be benign although, if severe, it can cause ulceration and gangrene of the digits. Raynaud's is nine times more common in women than in men, and is prevalent in approximately 10% of the population, although it may affect as many as 20–30% of women in younger age groups (Fitzgerald et al., 1988). There is also a familial predisposition which is more marked if the onset occurs in people under 30 years (Porter et al., 1976).

Raynaud's disease and phenomenon is classically described as episodic, vasospastic ischaemia of the small arteries and arterioles in the most distal part of the extremities in response to cold or emotional stress. The fingers and hands are most commonly affected although the feet and toes may also be involved. It is classically manifested by *pallor* of the affected digits, followed by *cyanosis* and *rubor* due to reactive hyperaemia. Blanching of the fingers and hand occurs when exposed to cold, and the nails may become fissured. Stimuli other than cold can also trigger an attack and include tobacco, hormones, and trauma (Belch, 1996).

Physical examination may be unremarkable in a young female presenting with Raynaud's disease as radial, brachial and axillary pulses are usually unaffected. Diagnosis may be confirmed by exposing the hands to cold until blanching, cyanosis and hyperaemia occurs.

A careful medical history will assist in identifying the aetiology of the phenomenon which can be classified into the following categories:

- *Immunological conditions* – systemic sclerosis, rheumatoid arthritis, cryoglobulinaemia, systemic lupus erythematosus.
- *Obstructive conditions* – atherosclerosis, embolism, vasculitis, e.g. Buerger's disease, and thoracic outlet syndrome (cervical rib).
- *Occupational hazards* – frozen food packers and vibrational pneumatic drill operators.
- *Other* – hypothyroidism, malignancy, drugs, e.g. ergotamine, beta-blockers, oral contraceptives.

Diagnosis of Raynaud's

Differential diagnosis can usually be determined from the clinical history and clinical signs. Investigations may include the following:

- Digital blood flow measurement using plethysmography.
- Digital temperature recovery time.
- Laser Doppler flowmetry.
- Chest X-ray to exclude cervical rib.
- Blood screening for full blood count, platelets, and glucose, to exclude anaemia, thrombocytosis and diabetes.
- Erythrocyte sedimentation rate (ESR) to help detect systemic disease.
- Immunological screening for rheumatoid factor for rheumatoid arthritis, and antinuclear factor (ANF), for systemic lupus erythematosus (SLE).
- Cryoglobulins, macroglobulins and cold globulins – these can coagulate in cool temperatures, and should be checked if other tests are negative.
- Angiography – this may be required if more proximal obstruction is considered, or if symptoms are localised to one hand only.

Management of vasospastic conditions

Management involves determining and addressing any underlying disorder. Raynaud's disease is not curable although there are many palliative and supportive care measures which can be of benefit:

- Patients should be advised to protect their limbs from the cold and to wear warm thermal clothing. Heated gloves and socks with a rechargeable battery are available from an appliance office.
- Smoking must be avoided as this will exacerbate the condition. The patient should be given advice on smoking cessation and referred to a support group if required.
- A change of occupation may be required if this is known to be an associated factor.
- Oral contraception should be stopped if there is a clear link with onset of disease (Belch, 1996).
- Calcium blocking drugs such as slow release nifedipine, or alpha-blockers such as thymoxamine, may benefit the patient by their vasodilatory effect (Belch, 1996). Unfortunately, the unpleasant side effects of vasodilatory drugs such as dizziness, flushing, palpitations, headache, and ankle swelling may require the treatment to be stopped. Administration of nifedipine SR at night will also help the patient to sleep through the vasodilatory side effects. Amlodipine has been found to produce fewer side effects and can be administered by a once daily dose to aid patient compliance (Bremner et al., 1993; La Civita et al., 1993).
- Stress reduction techniques or behavioural treatments using biofeedback training techniques, may be helpful in well-motivated patients whose symptoms are anxiety or stress induced (Freedman et al., 1991).
- Many patients with Raynaud's disease will feel very anxious about their condition and will benefit from self-help support groups such as the Raynaud's Association, Alsager, Cheshire, UK.

Prostaglandin therapy

Prostaglandin therapy (PGE2), has a potent vasodilatory effect and also reduces platelet aggregation. Iloprost, which is a stable analogue of prostaglandin and is currently unlicensed, has been used in the treatment of vasospastic conditions. It has also been used as an adjuvant therapy in distal vessel reconstructive surgery, and in patients with critical leg ischaemia (Dormandy and Loh, 1996).

Iloprost requires intravenous administration as an effective oral equivalent has not been developed (Dormandy and Loh, 1996). Side effects include facial flushing, headache, hypotension, bradycardia, tachycardia, nausea, vomiting, and abdominal pain. The unpleasant vasodilatory side effects, such as headache and flushing, usually pass off quickly when the infusion is completed, although the beneficial effects of iloprost therapy can last for a few weeks or months (Belch, 1996).

During iloprost infusions, the patient's blood pressure and pulse must be carefully monitored half-hourly whilst increasing the dose to the optimum rate tolerated. Infusions are normally administered for 6 hours daily, and the dose, which is weight related, is titrated to the vasodilatory effects. Iloprost 0.1 mg/ml, is prepared in a saline or dextrose solution of 50 ml or 500 ml volume, depending on whether a syringe driver, or volumetric infusion pump is used. The rate is then incrementally increased by 1 ml/10 ml half-hourly as tolerated, and can be reduced if unacceptable side effects occur.

If any of the following serious side effects occur, the infusion should be stopped, and restarted at the previous rate, after the situation has returned to normal for 1 hour:

- a persistent, clinically significant drop in blood pressure
- a persistent, clinically significant tachycardia
- vagal reaction, with bradycardia, nausea and vomiting

The infusion site should also be carefully monitored to avoid the pronounced inflammatory effects which can occur in the surrounding tissues. The recommended duration for infusions in vasospastic conditions is usually 6 hours daily over 3–7 days.

Sympathectomy

Surgical sympathectomy can be performed to relieve vasoconstriction, thereby improving small vessel perfusion to help reduce ischaemic pain, and ulceration in vasospastic conditions and Buerger's disease. Upper limb cervical sympathectomy is not recommended to relieve Raynaud symptoms due to the high relapse rate within 3–6 months (Johnson et al., 1965), although the development of transthoracic endoscopic techniques has resulted in renewed enthusiasm to the operation (Baker et al., 1994). In contrast, lumbar sympathectomy has been shown to be beneficial for treatment of Raynaud's disease affecting the lower limbs (Gifford et al., 1958; Belch, 1996).

The functions of the sympathetic nervous system include vasoconstriction, sweat gland stimulation, and pain transmission. According to environmental conditions, the sympathetic nervous system causes the peripheral vessels to vasodilate and vasoconstrict, to maintain the hands and feet at a comfortable temperature without overloading or underloading them with blood. The aim of sympathectomy is to remove a section of the sympathetic chain which will then reduce vasoconstriction to the small vessels of the skin. Current evidence indicates that sympathectomy has little value in the treatment of intermittent claudication as it does not improve muscle circulation (Tracy and Reid, 1992).

Axilla or palmar hyperhidrosis (excessive sweating) has been amenable to cervical sympathectomy which can also be performed by an open surgical, or endoscopic transthoracic approach.

Chemical lumbar sympathectomy, using phenol injection to destroy the nerves, is sometimes performed to relieve ischaemic rest pain and vasospasm of the lower limbs. Potential complications include psoas muscle weakness, lumbar plexus damage and male ejaculation dysfunction (Tracy and Reid, 1992).

Informed consent should be obtained and the patient warned of potential risks such as Horner's syndrome (eyelid droop and pupil constriction), following cervical sympathectomy.

Post-surgical care

- After cervical sympathectomy by open or endoscopic technique, a chest X-ray is taken immediately following surgery to check for pleural effusion or pneumothorax. A chest drain may be required.
- Limbs should be checked for colour, warmth and moistness.

Conclusion

Patients with intermittent claudication experience a decrease in their functional ability and quality of life, as well as having an increased mortality risk from cardiovascular and cerebral vascular disease. Drug therapy for symptom relief is currently limited. In comparison, exercise programmes are known to increase patients' functional ability and should constitute a major role in management. Nursing should focus on key aspects of risk factor modification including smoking cessation, reducing cholesterol levels, and diabetes control. Angioplasty can be performed for patients whose symptoms severely handicap their lifestyle or ability to work, whilst reconstructive surgery is generally reserved for those with very severe symptoms, or those who experience an acute on chronic episode who are unsuitable for radiological intervention.

In patients with small vessel disease and vasospastic conditions, it may not always be possible to control their symptoms satisfactorily and amputation may need to be considered in the longer term to improve a patient's quality of life.

References

Antiplatelet Triallists Collaboration (1994) Collaborative overview of randomised trials of antiplatelet therapy. British Medical Journal 308: 81–106.

Baker DM, Nicholson ML, Yusuf SW, Hopkinson BR (1994) Endoscopic transthoracic sympathectomy as adjuvant treatment for critical upper-limb ischaemia. British Journal of Surgery 81(2): 194.

Belch JJF (1996) Temperature-associated vascular disorders: Raynaud's phenomenon and erthromelalgia. In: Tooke JE, Lowe GDD (eds) A Textbook of Vascular Medicine. London: Arnold.

Belch JJF, Bell PRF, Creisen D, Dormandy JA, Kester RC, Mc Collum RD, Mizushima Y, Ruckley CV, Scurr JH, Wolfe JHN (1997) Randomized, double-blind, placebo-controlled study evaluating the efficacy and safety of AS-013, a prostaglandin E prodrug, in patients with intermittent claudication. Circulation 95(9): 2298–2302.

Belli A-M (1996) Percutaneous catheter procedures In: Tooke JE, Lowe GDO (eds) A Textbook of Vascular Medicine. London: Arnold.

Belli A-M, Buckenham T (1996) Vascular Intervention. In: Watkinson A, Adam A (eds) Interventional Radiology – A Practical Guide. Oxford: Radcliffe Medical Press.

Belli A-M, Cumberland DC, Proctor AE, Welch CL (1992) Follow-up of conventional versus laser thermal percutaneous angioplasty of total femoro- politeal artery occlusions: Results of a randomized trial. Journal of Vascular and Interventional Radiology (4): 485–488.

Bloor K (1961) Natural history of arteriosclerosis of the lower extremeties. Annals of the Royal College of Surgeons 28:36–52.

Bremner AD, Fell PJ, Hosie J et al. (1993) Early side effects of antihypertensive therapy: comparison of amlodipine and nifedipine retard. Journal of Human Hypertension 7: 79–81.

Buerger L (1908) Thrombo-angiitis obliterans: a study of the vascular lesions leading to pre-senile spontaneous gangrene. American Journal of Medical Science 136: 567–568.

Caprie Steering Committee (1996) A randomised, blinded, trial of clopidogrel versus aspirin in patients at risk of ischaemic events. Lancet 348(9038): 1329–1339.

Coffman JD (1986) Intermittent claudication: not so benign. American Heart Journal 112(5): 1127–1128.

Coffman JD (1991) Intermittent claudication – be conservative. New England Journal of Medicine 325(8): 577–578.

Coffman JD (1996) Intermittent claudication. In: Tooke JE, Lowe GDO (eds) A Textbook of Vascular Medicine. London: Arnold.

Conrad MC (1967) Large and small artery occlusion in diabetics and non-diabetics with severe vascular disease. Circulation 36 (1):83–91.

Creasy TS, Fletcher EWL (1991) Angioplasty for intermittent claudication. (editorial) Clinical Radiology 43(2): 81–83.

De Vries SO, Hunink MG (1997) Results of aortic bifurcation grafts for aortoiliac occlusive disease: a meta-analysis. Journal of Vascular Surgery 26(4): 558–569.

Dormandy JA (1991) Use of prostacyclin analogue iloprost in the treatment of patients with critical limb ischaemia. Therapie 46: 319–322.

Dormandy J, Heeck L, Vig S (1999) The natural history of claudication: risk to life and limb. Seminars in Vascular Surgery 12(2): 123–137.

Dormandy JA, Loh A. (1996) Critical limb ischaemia In: Tooke JE, Lowe GDO (eds) A Textbook of Vascular Medicine. London: Arnold.

Dormandy JA, Murray GD (1991) The fate of the claudicant, a prospective study of 1969 claudicants. European Journal of Vascular Surgery 5(2): 131–133.

Dotter CT, Judkins MP (1964) Transluminal treatment of arteriosclerotic obstruction. Description of a new technique and preliminary report of its application. Circulation 30(5): 654–670.

Duffield RGM, Miller NE, Brunt JNH, Lewis B, Jamieson CW, Colchester ACF (1983) Treatment of hyperlipidaemia retards progression of symptomatic femoral atherosclerosis: a randomized controlled trial. Lancet ii(8351): 639–642.

Edmonds ME, Blundell MP, Morris ME, Thomas EM, Cotton LT, Watkins PJ (1986) Improved survival of the diabetic foot: the role of a speculative foot clinic. Quarterly Journal of Medicine 60(232): 763–771.

Ericsson B, Haeger K, Lindell SE (1970) Effect of physical training on intermittent claudication. Angiology 21(3): 188–192.

European Concensus Document on Critical Limb Ischaemia (1989) In: Dormandy JA , Stock G (eds) Critical Leg Ischaemia – Its Pathophysiology and Management. London: Springer-Verlag.

Fiessinger JN (1990) Medical treatment of Buerger's disease. Critical Ischaemia 1(1): 23–26.

Fiessinger JN (1996) Buerger's disease or thromboangiitis obliterans. In: Tooke JE, Lowe GDO (eds) A Textbook of Vascular Medicine. London: Arnold.

Fiessinger JN, Schaffer M (1990) For the TAO study. Trial of iloprost versus aspirin treatment for critical limb ischaemia of thromboangiitis obliterans. Lancet (8689): 555–557.

Fitzgerald O, Hess EV, O'Connor GT, Spencer-Green G (1988) Prospective study of Raynaud's phenomenon. American Journal of Medicine 84(4): 718–726.

Fowkes FGR (1996) Epidemiology of peripheral arterial disease In: Tooke JE, Lowe GDO (eds) A Textbook of Vascular Medicine. London: Arnold.

Fowkes FGR, Housley E, Cawood EHH, Macintyre CC, Ruckley C, Prescott RJ (1991) Edinburgh Artery Study: Prevelance of Asymptomatic and Symptomatic Peripheral Arterial Disease in the General Population. International Journal of Epidemiology 20(2):384–392.

Freedman RR, Keegan D, Migaly P, Galloway MP, Mayes M (1991) Plasma catecholamines during behavioural treatments for Raynaud's disease. Psychosomatic Medicine 53(4): 433–439.

Gardner AW, Skinner JS, Smith LK (1991) Effects of handrail support on claudication and the hemodynamic responses to single-stage and progressive treadmill protocols in peripheral vascular occlusive disease. American Journal of Cardiology 68(1): 99–105.

Gibson JME, Kenrick M (1998) Pain and powerlessness: the experience of living with peripheral vascular disease. Journal of Advanced Nursing 27(4): 737–745.

Gifford RW, Hines EA, Craig WM (1958) Sympathectomy for Raynaud's phenomenon: follow-up study of 70 women with Raynaud's disease and 54 women with Raynaud's phenomenon. Circulation 17: 5–13.

Greenhalgh RM, Laing S, Ellis M, Walton J, Baxter K, Powell JT (1988) How can we detect early subclinical disease? In: Greenhalgh RM, Jamieson CW and Nicolaides AN (eds) Vascular Surgery Issues in Current Practice. London: Grune & Stratton.

Hiatt WR, Regensteiner JG, Hargarten ME, Wolfel EE, Brass EP (1990) Benefit of exercise conditioning for patients with peripheral arterial disease. Circulation 81(2): 602–609.

Hiatt WR, Wolfel E, Meier RH, Regensteiner JG (1994) Superiority of treadmill walking exercise versus strength training for patients with peripheral arterial disease. Circulation 90: 1866–1874.

Hill GL (1974) A rational basis for management of patients with Buerger syndrome. British Journal of Surgery 61(6): 476–481.

Horton BT (1938) The outlook in thromboangiitis obliterans. Journal of the American Medical Association 111(24): 2184–2189.

Housley E (1992) The non-operative treatment of lower limb ischaemia. In: Bell PRF, Crawford WJ, Vaughan Ruckley C (eds) Surgical Management of Vascular Disease. London: WB Saunders.

Housley E, Leng GC, Donnan PT, Fowkes FG (1993) Physical activity and risk of peripheral arterial disease in the general population: Edinburgh Artery Study. Journal of Epidemiology and Community Health 47(6): 475–480.

Jaap AJ, Tooke JE (1996) Diabetic angiopathy and the diabetic foot In: Tooke JE, Lowe GDO (eds) A Textbook of Vascular Medicine. London: Arnold.

Johnson EN, Summerly R, Birnstingl M (1965) Prognosis in Raynaud's phenomenon after sympathectomy. British Medical Journal i: 962–964.

Johnston KW, Rae M, Hogg-Johnston SA, Colapinto RF, Walker PM, Baird RJ, Sniderman KW (1987) 5 year results of a prospective study of percutaneous transluminal angioplasty. Annals of Surgery 206(4): 403–413.

Kallero KS (1981) Mortality and morbidity in patients with intermittent claudication as defined by venous occlusion plethysmography. A ten year follow-up study. Journal of Chronic Diseases 34(9–10): 455–462.

La Civita L, Pitaro N, Rossit M et al. (1993) Amlodipine in the treatment of Raynaud's phenomenon. British Journal of Rheumatology 32(6): 524–525.

Larsen AO, Lassen NA (1966) Effect of daily muscular exercise in patients with intermittent claudication Lancet ii: 1093–1096.

Lau H, Cheng SW (1997) Buerger's disease in Hong Kong: a review of 89 cases. Australian and New Zealand Journal of Surgery 67(5): 264–269.

Lehert P, Riphagen FE, Gamand S (1990) The effect of Naftidrofuryl on intermittent claudication: A meta-analysis. Journal of Cardiovascular Pharmacology 16(Suppl 3): S81–86.

Lie JT (1987) Thromboangiitis obliterans (Buerger's disease) in women. Medicine 66(1): 65–72.

McPherson JR, Juergens JL, Gifford RW (1963) Thromboangiitis obliterans and arteriosclerosis obliterans. Clinical and prognostic differences. Annals of Internal Medicine 59(3): 288–296.

Mills JL, Taylor LM, Porter JM (1987) Buerger's disease in the modern era. American Journal of Surgery 154(3): 123–129.

Missouris CG, Buckenham TM, Cappucio FP, MacGregor GA (1994) Renal artery stenosis: A common and important problem in patients with peripheral vascular disease. American Journal of Medicine 96: 10–14.

Mitchell JRA, Schwartz CJ (1965) Arterial Disease. Oxford: Blackwell.

Most RS, Sinnock P (1983) The epidemiology of lower extremity amputation in diabetic individuals. Diabetes Care 6(1): 87–91.

Murray S (1997) A nurse-led clinic for patients with peripheral vascular disease. British Journal of Nursing 6(13): 726–736.

Ohta T, Shionoya S (1988) Fate of the ischaemic limb in Buerger's disease. British Journal of Surgery 75(3): 259–262.

Patterson RB, Pinto B, Marcus B, Colucci A, Braun T, Roberts M (1997) Value of a supervised exercise program for the therapy of arterial claudication. Journal of Vascular Surgery 25(2): 312–319.

Perkins JMT, Collin JC, Morris PJM (1995) Angioplasty versus exercise for stable claudication: long-term results of a prospective randomized trial. Abstract. British Journal of Surgery 82(2): 557–558.

Porter JM, Bardana EJ, Baur GM, Wesche DH, Ruediger H, Andrasch RH, Rosch J (1976) The clinical significance of Raynaud's syndrome. Surgery 80: 756–764.

Porter JM, Cutler BS, Lee BY, Reich T, Reichle FA, Scogin JT, Strandness DE (1982) Pentoxifylline efficiency in the treatment of intermittent claudication: multicenter controlled double-blind trial with objective assessment. American Heart Journal 104(1): 66–72.

Raynaud M (1888) On Local Asphyxia and Symmetrical Gangrene of the Extremities. (Translated by T Barlow.) London: New Sydenham Society.

Regensteiner JG, Hiatt WR (1994) Medical Management of Peripheral Arterial Disease Journal of Vascular and International Radiology 5(5): 669–677.

Regensteiner JG, Gardner A, Hiatt WR (1997a) Exercise testing and exercise rehabilitation for patients with peripheral arterial disease: status in 1997. Vascular Medicine 2: 147–155.

Regensteiner JG, Meyer TJ, Krupski WC, Cranford LS, Hiatt WR (1997b) Hospital vs home-based exercise rehabilitation for patients with peripheral arterial occlusive disease. Angiology 48(4): 291–300.

Sasajima T, Kubo Y, Inaba M, Goh K, Azuma N (1997) Role of infrainguinal bypass in Buerger's disease: an eighteen-year experience. European Journal of Vascular and Endovascular Surgery 13(2): 186–192.

Tracy GD, Reid W (1992) Sympathectomy. In: Eastcott HHG (ed) Arterial Surgery. London: Churchill Livingstone.

Vorwerk D, Guenther RW, Schurmann K, Wendt G, Peters I (1995) Primary stent placement for chronic iliac artery occlusions: follow-up results of 103 patients. Radiology 194(3): 745–749.

Watson CJE, Phillips D, Hands L, Collin J (1997) Claudication distance is poorly estimated and inappropriately measured. British Journal of Surgery 84: 1107–1109.

Whyman MR (1998) Variation in management of intermittent claudication by vascular surgeons. European Journal of Vascular Surgery 15: 250–254.

Whyman MR, Fowkes FGR, Kerracher EMG, Gillespie IN, Lee AJ, Housley E, Ruckley CV (1996) Randomised controlled trial of percutaneous transluminal angioplasty for intermittent claudication. European Journal of Endovascular Surgery 12(2): 167–172.

Further reading

Kelley WN, Ruddy S, Harris ED, Sledge CB (eds) (1997) Textbook of Rheumatology, vols 1 and 2. London: WB Saunders.

Klippel JH, Dieppe PA (eds) (1995) Practical Rheumatology. London: Mosby.

MacVittie BA (1998) Mosby's Perioperative Nursing Series – Vascular Surgery. London: Mosby-Year Book.

CHAPTER 10

Critical Limb Ischaemia

CAROLYN NOCTON

This chapter outlines the nursing care and management required for patients who develop *critical limb ischaemia* and are at risk of limb loss. Critical limb ischaemia may arise *acutely* from an embolus, or *gradually* over the years from progression of chronic disease in the arteries. Care of these patients involves thorough assessment by practitioners to determine the appropriate treatment options. This may include conservative treatment, percutaneous radiological intervention, or surgical intervention.

Vascular surgery and radiological intervention are now recognised as a rapidly developing specialty, and this chapter demonstrates how skilled nurses can influence outcomes of care and treatment through the delivery of meticulous nursing care. The first part of the chapter will look at the care and management of patients with an acutely ischaemic limb. Care and treatment options for those with more gradual onset of chronic critical leg ischaemia will then be considered. Finally, care and management of patients presenting with upper extremity ischaemia will be discussed briefly.

Patients who present with critical limb ischaemia will usually fall into the following two clearly defined categories:

- acute ischaemia
- acute on chronic ischaemia

The clinical features of these can be seen in Table 10.1.

Table 10.1 Critical limb ischaemia – the difference between acute and acute on chronic ischaemia

	Acute ischaemia	Acute on chronic ischaemia
Cause	Thrombus or embolus sometimes in stenotic lesion. Often history of atrial fibrillation or recent myocardial infarction	Stenosis or occlusion, worsening stenotic lesion or thrombus in stenosis
Progress	Sudden onset	Gradual deterioration
Ulcers	Unlikely	Likely – usually develop following trauma to skin
Gangrene	Rarely	Often
Mobility	Usually mobile pre-event	Restricted – gradual deterioration
Diabetes	Rarely	High risk
Ischaemic heart disease	Sometimes	High risk
Skin	Usually healthy, no loss of hair	Often poor integrity, dry skin, hair loss
Oedema	Unlikely	Frequently – due to hanging limb downwards to help reduce ischaemic pain
Pain	Sudden extreme onset	Usual – gradually worsening. Opiates often required to relieve rest pain
Intermittent claudication	Sometimes a history of mild symptoms	Usual – gradual worsening pain-free walking distance
Other leg	Normal	Often both legs are symptomatic, sometimes differing amounts

Acute limb ischaemia

In the UK approximately 5000 patients present annually with acute lower limb ischaemia; usually the aetiology is thromboembolic (Golledge and Galland, 1995). Since 1975 thrombosis has replaced embolism as the principal cause of acute ischaemia, mainly due to improved cardiac management and reduction of cardiac risk factors, and now accounts for approximately 59% of all cases (Golledge and Galland, 1995).

Assessment and diagnosis of patients presenting with acute limb ischaemia

Patients with acute limb ischaemia classically present with the *six p's*: pain, pallor, pulselessness, paraesthesia, paralysis and perishing cold (Table 10.2).

Table 10.2 Symptoms and signs of acute limb ischaemia - the six P's

Characteristics	Nursing assessment guide
Pain	Is usually severe but often not in diabetics with neuropathy Ask how does the patient relieve the pain? Consider positioning of the limb Is analgesia effective? What makes the pain worse? Identify: • rest pain? • claudication? • painful or tender to touch or on movement? It should be noted that pain precedes paraesthesia
Pallor	A white limb indicates complete occlusion; however, more commonly the limb is mottled If blue mottling does not blanch under finger pressure, the small vessels have thrombosed and the ischaemia is often irreversible Is there colour loss on limb elevation or dependent rubor? This is as a result of 'pooling' of blood in the arteries as a result of chronic vasodilatation
Pulselessness	Foot pulses are more difficult to palpate in an obese patient Identify which pulses are present/absent using Doppler Ankle pressures (ABPI) are often too painful to undertake. It may be helpful to mark pulse site if located

Table 10.2 (contd)

Characteristics	Nursing assessment guide
Paraesthesia	Neuropathic diabetic patients mask this observation. Loss of sensation and absent pulses indicate the need to consider immediate vascular intervention Sensation is not always lost but it is important to assess the whole leg and foot
Paralysis	Failure of dorsiflexion of the foot is a poor sign that suggests immediate surgery is required with possible fasciotomy Indicate the degree of movement if any is present
Perishing cold	The extent of coldness is an unreliable indicator to the level of arterial occlusion. However, if the groin and buttocks are cold, aortic occlusion is likely. Skin temperature is a useful indicator in thrombolysis observations as the foot becomes reperfused

Source: McPherson (1992).

Acute thromboembolism requires prompt assessment and emergency treatment as any delay will increase the risk of irreversible tissue damage and limb loss. The aim of treatment is to remove the thrombus/embolus and restore blood flow to the limb.

As well as lower limb vessels, embolism may also occur in other major arteries such as cerebral, axillobrachial, superior mesenteric and renal which will produce sudden ischaemia to the organs supplied.

Diagnosis will depend on differentiating between an acute embolic episode and a thrombotic event in the presence of long-term chronic disease. It is important but often difficult for the assessing doctor and nurse to establish this (Table 10.3).

A full medical assessment will include history taking and physical examination which will identify previous symptoms and signs of peripheral vascular disease such as intermittent claudication, walking distance, lifestyle handicap/disability, as well as cerebro/cardiovascular, renal or respiratory disease (Table 10.4).

Familial history and other risk factors also need to be documented such as:

- smoking
- hyperlipidaemia

Table 10.3 Identification of acute arterial occlusion

	Embolism	Thrombus
Source	Moved from somewhere else – often cardiac source which becomes 'lodged' in an artery. Dislodged from a proximal source, e.g. abdominal aorta	Always a blood clot, often superimposed on an atheromatous stenosis or plaque
History	Atrial fibrillation/ myocardial infarction	Claudication/graft in situ
Treatment urgency	Within 6 hours but as soon as possible to avoid irreversible skin damage/ tissue loss	As soon as possible for acute or acute on chronic

Table 10.4 Identification of thromboembolism

Cardiac	Non-cardiac
Myocardial infarction/atrial fibrillation/ congestive cardiac failure	Aneurysm (aorta, femoral, popliteal)
Poor left ventricular function	Atherosclerotic plaque
Mitral valve stenosis/disease	Tumour
Cardiac valve prosthesis	Bullet
Endocarditis	Caused by intervention
Cardioversion	Venous thrombosis

Source: Adapted from Fahey and McCarthy (1994).

- hypertension
- obesity
- diabetes
- clotting disorders

These risk factors must be fully explored. The nurse should identify and set realistic goals with the patient regarding areas of risks which are modifiable.

An anaesthetic opinion will be required if surgery is indicated. Cardiology review may also be urgently required as myocardial infarction is considered the primary cause of perioperative morbidity and mortality in these patients (Weitz, 1993).

The following areas also need to be thoroughly assessed and are discussed in more depth in Chapter 4.

History of symptoms

This includes identifying the onset, and how the symptoms developed and resulted in handicap and/or lifestyle adjustment. It is important to gain a measure of the patient's walking distance and to determine if mobility is reduced because of claudication, or for other reasons such as angina, arthritis or shortness of breath.

Limb assessment

This should be undertaken as discussed in Chapter 4 and it can be helpful to mark on the patient's skin, lines of demarcation to monitor treatment progress. Limb temperature, sensation, movement and pedal pulses should also be documented accurately and verbally communicated to colleagues taking over the patient's care. It is recommended that nurses should assess the limb together at shift handover times to aid continuity.

Pressure areas

This is a major priority of care for patients with critical ischaemia who are high risk for developing sacral and heel sores. A pressure sore risk assessment score should be immediately undertaken and the appropriate pressure-relieving mattress and heel protectors provided before the patient is sent for any necessary intervention.

Nutrition

A food intake chart should be commenced as soon as possible to assess nutritional intake and a referral to the dietician may be needed to calculate dietary requirements accurately and provide high protein supplements.

Ulcer /wound care

Any ulcerated lesions or wounds should be measured, described and ideally photographed to provide baseline documentation and allow progress to be monitored (see Chapter 14).

Bowel function

Constipation is not uncommon due to immobility and opiate analgesic requirements.

Psychosocial

The patient with a critically ischaemic leg will often fear limb loss and these fears may be intensified in patients with acute on chronic disease by the presence of offensive ulceration/gangrene, and the possibility of a disabled lifestyle. Furthermore, the presence of other patients on the ward with major lower limb amputations often exacerbates these anxieties. The patient's expectation of the outcome of intervention should be discussed and the nurse should identify realistic outcomes with the patient and their family.

Health education

It is not always appropriate to initiate discussion on health promotion when a patient is admitted with an acutely ischaemic event. However, following emergency intervention the nurse will need to provide advice based on identified risk factors in relation to smoking, diabetes, cholesterol and blood pressure control, foot care and exercise. This is discussed in detail in Chapter 3. Patients with acute limb ischaemia may require long-term anticoagulation and the importance of this therapy will need to be stressed.

Pain assessment

Assessment of ischaemic limb pain should include establishing when the pain first occurred, whether it came on gradually or suddenly, what makes it better or worse. Is the analgesia effective and does it provide total pain relief? Is the patient able to relieve the pain by limb positioning and/or level of activity?

Characteristics of critical limb pain include:

- sharp, stabbing, burning 'like a hot poker or sharp knife'
- aching, heaviness
- pins and needles
- numbness
- extreme sensitivity to touch (requires a bed cradle to relieve weight of bed linen)

The pain can be constant or intermittent and is usually exacerbated by mobility and limb elevation. The patient is likely to require regular opioid analgesia and epidurals should be considered whenever possible (see Chapter 6).

Investigations

Preliminary investigations required to determine the site and nature of the thrombus and/or the embolic source may include the following:

- ECG/echocardiogram to determine cardiac source if embolic
- full blood screening
- Doppler assessment to assess pedal pulses and ankle brachial pressure index (ABPI)
- duplex scan
- angiogram – to view run-off vessels and collaterals

It is essential to minimise any delays in treating the limb occlusion. Therefore an angiogram may not need to be performed preoperatively if surgical embolectomy or thrombectomy has been decided upon.

Treatment of acute ischaemia

Initial anticoagulation therapy using *intravenous heparin* is immediately commenced and *analgesia* administered to help relieve the pain before treatment is commenced.

Thrombolysis (clot breakdown)

The aetiology of acute lower limb ischaemia is usually thromboembolic disease, the primary cause being thrombosis (Golledge and Galland, 1995). As a consequence, intra-arterial thrombolysis is being increasingly used as first-line treatment as an alternative to surgery, and this change in practice has led to evaluation of alternative thrombolytic agents and techniques (Buckenham, 1998).

The aim of thrombolysis is to return patients to their pre-thrombotic or pre-embolic state. Frequently after successful thrombolysis an underlying atherostenotic lesion is identified which requires further treatment by angioplasty, surgery or anticoagulation.

Any contraindications to thrombolysis should be reviewed as a risk assessment (Table 10.5) and careful patient selection is of paramount importance to reduce complications (Buckenham, 1998). The risk of no treatment could be threatening to life or limb and therefore the risk/benefit ratio needs careful consideration. A randomised trial revealed that, as an initial therapy for acute leg ischaemia, thrombolysis reduces the magnitude of any subsequent surgical procedure in 40–60% of patients, and provides improved limb salvage for patients with acute bypass graft occlusions (STILE Trial, 1994).

Patient selection for thrombolysis

This is based on careful assessment by the vascular team and successful thrombolysis is dependent upon the time of onset of symptoms (Buckenham, 1998). A patient with a short history of symptoms and a clinically viable limb is more likely to respond to thrombolysis than a patient who has a limb with more advanced ischaemia and a history of chronic disease. Any patient who has a haemorrhagic disorder or lesion which may bleed is not suitable for thrombolysis. Contraindications to thrombolysis can be seen in Table 10.5.

Table 10.5 Criteria and contraindications for thrombolysis

Criteria for thrombolysis	Contraindications
Patients with acute onset of critical ischaemia with a thrombus as identified on duplex scan or angiogram	Recent stroke or transient ischaemic attack in previous 2 months Any bleeding tendency or recent haemorrhage, e.g. gastric ulcers Recent surgery/trauma - 6 weeks considered as danger period History of carotid disease, severe hypertension, acute pancreatitis/severe liver disease or renal failure Confused patients who will be unable to tolerate lying flat/still Patients on oral anticoagulant therapy (warfarin must be stopped)

Source: Buckenham (1998).

Thrombolysing agents

There are a variety of thrombolytic agents available including alteplase (rt-PA), streptokinase and urokinase. Recombinant human tissue-type plasminogen activator (rt-PA) is the agent most commonly used for thrombolysis in the UK, and will be the thrombolytic agent discussed here.

Unlike other lytic agents, rt-PA has a clot-specific action which leaves the systemic coagulation system almost completely intact at the same time having the ability to produce a powerful lytic effect on contact with fibrin, which rapidly breaks down the clot (Murray, 1992). It may be helpful to consider this process as a blood clot held together by a fishing net type structure (i.e. fibrin) with the rtPA dissolving the net, thus breaking down the blood clot (Figure 10.1). Another benefit of rt-PA is that, unlike streptokinase, it does not stimulate antibody formation.

Thrombolysis works best with fresh thrombus and unless contraindicated should be considered as first-line treatment for the following conditions:

- acute limb ischaemia
- acute on chronic limb ischaemia
- limb bypass graft occlusion

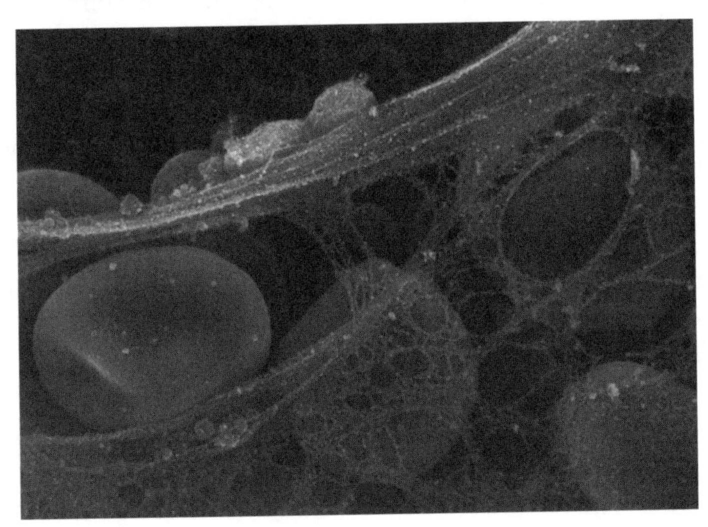

Figure 10.1 Structure of a thrombus demonstrating fibrin strands. Reproduced by kind permission of Boeringher Ingleheim.

Although peripheral thrombolysis is advocated by some as the best treatment for acute leg ischaemia, it is associated with a substantial risk in the elderly, with high complication rates (Braithwaite et al., 1998; Buckenham, 1998). Patients receiving thrombolysis should be considered 'high-risk' patients and this treatment should only be undertaken in a safe nursing environment (Murray, 1992).

Methods of rt-PA administration

The methods of intra-arterial thrombolysis will vary slightly according to local protocols and resources. Some centres nurse patients receiving low-dose thrombolysis on an intensive care/high dependency unit and others on vascular or surgical wards.

Doses of thrombolytic agent will vary according to local policy and are often dependent upon the availability of the rescreening angiography sessions; for example, high-dose thrombolysis is not indicated if 2–4-hourly rescreening is unavailable. Other centres will use high-dose bolus infusion or a pulse spray technique which has a more rapid lysis effect, whilst the patient remains in the radiology department (Yusuf et al., 1995; Armon et al., 1997; Braithwaite et al., 1997).

Wherever the setting for administration of thrombolysis, and when considering the associated risks, it is clear that the nurse makes a unique contribution to patient care and treatment outcomes. He/she will need to establish a therapeutic relationship with the patient and be highly skilled to supervise the treatment, and make clinical decisions based on nursing observations. Benner (1984) suggests that drugs can be used safely only if their effects are observed and if possible incompatibilities, contraindications and adverse reactions are detected early. The patient should be managed by an experienced team of radiologists, vascular surgeons, and nurses who will need to maintain close communication with the team throughout the infusion, adhering to local management protocols.

The following recommended nursing care relates to low-dose infusions but the principles of care are the same for all methods of thrombolysis.

Nursing care and responsibilities

Many hospitals utilise vascular nurse specialists to supervise nursing care of this high-risk patient group, as they can ensure the smooth administration of the treatment. They are uniquely placed to understand the difficulties and priorities of thrombolysis and can act as problem-solvers and plan care and intervention to prevent complications occurring (Dawson and Hamilton, 1994).

Nursing care for patients receiving thrombolysis focuses on prevention and early detection of complications which could be life-threatening (Table 10.6).

Table 10.6 Complications of thrombolysis

1. Bleeding – puncture site, groin haematoma, cerebrovascular event, retroperitoneal haemorrhage, muscle haematoma, other haemorrhage
2. Pericatheter thrombus
3. Reperfusion syndrome
4. Distal embolisation
5. Allergic reactions
6. Arterial/graft perforation
7. Catheter related problems

Source: Dawson and Hamilton (1994).

Nursing responsibilities include:

- Knowledge of the drug and potential complications.
- Strict observation of the patient throughout the infusion.
- Maintaining accurate documentation of observations and care throughout treatment and during the acute post-thrombolysis period.
- Immediate reporting of potential complications to ensure prompt intervention to reduce this risk.

Although haemorrhage is the most serious complication of thrombolysis, it is generally minor and should be considered against the risks of surgery or no treatment and potential limb loss. Berridge et al. (1989) identify the risks of haemorrhagic complications of thrombolysis as stroke 1%, major haemorrhage 5%, and minor haemorrhage 14.8% (major haemorrhage requires blood transfusion; minor haemorrhage resolves without specific treatment). These complications can be reduced by vigilant nursing care and careful patient selection.

Pre-thrombolysis care:

- Baseline bloods – full blood and platelet count, urea and electrolytes, clotting screen.
- ECG recommended.
- Site large bore (16 gauge) peripheral cannula.
- Nil-by-mouth for 4 hours prior to procedure in case surgical intervention is required.
- Observe and document the patient's observations as follows:
  - blood pressure in both arms, pulse and temperature
  - pedal pulse and limb perfusion observations
  - oxygen saturation on room air
  - urinalysis
  - pressure area risk assessment (provide appropriate pressure-relieving mattress/heel pads)
  - blood glucose in diabetic patients: a sliding scale insulin regime may be required in insulin/tablet controlled diabetics until normal diet resumed
- Informed consent and full explanation of treatment and care and risks – the nurse should reiterate this to the patient and his/her family to ensure that they are clear about the intensity of nursing observation, implications of care, e.g. flat bedrest and likely duration of treatment.
- Reassess pain relief and administer analgesia as required.
- Safely escort patient to radiology department for angiogram and thrombolysis.

Once the thrombus is identified in the angiogram room, the catheter is embedded into it if possible, or the clot is agitated to permit accelerated penetration of the thrombolytic agent. The infusion must begin immediately to prevent further risk of thrombus and the catheter will be firmly secured with an occlusive transparent dressing at the groin site. This allows the nurse to inspect the groin site easily. The catheter enters the artery via a sheath with a side arm. Both must be clearly labelled to ensure correct identification for drug administration. The sheath is used either to run a concurrent heparin infusion, or for bolus dose flushes of heparin or saline to maintain patency of the sheath. The infusion of rt-PA must run via the catheter directly to the thrombus. The sheath must be regularly checked to ensure it does not become dislodged or kinked.

Nursing care during thrombolysis

Careful observation of the patient is essential throughout the treatment as these patients have high dependency needs. The nurse must ensure that the infusion is running via an infusion pump and that the solution does not run out. This would cause back bleeding and thrombosis of the infusion line. The next syringe should be ready for immediate reconnection. The nurse should ask the advice of the doctor immediately if there are any concerns. A suggested nursing care plan for patients receiving thrombolysis can be seen in Table 10.7.

Haemorrhage

Although this is the most worrying complication during thrombolysis, close nursing observation will ensure immediate detection of haemorrhage and prompt intervention. In the case of major haemorrhage the doctor must be called immediately and the infusion stopped. Direct, firm pressure should be applied to the site of haemorrhage (often at the arterial catheter puncture site) and standard treatment for shock should be implemented.

It should be noted that haemorrhage is not always as obvious as a large blood loss (e.g. haematemesis/groin bleed). Bleeding can occur internally, e.g. retroperitoneally, gastrointestinal, renal. This is not always immediately evident through observation of clinical signs and the nurse must observe the patient closely for restlessness, agitation, discomfort and haematoma formation.

Some bleeding around the sheath is not uncommon. Minor oozing can be dealt with by local digital pressure and thrombolysis can continue. Extra dressing pads should not be continually added to the site as this will occlude vision of the site. Any oozing should be cleansed away and replaced with clean gauze or a light dressing pad. Uncontrolled hypertension should be treated to reduce the risk of bleeding, particularly at the groin puncture site. Patients should continue their usual cardiac/anti-hypertensive medication.

Pain

Successful thrombolysis and revascularisation of the limb can cause severe limb pain. The patient must be warned about this as patients may associate pain with worsening threat of limb loss.

Table 10.7 Nursing care for patients receiving thrombolysis

Problem/need	Goal	Nursing intervention
Risk of haemorrhage	To detect early signs and minimise effect	• Half-hourly pulse, blood pressure for 4 hs, thereafter l-hourly if stable • Report hypotension and tachycardia • Observe catheter site for bleeding, bruising and haematoma – report immediately • Report any groin, abdominal or back pain • Mark any haematoma or bruising on the skin/dressing • Observe other puncture sites for bleeding • Avoid IM injections/venepuncture • Hourly IV pump checks to ensure correct dose is delivered
Risk of dislodging the catheter	To maintain correct catheter position	• Flat bedrest/minimal patient movement – use of slide boards and slipper bed pans • Ensure dressing is secure • Check catheter position hourly. Mark catheter position • Explain to the patient the need for flat bedrest to promote their compliance
Risk of catheter thrombosis	To prevent thrombosis and further deterioration of limb	• Do not allow the infusion to stop • Check pump and arterial infusion lines hourly • Correct labelling of lines • Foot observations hourly – record colour, warmth, sensation and movement. Locate pedal pulses with Doppler and document their presence/absence

Table 10.7 (contd)

Problem/need	Goal	Nursing intervention
		• Immediate reporting of any deterioration in the limb • Ensure heparin or saline flush to sheath is delivered as prescribed
Risk of dehydration	For patient to be fully hydrated	• Assist the patient with diet and fluids – keep nil-by-mouth prior to rescreening if complications suspected • Maintain fluid balance chart • Review need for intravenous infusion • Provide mouthcare
Painful limb and potential risk of developing compartment syndrome	To keep patient comfortable and detect early signs of compartment syndrome	• Provide regular analgesia, e.g. oral/IV morphine and review effectiveness • Identify site of pain and degree of pain using assessment tool • Relieve anxiety • Careful positioning of limb and use of bed cradle • Observe calf for increased pain/swelling, muscle tightness and shiny skin – report immediately if this occurs

IM, intramuscular; IV, intravenous.

Opiate intravenous or oral analgesia is required and possibly midazolam or diazepam if the patient becomes anxious. Intramuscular injections must not be given due to the risk of haematoma formation.

Foot observations

As lysis commences, the thrombus will break up and the nurse should observe for signs of *trash foot*. Small areas of mottling or necrosis can occur. These microthrombi often disperse with continuing thrombolysis or the dose may need to be increased. Limb perfusion should be carefully observed (see Table 10.7).

Fluid balance

Fluid and dietary intake during thrombolysis will vary according to local policy, the condition of the patient and the possible need for emergency surgical intervention. Due to the unpredictability of thrombolysis, it may be advisable to restrict the patient to fluids only and this will be necessary for 2 hours prior to rescreening. If the nurse suspects complications during treatment, nil-by-mouth status should be introduced. A fluid balance record should be maintained and action taken according to observations. The nurse will need to observe the patient's output carefully and catheterisation may occasionally be required. Patients will require assistance to eat and drink whilst lying flat.

Rescreening

The patient must be safely escorted to radiology for repeat angiogram by a trained nurse who is competent in emergency action if necessary. The infusion must continue via a battery-operated pump. The catheter will clot if the infusion is not maintained.

Lysis is confirmed by angiogram and the infusion can be stopped immediately and the catheter withdrawn. The sheath can be removed 2 hours afterwards according to local policy. It is essential that continuous firm, direct pressure is applied over the arterial puncture site for 15–20 minutes, and the direction of sheath entry considered so pressure can be specifically applied. Whilst applying this pressure, the nurse or doctor should closely observe for haematoma development around the site. A clear film dressing is sometimes applied to the skin puncture and observations commenced as per post-angioplasty care (see Chapter 9). Flat bedrest is maintained for 4–6 hours and usually full bedrest for a further 6 hours (12 hours total). Minimal disturbance to the groin is required to reduce the risk of bleeding. An intravenous heparin infusion will commence after sheath removal and the patient will then be converted to warfarin. The duration of warfarin therapy will be determined by the vascular surgeon/radiologist. Low-dose aspirin therapy should be commenced for long-term use (Working party on thrombolysis in the management of limb ischaemia, 1998).

It is important for the patient to understand that successful lysis will often reveal underlying chronic atherosclerotic disease which may require follow-up angioplasty or surgical intervention. Providing initial lysis is achieved and underlying stenosis is corrected, thrombolysis produces long-term patency rates comparable to that of surgical reconstruction (Berridge, 1998).

Anticoagulation

All patients receiving anticoagulation therapy to prevent a further thromboembolic event should be advised by the nurse, and be able to demonstrate a clear awareness of potential side effects, how to recognise these and when to seek medical attention.

Vascular patients require anticoagulation with intravenous heparin for treatment of the following:

- acute arterial or graft occlusions (often after thrombolysis)
- intraoperatively to flush artery/graft
- postoperatively, e.g. repetitive graft failure
- treatment of DVT
- cerebrovascular embolic disorders and distal emboli, e.g. trash foot

Warfarin is used in the longer term to prevent graft occlusion and thrombus in high-risk patients. The dose of warfarin will be managed by the GP/anticoagulation clinic on discharge from hospital. Anticoagulation therapies are briefly reviewed in Table 10.8.

Table 10.8 Anticoagulation therapy

Drug	Dose	Considerations
Aspirin – orally	75 mg daily with food	Antiplatelet drug with immediate effect of reducing platelet aggregation which minimises the progression to clot formation. Does not have direct effect on coagulation cascade. A preventative measure, not curative. Side effects are rare but more frequently affect the gastrointestinal tract
Dipyridamole	100 mg three times a day	These can be used in patients where aspirin is contraindicated or cannot be tolerated
Clopidogrel	75 mg once a day	
Warfarin – orally	1-10 mg usually	Anticoagulant drug titrated to patient's blood clotting results. Takes 48 hours for full absorbency
Heparin or low molecular weight heparin, e.g. Fragmin – intravenously/ subcutaneously	according to patient's weight	Anticoagulant drug. Usually given via intravenous infusion until oral anticoagulants have produced a therapeutic effect for long-term use or until the cause of the embolus is determined and treated. It does not break down a thrombus but acts to accelerate antithrombin III. It prevents extension and embolisation of a thrombus. It is contraindicated with epidurals

Embolectomy/Thrombectomy

This is an emergency surgical procedure, required when patients are not suitable for thrombolysis, including early postoperative graft failure, and is usually performed under local anaesthetic (McPherson, 1992). In some centres percutaneous clot aspiration is a developing radiological technique, particularly for treating catheter-induced thrombosis during angiography (Buckenham, 1994).

Preparation for theatre

Preparation includes explaining the type of surgery, and associated risks (including possible limb loss) to the patient. Close liaison with the surgeon and anaesthetist is required with regard to the heparin infusion, which may need to stop temporarily prior to surgery to prevent haemorrhage. Local protocols should be followed. Blood screening, e.g. full blood count (FBC), urea and electrolytes (U&Es) and clotting, should be undertaken. An ECG is required and opiate analgesia should be given for limb pain.

Operative procedure

The thrombus is removed via a femoral incision using a Fogarty balloon catheter. This is passed through the thrombus and the balloon is inflated, then carefully withdrawn back up the artery, withdrawing the thrombus. The balloon must be inflated with great care to avoid over-inflation, which could cause damage/rupture of the arterial wall. After thrombus removal, the vessels will be irrigated with heparinised saline and a check on-table angiogram will be performed to review the arterial flow and the run-off vessels.

Postoperative care

This includes accurate assessment and documentation of pedal pulses and foot observations. Early recognition of re-occlusion requires urgent medical review.

Care should include:

- Wound care – observe for haemorrhage/infection.
- Observation for signs of compartment syndrome (see below).
- Oedema reduction with limb elevation (vascular reperfusion).
- Anticoagulation management.
- Cardiology review requested if the embolic source is thought to be cardiac.
- Health promotion regarding identified risk factors to prevent recurrence of thrombus.

Compartment syndrome

Compartment syndrome can occur in any patient with acute limb ischaemia. Acute ischaemic events or surgical intervention can produce excessive swelling. The fascia is a fibrous (non-expandable) tissue surrounding each muscle group in the extremities. This results in a closed space (i.e. compartment), containing muscle, bone, nerves, arteries and veins. If the pressure caused from the swelling increases in a compartment, the circulation and neuromuscular function within the space can become compromised as blood flow will be restricted to the tissues. Blood flow to the tissues decreases as the pressure nears diastolic pressure. Causes of compartment syndrome are shown in Table 10.9.

Table 10.9 Causes of compartment syndrome

Decreased compartment size	Increased compartment size
Closure of fascial defects Tight dressings Localised external pressure	Bleeding • major vascular injuries • bleeding disorders Increased capillary permeability • post-ischaemic swelling • exercise • seizures/eclampsia • trauma • burns • orthopaedic surgery • intra-arterial drugs Increased capillary pressure • exercise • venous obstruction Muscle hypertrophy Infiltrated infusion Nephrotic syndrome

Source: Mravic and Massey (1992).

Signs and symptoms of compartment syndrome

The nurse must be familiar with these to ensure prompt medical treatment. Nursing observation should focus on circulatory and neuromuscular function of the limb. Diligent nursing assessment and prompt reporting of symptoms can prevent irreversible complications (Payne, 1994). The signs and symptoms to observe for are as follows (Mravic and Massey, 1992):

- Pain greater than anticipated from the clinical situation, not relieved by opiates.

- Pain on passive stretching of muscles (unique sign).
- Reduced sensation in sensory nerves.
- Weakness of muscles and nerves.
- Tenseness/tightness of muscles and shiny skin.

It is important to compare the strength and tightness of both limbs as the patient is likely to be resting in bed and these symptoms may not always be obvious. It can be helpful to record and repeat calf circumference measurements. The nurse should also be aware of the masking effects of epidural analgesia in this situation. As the duration of compartment syndrome progresses, the complications become more serious (Table 10.10).

Table 10.10 Onset of complications with compartment syndrome

Time	Tissue damage
<30 minutes	Nerve damage
2–4 hours	Muscle function changes
>4 hours	Muscle death
<12 hours	Permanent damage to nerves and muscles
>12 hours	Maximum muscle contracture

Complications of compartment syndrome

Prolonged ischaemia can cause the following complications:

- Infection, often in the presence of necrosis, and skin breakdown.
- Significant loss of neuromuscular function.
- Post-ischaemic contracture – by shortening of the damaged muscles and nerves where necrotic tissue is replaced by fibrous tissue. The application of foot splints can help to minimise this. Passive stretching exercises will help maintain muscle length and movement.
- Myoglobinuric renal failure/rhabdomyolysis – myoglobin is released from damaged muscle tissue into the circulation which can precipitate in and cause blockage of the renal tubules, resulting in renal failure. After 4 hours of muscle ischaemia, significant myoglobinuria can occur (Matsen, 1980). Urine testing is recommended for blood and is commonly a reddish brown colour. Blood urea and nitrogen will be raised.

Nursing action/treatment

- Remove circumferential dressings which could produce additional pressure.
- Elevate limbs no higher than the heart. This reduces local arterial pressure and therefore the accumulation of fluid in interstitial space. To position the limb higher than the heart could reduce arterial blood flow and increase the risk of ischaemia.
- Provide effective analgesia.

If tissue pressure remains elevated and immediate relief is not apparent, then the surgeon will need to perform a *fasciotomy*, which provides immediate relief of pressure.

Fasciotomy

This procedure is usually carried out as an emergency following surgery to minimise tissue damage/ischaemia in compartment syndrome, although it may also be performed prophylactically in some patients. Fascial compartments are opened with an incision (usually on both sides of the calf), which allows the compartments to expand and thus relieve pressure on the microcirculation (Figure 10.2). Muscle debridement is indicated if muscle necrosis has occurred. The incisions are left open and aseptic dressings applied, e.g. paraffin gauze, alginate or transparent film (see Chapter 14). These are usually low exudate wounds, although haemorrhage can occur. As the swelling reduces, the incision may be sutured and occasionally skin grafting is required. Many fasciotomy wounds can be left to heal by secondary intention using dressings only.

In addition to its use in compartment syndrome, fasciotomy may also be required at the time of clot lysis, surgical embolectomy/thrombectomy, or bypass surgery as a preventative measure in the cases of:

- Prolonged period between compromised blood flow to the limb and surgery.
- Extensive preoperative swelling.

Prevention of footdrop

Footdrop can occur after prolonged periods of immobility, bedrest without limb exercises and following fasciotomy.

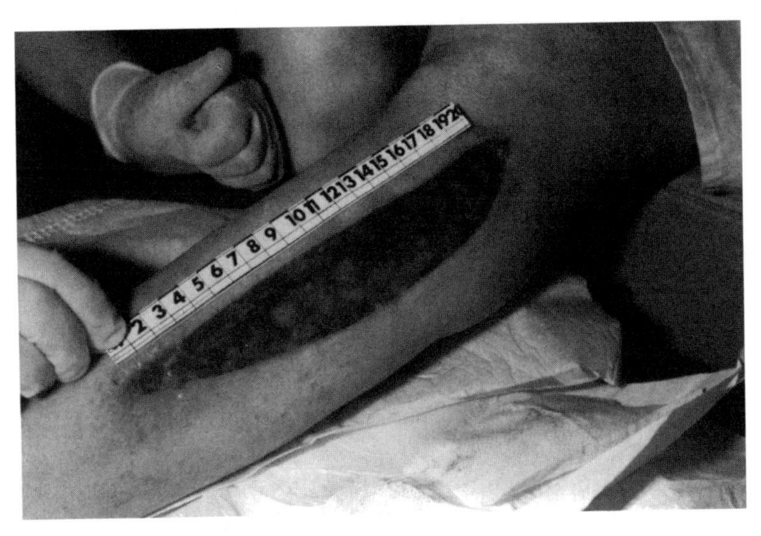

Figure 10.2 Fasciotomy wound.

The nurse should liaise closely with the physiotherapist to ensure that all vascular patients are encouraged and supervised with limb and foot exercises to prevent loss of muscle tone and function in the calf, which can result in loss of ankle movement. It is advisable that a foot support splint, such as a Roylan split, accompany the patient to theatre, so that it can be applied immediately following surgery. Footdrop can also be prevented by regular simple flexion and extension exercises for the foot/ankle with the aid of elastic bands/bandages placed around the sole of the foot and pulled by the patient to support the foot and aid movement. The nurse must ensure the patient receives effective analgesia to permit limb exercises.

If footdrop occurs, the toes and forefoot drop away from the ankle and become fixed in an extension position. This will affect limb function and will reduce the rehabilitation/mobility potential for the patient. In severe cases the patient may need to have a walking foot splint fitted to aid correct positioning of the foot to permit mobility.

Chronic critical limb ischaemia

The term *critical limb ischaemia* was first defined in 1981 at the International Vascular Symposium in London and has since been redefined in the second European Consensus document (European Working Group, 1991) (Table 10.11).

Table 10.11 Definition of critical leg ischaemia (CLI)

- Persistently recurring rest pain requiring regular adequate analgesia for more than 2 weeks

or

- Ulceration or gangrene of the foot and toes

plus

- Ankle systolic pressure ≤50 mmHg (non-diabetics)
- Toe systolic pressure ≤30 mmHg (diabetics)

Source: European Working Group (1991).

The guidelines recommend that the toe systolic pressure is measured in diabetic patients as calcification of the arteries makes ankle pressure measurements inaccurate and therefore an unreliable aid to assessment. This is discussed fully in Chapter 4.

Rest pain is often misinterpreted as general leg pain or night cramps at rest. However, it is more specifically defined as severe, persistent pain usually localised in the forefoot and/or toes, which is characteristically intensified when the limb is horizontal and eased by letting the foot hang down. Rest pain often disturbs sleep and patients frequently report that they sleep in an armchair with their legs down. Usually strong opiate analgesia is required to relieve ischaemic rest pain.

When considering these definitions it is clear that nurses can play a crucial role in instigating prompt referral to a vascular surgeon for this patient group. With the developing role of vascular nurse specialists who are able to liaise closely with community nurses and vascular surgeons, patients with limb-threatening disease are more likely to be referred promptly to specialist vascular teams.

Treatment objectives for patients with chronic critical leg ischaemia are to:

- Ensure an early vascular referral
- Save the limb and promote patient wellbeing and independence
- Preserve a functional limb
- Treat the patient in such a way that provides minimal risk to life and limb

- Optimise wound healing and maintain skin integrity (ulcer healing is often unlikely without revascularisation)

Reconstructive surgery and/or radiological intervention for critical ischaemia is often a palliative not curative measure (Ronayne, 1985). The nurse plays a key role in explaining this to patients to ensure that they have a realistic expectation of any procedure.

Patients with chronic critical leg ischaemia present a huge nursing challenge as this group of patients are largely elderly (Figure 10.3). Approximately 62% of patients undergoing femoro-popliteal bypass are over 70 years, and 71% of patients undergoing thrombectomy for acute ischaemia are over 70 years (Haiart et al., 1991). The projected increase in the elderly population is likely to increase vascular workload in the future. Many of these elderly patients have additional risk factors and other concurrent diseases which reduce their fitness for surgery. These include: cardiovascular disease, cerebrovascular disease, renal disease, respiratory disease, diabetes and arthritis. The vascular team must work in close collaboration with the patient, community nurses, general practitioners, chiropodists and other specialist practitioners to reduce any associated risk factors for the patient (see Chapter 3). Appropriate referrals and communications with other teams such as cardiologists, anaesthetists and diabetic teams are essential to obtain specialist input. In some cases, owing to multiple or single severe risk factors and/or failed previous surgical bypass, further intervention may not be possible and palliative management only can be considered. Community/palliative care/vascular specialist nurses will need to work closely with the patient in this situation to maximise their independence, provide symptom relief and health education to reduce the impact of peripheral vascular disease on their daily life (see Chapter 15).

Percutaneous transluminal angioplasty (PTA) for chronic critical leg ischaemia

Angioplasty is a less invasive procedure which can be performed for chronic critical leg ischaemia, although many of these patients have multilevel stenoses which often involve distal vessels. Specialist vascular centres are now successfully performing angioplasties of distal vessels in patients with limb-threatening disease. Temporary

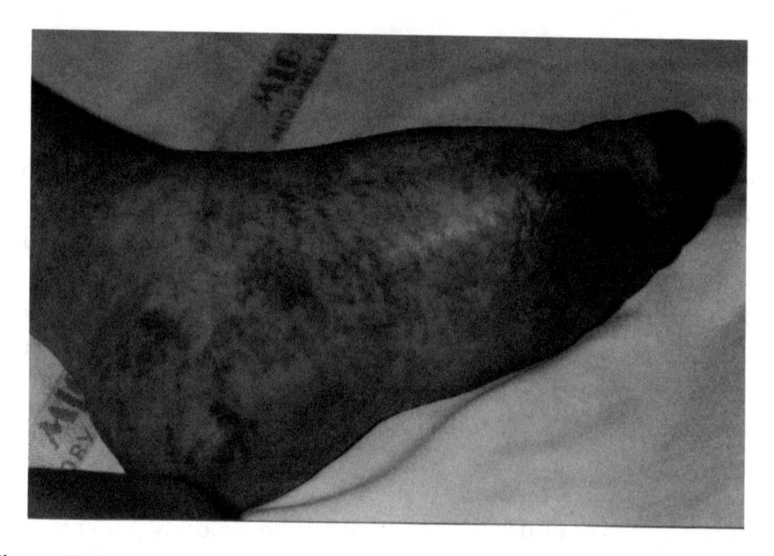

Figure 10.3 Chronic ischaemia, left foot; see Plate 9.

spasm of these small vessels during angioplasty is recognised as a problem and can be treated effectively with vasodilators. Percutaneous reopening procedures are now well established in this group of patients, particularly for patients who are considered too unfit for major bypass surgery or where long-term graft patency is a concern. Angioplasty can also be performed for bypass graft occlusion in combination with thrombolysis, although vein grafts generally respond better to angioplasty than do synthetic grafts (Greenspan et al., 1985).

Stent insertion may also be performed in iliac vessels to prevent restenosis following angioplasty. Care of the patient undergoing angioplasty is described in Chapter 9.

Endarterectomy

This surgical procedure is now rarely performed due to improved medical management of vascular patients and advances in angioplasty and bypass grafting. Endarterectomy involves opening a stenotic artery and excision of the atherosclerotic lesion on the inner arterial wall. This surgery carries a high risk as emboli from the atherosclerosis can pass to distal vessels and cause occlusion. The procedure requires meticulous dissection and can result in considerable blood loss, particularly in aortoiliac lesions.

Arterial reconstructive bypass surgery

Indications and rationale for performing arterial bypass surgery are identified as follows:

- Patients with severe ischaemic rest pain and/or ulceration/ gangrene where the arterial lesion is unsuitable for percutaneous angioplasty.
- The patient has severe claudication and lifestyle handicap and the lesion is unsuitable for percutaneous angioplasty.
- The patient is suitable for general anaesthetic after careful assessment.
- Risk of surgery is less than the risk to life and limb of no surgery.
- Good arterial inflow and run-off vessels demonstrated on duplex/angiogram.
- The limb is salvageable and is expected to be functional postoperatively.

Additional considerations:

- Infection risk if leg ulcer present. Ensure topical wound management is optimal and all other wound healing factors are maximised.
- Local and national mortality rates.
- Effective cardiology, respiratory, renal and diabetic management to reduce operative risks.

Specific preoperative investigations

Patients requiring bypass surgery may already be inpatients having undergone investigations and pain management or they may be admitted electively and will undergo pre-admission assessment. Investigations will need to include:

- Duplex/angiogram/digital subtraction angiogram (DSA) to identify stenosis/occlusion and inflow and outflow of arterial blood supply.
- Full blood screening: FBC/clotting/U&Es/blood glucose.
- Blood cross matching.
- Chest X-ray, blood gases and lung function tests are needed in patients with chronic obstructive pulmonary disease (COPD)/ chest infection.

- ECG/echo to review cardiac status; exercise ECG may be needed.
- MUGA scan – this reviews left ventricular ejection fraction. If <30%, surgery should be reconsidered.
- ABPI/toe systolic baseline pressures in both legs to assess/compare postoperative progress.
- Duplex vein mapping – if vein required for femoro-popliteal or femoro-distal graft.
- Referral to appropriate teams to reduce perioperative risks, e.g. anaesthetic, cardiology, respiratory, renal and diabetic.

Preparation for surgery

Nursing assessment, as discussed at the beginning of the chapter, needs to be thorough to aid accurate pre- and postoperative care planning. The patient and family/carers should be involved in all discussions wherever possible and discharge planning arrangements should also be discussed at this stage.

The medical staff, physiotherapist, occupational therapist and social worker will need to assess the patient's preoperative fitness, independence, mobility and social circumstances and assess the need for a postoperative home assessment.

Specific areas of focus should include the following issues:

Informed consent – a senior surgeon should discuss any associated risks of surgery with the patient and family, e.g. local/national morbidity/mortality risks, graft patency rates and risks of haemorrhage/thrombus/graft infection. The type of surgery should be explained with the aid of diagrams/leaflets to demonstrate bypass grafts.

Rehabilitation – provide a realistic explanation of the rehabilitation process and explain what the patient should expect postoperatively; e.g. immediate postoperative mobility may be worse initially than preoperatively. Discuss postoperative limb movement/swelling and mobilisation.

Pain control – review and discuss with the patient/pain management team, and explain postoperative pain management plan, e.g. patient-controlled analgesia (PCA)/epidural.

Tissue viability/ulcer healing/wound care – discuss the aims of revascularisation to aid ulcer healing and explain postoperative wound care needs/limb swelling etc. Reassess the patient's pressure sore risk and review pressure-relieving aids.

Respiratory status – oxygen saturation levels on room air should be checked and the physiotherapist will need to assess the patient and demonstrate deep breathing exercises.

Nutrition/hydration – provide high protein supplements and maintain a food intake chart if required. The patient should only be fasted for a minimum period preoperatively following local policy. An intravenous infusion may be needed to prevent dehydration in some cases where theatre cancellation has been necessary.

Diabetic review – blood glucose control should be optimised preoperatively and the diabetic team/specialist nurse should be asked to review the patient if necessary before surgery. Insulin-dependent diabetics and those on oral hypoglycaemics will require a sliding scale insulin regime and blood glucose monitoring throughout the fasting period and until they are able to resume a normal diet.

Skin preparation – thorough skin cleansing is essential. Many patients are smokers, diabetic, elderly and some may be malnourished and have a high risk of impaired wound healing and graft infection, with potentially serious consequences. Any ulcerated lesions should be swabbed and the swab sent for culture and sensitivity. Preoperative showers or baths with povidone iodine or chlorhexidine antiseptics will help to reduce skin bacteria. Any skin shaving that may be required should preferably be performed immediately before surgery.

Prophylactic intravenous antibiotics – these will be prescribed and administered according to local protocol immediately before surgery.

Types of graft material used

Arterial revascularisation can be performed using either autologous vein graft or prosthetic graft material.

Prosthetic grafts (Figure 10.4): these include terephthalate (Dacron) and expanded polytetrafluoroethylene (ePTFE). The latter (ePTFE) is a popular graft material due to ease of handling and tight interstices that do not require pre-clotting, and is used if a vein is either unavailable, i.e. already harvested for cardiac or peripheral use, varicosed or not long or wide enough. For bypass operations using larger proximal vessels such as the aorta, iliac or common femoral arteries, a synthetic graft is the preferred material. These are also required if there is local skin breakdown or infected ulceration which would make vein grafting unsuitable.

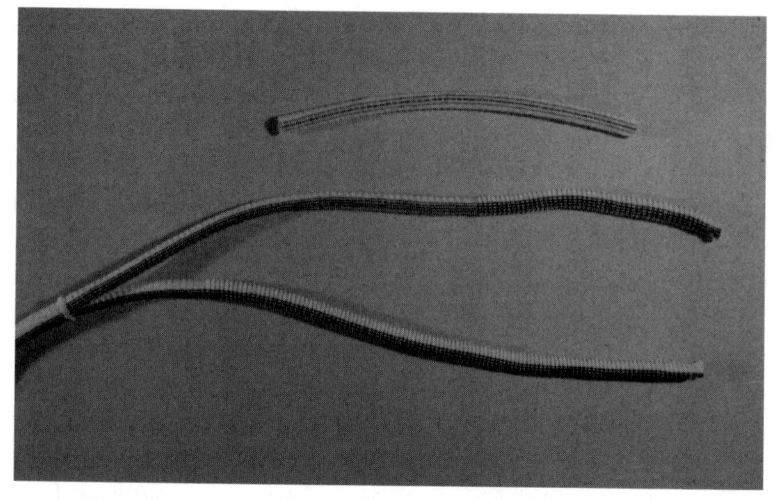

Figure 10.4 Example of prosthetic bypass graft material.

Vein grafts – this is the preferred choice of material for infra-inguinal (below the groin) bypass surgery due to higher patency rates and lower infection risk. The saphenous or cephalic vein provides greatest patency rates and is identified with a duplex scan and marked on the leg for identification prior to surgery. An in situ autologous vein graft is commonly used and the valves of the vein are stripped to prevent arterial occlusion (the valves would close with arterial flow) and all tributaries are dissected to prevent arteriovenous fistulae. The vein is then anastomosed to the proximal and distal artery to create a bypass. Reversing the vein to deactivate the valves results in a narrowed vein end at the proximal artery because of the size disparity between the vein and the native artery, often requiring a patch to widen it. This in itself can increase the risk of complications. Grafts are anastomosed to the artery proximal and distal to the atherosclerotic stenosis or occlusion. Positions of grafts are demonstrated in Figure 10.5.

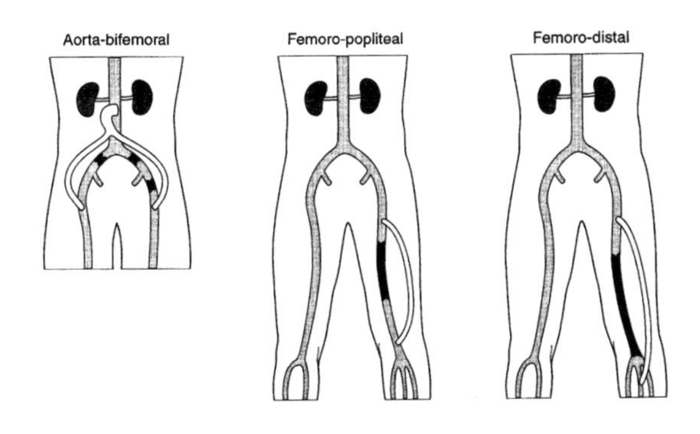

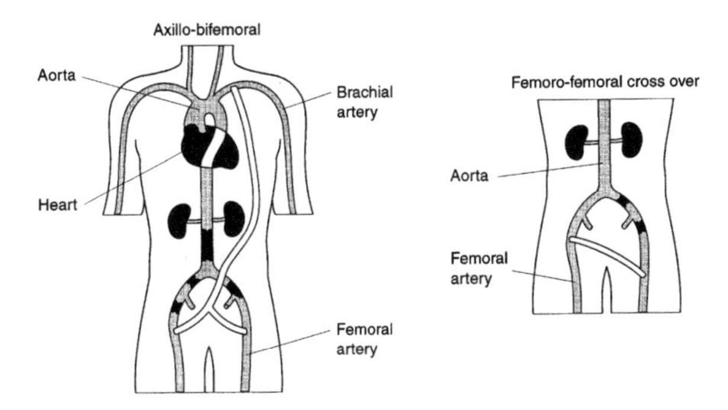

Figure 10.5 Sites of stenosis/occlusion and position of bypass grafts.

Postoperative nursing care

Patients with severe vascular disease carry a high operative risk of myocardial infarction, cerebrovascular event, or respiratory complications and will therefore need close monitoring for the first 48 hours. Specific areas of care should focus on early detection and prevention of complications, working closely with the patient and the surgeon to promote safe and well-planned discharge from hospital. The nurse needs to frequently review and critically analyse care using his or her skill and judgement to report abnormalities to the vascular team. Every opportunity to provide health education to the patient should be taken, focusing on risk factors and areas specific to individual needs (see Chapter 3). Postoperative complications can be identified as early and late onset and are shown in Table 10.12. The nursing care required in this postoperative period is outlined in Table 10.13 (pages 303–5).

Table 10.12 Complications of arterial bypass surgery

Early	Late
Bleeding (anastomosis) often technical reasons	Graft infection
Wound infection (haematoma)	Graft stenosis (recurring symptoms)
Occlusion	Anastomotic aneurysm, i.e. false aneurysm
Peri/post operative myocardial infarction	Arteriovenous fistula in vein graft
Graft infection	
Internal hyperplasia	
Pressure sores (heels are very high risk areas)	
Groin lymphatic fistulae or lymphocele	
DVT – rare due to intraoperative heparin	

Discharge planning

Discharge planning must involve the patient, their family/carers, and the multidisciplinary team to ensure that any required support services are organised.

Verbal and written leaflet information should be provided by the nurse on the following points:

- Explain what is normally expected during the postoperative period and what the patient should expect, e.g. some wound discomfort /tightness/leg swelling.
- Abnormal signs that require prompt medical attention, e.g. sudden onset of pale, cold or painful leg, or increased leg/foot pain.
- Wound/ulcer care:
  - agree aims of wound management with the patient and community nurses and consider short-term and long-term goals
  - keep suture line clean and dry following baths/shower
  - avoid perfumed creams/soap/talc. Advise the patient to report any abnormal wound pain/swelling/inflammation/ offensive exudate and/or new skin breakdown to the community nurse or GP.
- Foot care advice – explain the importance of meticulous foot care, especially in diabetic patients. It may be necessary to instruct the spouse/carer to examine and moisturise the feet daily. Chiropody referral is recommended for follow-up care.

Table 10.13 Potential complications of bypass graft surgery and the nursing care required

Potential complications	Nursing observation and care
Haemorrhage from rupture at site of anastomosis or inadequate ligation of vessels	Haemodynamic observation: blood pressure and pulse $^{1}/_{2}$ hourly for 4–6 h, 1 hourly for 4–6 h and thereafter 4-hourly. Monitor urine output hourly and report if <30 ml/h
Wound bleeding, haematoma	Check blood results to ensure patient is not receiving excessive antgicoagulation. Observe wounds for bleeding/haematoma. Measure and record blood loss into drains and ensure vacuum is maintained
Graft occlusion due to 'kinking' of graft, inadequate size of vein graft, inadequate graft inflow/outflow due to poor anastomosis construction, arterial thrombus, trash foot from microthrombotic emboli, compartment syndrome, or a hypercoagulable state	Document hourly limb perfusion observations for 18 h, then 4-hourly for 48 h, thereafter daily. Observe colour, warmth, sensation, movement and locate pedal (DP/PT) pulses using Doppler. Report any deterioration/changes in foot observations – these could be sudden or gradual
Increase in limb pain due to limb ischaemia/onset of compartment syndrome	Assess pain regularly and ensure effective administration of patient controlled analgesia (PCA)/epidural or regular oral analgesia. Ensure effective use of PCA/epidural/oral analgesia Observe calf for swelling, tightness/shininess to the skin. Report uncontrolled or sudden increase of limb pain/swelling to doctor
Wound/graft infection	Remove wound dressing 48 h postoperatively and leave exposed if dry. Remove wound drain as instructed usually when <50 ml in 24 h. Observe exposed wounds each shift for signs of inflammation/

(contd)

Table 10.13 (contd)

Potential complications	Nursing observation and care
	erythema/exudate/breakdown or lymphatic leakage from groin. Check and record 4-hourly temperature. Special attention to groin hygiene is essential, especially in obese patients as the groin can become moist from perspiration and is more likely to become infected. Showers are advised after 48 h. Administration of prophylactic intravenous antibiotics required if prosthetic graft in situ. Remove sutures/staples 12–14 days after operation as directed
Chest infection	Liaise with physiotherapist Encourage early mobility and chest exercises/expectoration Monitor O_2 saturation levels for 24 h and administer humidified O_2 /nebulisers if required. (It is essential that the ischaemic limb receives maximum O_2 delivery via the new arterial blood supply)
Reperfusion oedema of limb – reduces capillary circulation and could occlude distal graft	Keep leg elevated to the level of the hip and on a foot stool whilst sitting out Discourage the patient from hanging limb out of the bed or sitting with knee bent (if graft extends below knee) Encourage/supervise limb/foot and ankle exercises
Deterioration in skin integrity/development of pressure sores	Observe sacrum, feet and heels 4-hourly, keep well moisturised and review pressure-relieving mattresses/heel pads. Ensure good foot care/hygiene is maintained Encourage foot/limb movement and early mobility as soon as patient is able Do not use adherent tape on ischaemic tissue as skin can be easily damaged upon dressing removal

Table 10.13 (contd)

Potential complications	Nursing observation and care
Reduced mobility (and associated complications)	Increase level of mobility daily: 24 h after operation the patient can usually sit out of bed with legs elevated to avoid oedema and below-knee graft occlusion and begin gentle, short distance mobilisation with assistance/supervision Review/provide suitable footwear to prevent foot damage Liaise with physiotherapist to assess patient and supervise walking. Encourage regular walks and assist with balance until confident Do not apply anti-embolic stockings unless directed by surgeon. These can cause further occlusion in atherosclerotic arteries Deep vein thrombosis is unlikely due to heparin intraoperatively and prophylactic subcutaneous heparin injections pre- and postoperatively

- Medication compliance – explain importance of taking medications, e.g. antiplatelet, lipid-lowering, diabetic and hypertensive therapy, and the need to reduce stress levels.
- Exercise guidelines – increasing distance gradually as tolerated.
- Dietary advice, e.g. diabetic, reducing/low fat.
- Follow-up outpatient/graft surveillance duplex appointments.
- Contact numbers, e.g. vascular nurse specialist/ward for direct patient referral if they have any concerns following discharge.

Postoperative complications

These can be defined as early and late onset complications (Table 10.12).

Graft surveillance programme

Duplex scanning, as discussed in Chapter 4, is recommended for all patients who have undergone limb bypass surgery to ensure early detection of failing bypass grafts. This will enable early treatment to avoid further complications. It is desirable to scan the graft prior to discharge, then repeat at 6 weeks, 3, 6 and 9 months, and thereafter annually.

Distal venous arterialisation

This is a new procedure in vascular surgery for limb-threatening distal vessel disease whereby patients with non-reconstructable arterial disease can be revascularised via the venous system (Taylor et al., 1999). Figures 10.6 (a and b) demonstrate wound healing following this type of surgery.

Upper extremity ischaemia

Acute

This is not as common as lower limb ischaemia due in part to extensive collateral circulation around the shoulder from the vertebral arteries. There are no randomised or controlled trials on acute arm ischaemia. However, it was found in a recent UK study reviewing data on acute arm ischaemia that the incidence of acute arm ischaemia is one-fifth that of acute leg ischaemia (Eyers and Ernshaw, 1998). Most patients were treated with embolectomy under local

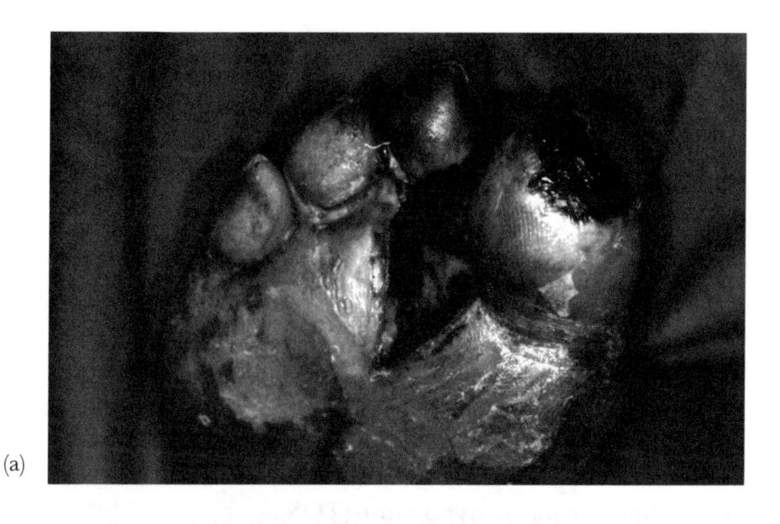

(a)

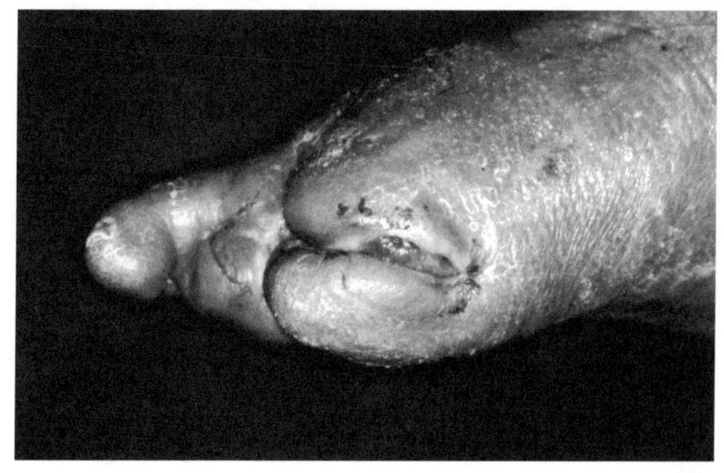

(b)

Figure 10.6 (a) Foot prior to distal venous arterialisation. (b) Healing foot following distal venous arterialisation. Courtesy of Mr R.S. Taylor, St George's Hospital, London. See Plate 10

anaesthetic and successful revascularisation was achieved in 65–94% of patients, with amputation rates of only 0–18%. Although local anaesthetic was largely used, the mortality rates ranging from 0 to 19% were due mostly to associated heart disease.

Pentti et al. (1995) reviewed 547 thrombectomies undertaken for acute upper limb ischaemia over a 26-year period and only 17.7% of these were for acute upper limb ischaemia, with an age range of 17–92 years. Main symptoms of the affected arm/hand included:

pulselessness (96%)
coldness (94%)
pain (85%)
paraesthesia (45%)
dysfunction (45%)

Coronary embolism was the main cause of occlusion in patients with local thrombus. The mortality rate following embolectomy was related to the patient's general condition (e.g. recurrent embolism), not to duration of ischaemia. The study suggests significantly better clinical results in upper limb ischaemia caused by embolism than by local thrombosis.

Chronic – thoracic outlet syndrome (TOS)

This is a relatively rare condition which is more common in young adults, especially females who are otherwise fit and healthy, and is caused by compression of the subclavian artery, vein or nerves (brachial plexus) at the point where they cross the first rib (Williams et al., 1994; MacVittie, 1998). Thoracic outlet syndrome can cause arterial post-stenotic dilatation, embolisation and acute arm claudication. Compression is often exacerbated upon arm elevation.

The compression can also be caused by a congenital cervical rib (bone or multiple fibrous bands), abnormal muscle formation following trauma, injury or a tumour (Williams et al., 1994; MacVittie, 1998). In many patients aetiological factors cannot be identified.

Presentation

This can be one or more of the following symptoms, which can be constant or intermittent, of varying severity and worse on arm elevation:

- Pain
  - dull ache from shoulder to arm and hand
  - neck pain
  - sharp pain in specific muscle groups.
- Numbness and paraesthesia
  - in hand/arm.

- Upper limb ischaemia
  - pallor.
- Weakness of upper arm and muscle wasting in the long term, e.g. difficulty in writing, gripping.
- Splinter haemorrhage of finger nails.

Patients with thoracic outlet syndrome are otherwise generally healthy.

Complications

As a result of disturbed blood flow in the subclavian artery, post-stenotic dilatation (i.e. aneurysm), thrombosis and embolism can occur. These can have potentially fatal consequences if left untreated.

Investigations to confirm diagnosis

- Positive Rous test – absent pulses on arm elevation and skin discoloration.
- Chest X-ray – to visualise cervical rib/cervical spine.
- Arch aortogram (either femoral or brachial access) or duplex – to examine blood flow with arm in different positions including hyperabduction.

Treatment

The aim is to restore arterial blood flow by decompression and surgery is not always the first choice of treatment. Conservative treatment is the first-line management of choice and includes the following:

- Physiotherapy – cervical traction, heat application, posture correction and exercise to elevate shoulder girdle.
- Activity restriction to avoid compression (avoidance of upper limb activity which may entail job retraining).
- Wrist/neck splints.
- Muscle relaxants.
- Avoidance of sleeping with arm above/under the head.
- Referral to pain clinics/and neurology opinion if required.

Surgical repair

This is indicated promptly for subclavian aneurysm, emboli and thrombus removal (with or without thrombolysis). Surgery is also reserved for those with severe incapacity, i.e. muscle wasting/pain where conservative therapy has failed to improve symptoms. First rib resection is now a rare operative procedure. It is accessed via a small incision (<6 cm) above the clavicle over the sternocleidomastoid muscle. The anterior scalene muscle is divided and after identification of the brachial plexus and subclavian artery the entire lower muscle attached to the first rib is removed. The first rib is then freed from any fibrous bands and excised with bone cutters.

Postoperative care and observations

- Limb perfusion observation – document presence/absence of brachial, radial and ulnar pulses.
- Respiratory monitoring – risk of pneumothorax – check if chest X-ray required.
- Observation of skin colour, temperature, swelling, movement of fingers and hands (risk of nerve damage).
- Support hand and arm at the same level as the heart. Avoid hyperabduction/extension of the arm.
- Wound care – observe for haematoma, haemorrhage.
- Early mobilisation.
- A support sling may be required once the patient is mobile.
- Postoperative physiotherapy – may require outpatient follow-up physiotherapy.
- Provide regular analgesia to permit limb movement and exercises.

Summary

Critical limb ischaemia requires prompt recognition to enable urgent specialist multidisciplinary care. The aim of assessment is to determine the site and likely cause of the occlusion, and coexisting medical and nursing problems. The aim of treatment is to revascularise the limb with appropriate percutaneous or operative intervention where possible. These patients are usually elderly and treatment carries considerable morbidity and mortality risks. Furthermore, these vulnerable patients may have many anxieties exacerbated by the threat of limb loss. Sensitive and skilled nursing care is therefore essential to enhance the patient's wellbeing.

References

Armon M, Yusuf S, Whitaker S, Gregson R, Wenham P, Hopkinson B (1997) Results of 100 cases of pulse spray thrombolysis for acute and subacute leg ischaemia. British Journal of Surgery 84(1): 47–50.

Benner P (1984) From Novice to Expert. California: Addison Wesley.

Berridge DC (1998) Peripheral arterial thrombolysis. Care of the Critically Ill 14(5): 172–175.

Berridge D, Makin G, Hopkinson B (1989) Local low dose intra-arterial thrombolytic therapy: the risk of stroke or major haemorrhage. British Journal of Surgery 76: 1230–1233.

Braithwaite B, Buckenham T, Galland RB, Heather BP, Earnshaw J (1997) Prospective randomised trial of high-dose bolus versus low-dose tissue plasminogen activator infusion in the management of acute limb ischaemia. British Journal of Surgery 84(5): 646–650.

Braithwaite B, Davies C, Birch PA, Heather BP, Earnshaw J (1998) Management of acute leg ischaemia in the elderly. British Journal of Surgery 85(2): 217–220.

Buckenham T (1994) Graft thrombolysis. In: Earnshaw JJ, Gregson RHS (eds) Practical Peripheral Arterial Thrombolysis. Oxford: Butterworth Heinemann.

Buckenham T (1998) Thrombolysis for acute limb ischaemia – a reliable recipe at last. RAD Magazine 24(272): 42.

Dawson K, Hamilton D (1994) Avoiding the complications of thrombolysis. In: Earnshaw JJ, Gregson RHS (eds) Practical Peripheral Arterial Thrombolysis. Oxford: Butterworth Heinemann.

European Working Group (1991) 2nd European Consensus Document on Critical Leg Ischaemia. Circulation (Suppl) 84(4).

Eyers P, Ernshaw J (1998) Acute non-traumatic arm ischaemia. British Journal of Surgery 85(10): 1340–1346.

Golledge J, Galland R (1995) Lower limb intra-arterial thrombosis (review). Postgraduate Medical Journal 71(883): 146–150.

Greenspan B, Pillari G, Schulman ML, Badhey M (1985) Percutaneous transluminal angioplasty of stenotic deep vein arterial bypass grafts. Archives of Surgery 120: 492–495.

Haiart D, Callam M, Murie J (1991) Vascular surgery in the elderly. Care of the Elderly 3(1): 23–26.

MacVittie BA (1998) Thoracic outlet surgery. In: Vascular Surgery – Perioperative Nursing Series. St Louis: Mosby-Yearbook.

Matsen FA (1980) Compartmental syndromes. Hospital Practice 15(2): 113–117.

McPherson GAD (1992) Acute ischaemia of the leg. In: Wolfe JH (ed.) ABC of Vascular Disease. London: British Medical Journal.

Mravic P, Massey D (1992) Compartment syndrome. Journal of Vascular Nursing 10(1): 9–11.

Murray S (1992) Caring for patients undergoing treatment for vascular occlusion. British Journal of Nursing 2(1): 17–19.

Payne J (1994) Vascular trauma. In: Fahey V (ed.) Vascular Nursing, 2nd edn. Philadelphia: WB Saunders.
Pentti J, Salenivis JP, Kuukasjarvi P, Tarkka M (1995) The outcome of surgical treatment in upper limb ischaemia. Annales Chirurgiae et Gynaecologie 84(1): 25–28.
Ronayne R (1985) Feelings and attitudes during early convalescence following vascular surgery. Journal of Advanced Nursing 10(5): 435–441.
STILE Trial (1994) Results of a prospective randomised trial evaluating surgery *versus* thrombolysis for ischemia of the lower extremity. Annals of Surgery 220(3): 251–268.
Taylor RS, Belli A-M, Jacob A (1999) Distal venous arterialisation for salvage of critically ischaemic inoperable limbs. Lancet 354: 1962–1965.
Weitz HH (1993) Cardiac risk stratification prior to vascular surgery. Medical Clinics of North America 77(2): 377–396.
Williams L, Lee J, Ekers M (1994) Upper arm extremity arterial problems. In: Fahey V (ed.) Vascular Nursing, 2nd edn. Philadelphia: WB Saunders.
Working party on thrombolysis in the management of limb ischaemia (1998) Thrombolysis in the management of lower limb peripheral arterial occlusion – a consensus document. American Journal of Cardiology 81: 207–218.
Yusuf SW, Whitaker SC, Gregson RH, Wenham PW, Hopkinson BR, Makin GS (1995) Immediate and early follow-up results of pulse spray thrombolysis in patients with peripheral ischaemia. British Journal of Surgery 2(3): 338–340.

Further reading

Buckenham T (1997) Thrombolysis for peripheral arterial occlusive disease: consensus or controversy? Interventional Radiology Monitor 1(2): 2–4.
Buckenham T, George CD, Chester JF, Taylor RS, Dormandy JA (1992) Accelerated thrombolysis using pulsed intrathrombus recombinant human tissue-type plasminogen activator. European Journal of Vascular Surgery 6: 237–240.
Dormandy JA, Ray S (1996) Natural history of peripheral arterial disease, In: Tooke JE, Lowe DO (eds) A Textbook of Vascular Medicine. London: Arnold.
Fahey V, McCarthy WJ (1994) Arterial reconstruction of the lower extremity In: Fahey V (ed.) Vascular Nursing, 2nd edn. Philadelphia: WB Saunders.
Palfreyman SJ, Michaels JA (1999) Vascular Surgical Society of Great Britain & Ireland: Systemic review of intraarterial thrombolytic therapy for peripheral vascular occlusions. British Journal of Surgery 86(5): 704.
Pederson WC (1997) Management of severe ischaemia of the upper extremity. Clinics in Plastic Surgery 21(1): 107–120.
Soong CV, Barros D'Sa AAB (1998) Lower limb oedema following arterial bypass grafting. European Journal of Vascular and Endovascular Surgery 16: 465–471.
The Vascular Surgical Society of Great Britain and Ireland (1995) Critical limb ischaemia: management and outcome. Report of national survey 10: 108–113.

Chapter 11

Lower Limb Amputation

SAMANTHA DONOHUE AND PENNY SUTTON-WOODS

Introduction

Lower limb amputation has decreased in incidence during the past half century, partly due to increased knowledge concerning the treatment of infection, but predominantly as the result of developments in vascular surgery and revascularisation techniques (Helt, 1994). However, vascular insufficiency paired with poorly controlled diabetes or infection still often necessitates amputation, so by providing information on health promotion and illness prevention to these patients, the vascular nurse has an important role in reducing the need for amputation (Donohue, 1997a).

This chapter will outline the causes of lower limb amputation and the factors to be considered when a decision to amputate is made, then review the method of level selection and the different types of amputation. It will discuss the pre- and postoperative care involved, including the patient's rehabilitation to as much functional independence as possible. Finally, the ethical issues concerning a patient's decision to refuse amputation will be briefly discussed.

Indications for lower limb amputation

Amputation results from a multitude of pathologies. In the past, most amputations were the result of trauma to the lower limb, but as the incidence of war casualties has diminished in the Western world, so the cause of amputations has altered. In Britain, amputations are now predominantly performed on people with irreversible tissue ischaemia caused by vascular disease, diabetes, or occasionally, infection (Ham and Cotton, 1991).

The indications for amputation can be divided into five broad categories: vascular disease; trauma; malignant disease; congenital limb deformity; and infection (Table 11.1).

Table 11.1 Approximate percentage of cause of lower limb amputation in developed world

Cause of lower limb amputation	Approx. %
Peripheral vascular disease (≈25–50% have diabetes mellitus)	85–90
Trauma	9
Malignant disease	4
Congenital limb deficiency	3
Infection	1

Peripheral vascular disease

Many amputees previously had longstanding arterial or venous problems, and may have had vascular reconstruction in the form of bypass surgery. It tends to be the coexistence of pathologies such as diabetes, rest pain, ischaemic ulceration and infection that indicates the need for an amputation (Donohue, 1997a).

It is estimated that one-third of dysvascular amputees die within 6 months of primary amputation mainly due to multisystem disease, one-third have a major amputation of the other leg within 2-3 years, and only one-third survive longer than 3 years with only the primary amputation (Dormandy and Ray, 1994).

Atherosclerosis

This is a gradual and progressive narrowing of the arteries which eventually leads to total occlusion, and is the most common reason for amputation. It is the primary cause of chronic arterial ischaemia, and accounts for more than half the deaths in the Western world (Ham and Cotton, 1991). Patients with atherosclerosis requiring amputation may initially present with *intermittent claudication* (see Chapter 9). *Rest pain* (see Chapter 6) may then develop, indicating severe tissue and nerve ischaemia, and characterised by a burning pain in the feet and toes. Local trauma may result in ischaemic ulceration and tissue necrosis. Ischaemic rest pain is often debilitating and indicates the need for an amputation if bypass surgery, or other radiological intervention such as angioplasty, is not possible.

Acute arterial occlusion

Acute arterial occlusion may be caused by an embolism, thrombosis, or trauma, which results in lower limb ischaemia (see Chapter 10), and is a limb-threatening and life-threatening situation. It differs from chronic occlusive disease in that there is no time for a sufficient collateral circulation to develop. Treatment such as surgical embolectomy or thrombolysis may fail, resulting in irreversible ischaemia and lower limb amputation.

Raynaud's disease

This predominantly affects women and is characterised by bilateral attacks of ischaemia, usually affecting the fingers and toes. The skin becomes pale and the sufferer experiences burning and pain in the digits. The disease rarely extends beyond the metacarpophalangeal joint, but in severe cases it can cause digital gangrene which requires amputation (see Chapters 2 and 9).

Arteritis

This is the inflammation of an artery and is often caused by an autoimmune response. Buerger's disease, or thromboangiitis obliterans, is one type of arteritis (Chapter 9). It is a rare condition which occurs predominantly in males under 50 years of age, and is thought to be caused by heavy smoking (Graham and Ford, 1994).

Venous disease

Leg ulceration, whether venous, arterial or of mixed aetiology, can cause immense discomfort and disability to the sufferer (see Chapter 7). Uncontrolled pain, unpleasant odour, infection, and the need for frequent dressing changes are all common complaints voiced by patients with ulcers. If the pain remains untreatable due to the mixed aetiology of the ulcers then amputation may be an option.

Diabetic vascular disease

Patients with diabetes mellitus are extremely susceptible to peripheral occlusive disease (see Chapter 2), and twenty years after their initial diagnosis, over 80% of diabetics have some form of vascular disease (Graham and Ford, 1994). Diabetics are more prone to lower limb lesions and ischaemia for many reasons, especially peripheral neuropathy, tissue perfusion, and atherosclerosis.

Peripheral neuropathy

In 1993 the Diabetes Control and Complications Trial (DCCT) demonstrated a clear connection between poorly controlled diabetes and the onset of peripheral neuropathy and decreased peripheral circulation. Peripheral neuropathy is characterised by the loss of proprioception and sensation in the peripheral tissues, which increases the risk of pedal trauma and of the injury going unnoticed. The healing of the lesion is impaired further by the increased risk of infection due to hyperglycaemia and decreased tissue perfusion (Donohue, 1997a).

Tissue perfusion

Diabetics are also vulnerable to peripheral tissue hypoxia as their circulating haemoglobin is prevented from delivering an adequate oxygen supply due to the accumulation of glucose on the blood cell, i.e. their glycosylated haemoglobin (HbA_{1c}) is raised.

Atherosclerosis

Diabetics tend to have a higher serum concentration of low density lipoproteins (LDLs) and a lower concentration of high density lipoproteins (HDLs) that carry the LDLs to the liver to be removed. The aetiology of vascular disease does not differ, but the prevalence is higher in diabetics.

Trauma

Amputation remains a life-saving procedure following industrial, farming and road traffic accidents (Ham and Cotton, 1991). Any accident can involve extensive burns, tissue destruction, vascular impairment, bone non-union, and neurological damage, and surgery is often required immediately with no time allowed for any psychological preparation. Since the development of rapid-freezing procedures it is now possible to implant severed limbs, but severe crush injuries tend to result in amputation.

Malignant disease

Approximately 3% of amputations are performed due to the presence of malignant tumours such as osteosarcoma (Herbert, 1997). These amputations are performed on a much younger age group as these tumours rarely occur after 20 years of age (Macleod, 1986).

Congenital limb deformity

Approximately one in every 1000 children in the West is born with a major deformity (Vitali et al., 1986). Of these, 63% have upper limb defects, 19% have lower limb defects, and 18% have bilateral defects. Lower limb amputation may be considered for children born with grossly deformed limbs if a prosthesis is deemed suitable for future use.

Infection

Hyperglycaemia causes tissue hypoxia, changes in the body's glycoproteins, nutritional changes, and generally impairs healing in infected limb lesions (Faris, 1991). Consequently, diabetic patients are extremely prone to all types of uncontrolled infection, whether the infection is a localised lesion, diffuse infection such as cellulitis, or systemic infection. Ischaemic ulceration often leads to gangrene, and a patient with gas gangrene will exhibit the typical signs of infection, with a foetid odour to the wound and a coppery discolouring of the skin. Once this occurs, the primary task is to minimise damage by removing the necrotic, infected tissue and administering broad-spectrum antibiotics, and the limb will require immediate amputation. On X-ray, gas gangrene shows up as bubbles of air, which may be felt when touching the subcutaneous tissues. Scrupulous care with hygiene should be taken with patients post-amputation, as faecal contamination of the stump wound will increase the risk of infection. Prophylactic antibiotics are usually advocated, predominantly penicillin and metronidazole (Campbell, 1982). Cefuroxime can be given if the microorganism is resistant to penicillin, or if the patient has an allergy (Donohue, 1997a).

The decision to amputate

Once it has been decided that the only possible surgery is amputation, there are a number of factors to consider. Of prime importance is that the patient and his/her family feel psychologically and physiologically prepared for the operation, and understand the necessity for amputation and its implications for the future.

It is essential to emphasise that amputation is not considered to be the result of 'failure' of medical interventions, but should be viewed as the most effective means of relieving the pain and suffering that a patient may have been living with for years (Donohue, 1997b).

Some patients see amputation as a positive step towards achieving some kind of quality of life for the first time in years, whilst others take a different view. For example, a patient with a long history of non-healing, painful ulcers, may view amputation as a means of going out in public for the first time in years without worrying about the pain or the smell of the ulcers. Conversely, a patient who has spent the past 10 years with progressively worsening chronic ischaemia, undergoing multiple operations, may view amputation as the last stage before death, and may have spent these years dreading the moment when amputation would be necessary (Donohue, 1997b).

The next decision to be made is the optimal level of amputation.

Level selection

The primary object of limb amputation is to remove sufficient diseased, infected and gangrenous tissue to allow the stump to heal, whilst at the same time retaining adequate limb length for a prosthesis (Ham and Cotton, 1991). The level of amputation chosen should provide a residual limb that is suitable for prosthetic fitting, function, and cosmesis, and this may mean performing a higher level of amputation than is required simply to remove dead tissue. Amputations should not be performed by relatively junior medical staff, but by a skilled vascular surgeon, because if an incorrect level of amputation is selected or the stump is not formed sufficiently, then the fitting of any prosthesis will be problematic.

A variety of techniques may be used to predict the optimum level of amputation, e.g. angiography, segmental ankle brachial pressure indices, laser Doppler flowmetry (see Chapter 4). However, Helt

(1994) believes that none of these tests have proved to be consistently more reliable than clinical judgement in predicting wound healing at a given level.

The most successful method appears to be combining functional tests with simple examination of the limb for ulceration and skin friability, assessment of the general state of the patient and the possibility of a prosthesis, and ascertainment of the patient's wishes. Preservation of the knee joint where possible gives far greater success with functional prosthetic use, provided that the joint is functional preoperatively. Indeed the increase in oxygen consumption varies almost exponentially with the level of amputation (Huang et al., 1979; Murray and Fisher, 1982) (Table 11.2 and Figure 11.1).

Table 11.2 Increase in oxygen consumption during ambulation

Level of amputation	Increased oxygen Consumption (%)
Transtibial (BKA)	9–20
Transfemoral (AKA)	45–70
Bilateral AKA	280
Hip disarticulation	>300

BKA, below-knee amputation; AKA, above-knee amputation.

Foot and partial foot amputation

Auto-amputation has been documented in the writings of the ancient Greeks (Helt, 1994). The gangrenous part of the limb demarcates, and once mummified, falls off. Auto-amputation of digits is still promoted provided there is no secondary infection present. The main amputations of the foot are Ray, transmetatarsal and Syme's (Figure 11.2).

- Ray amputation. This is the amputation of an individual toe with its corresponding metatarsal. Amputation of the first ray (hallux) will cause the patient to weight-bear on the lateral border of the foot, which may result in breakdown and ulceration of the skin. Amputation of any other ray will leave the foot fairly stable, and is usually more successful.

- Midtarsal amputation (Chopart): This is the disarticulation between the talus and calcaneous proximally, and the navicular and cuboid distally.
- Tarso-metatarsal amputation (Lisfranc): This is the disarticulation of the forefoot at the tarso-metatarsal line. These amputations are now very rarely carried out other than for severe crush injury or frostbite of the digits.
- Transmetatarsal: This involves amputation of the toes, proximal to the metatarsal heads (Figure 11.3). After an initial period, weight bearing on the amputated foot can be achieved.
- Syme's amputation: This involves a disarticulation of the ankle joint, normally at the lower end of the tibia. This level of amputation is rarely used today, as a below-knee level allows better prosthesis use. It was previously used in trauma surgery, for congenital shortening of the leg, or in the presence of chronic infection of the foot, with the amputee able to use a prosthesis for weight bearing.

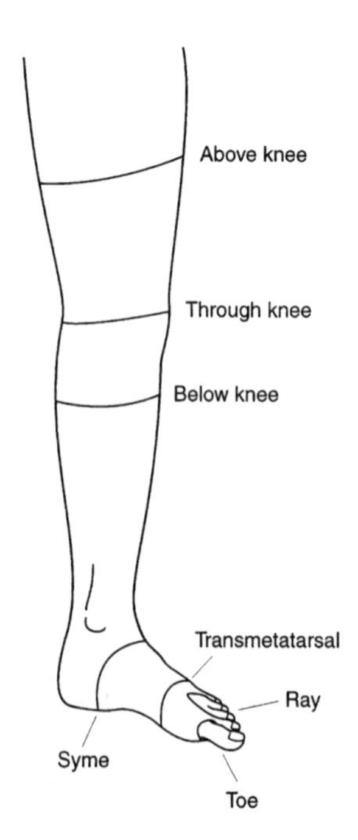

Figure 11.1 Levels of lower limb amputation.

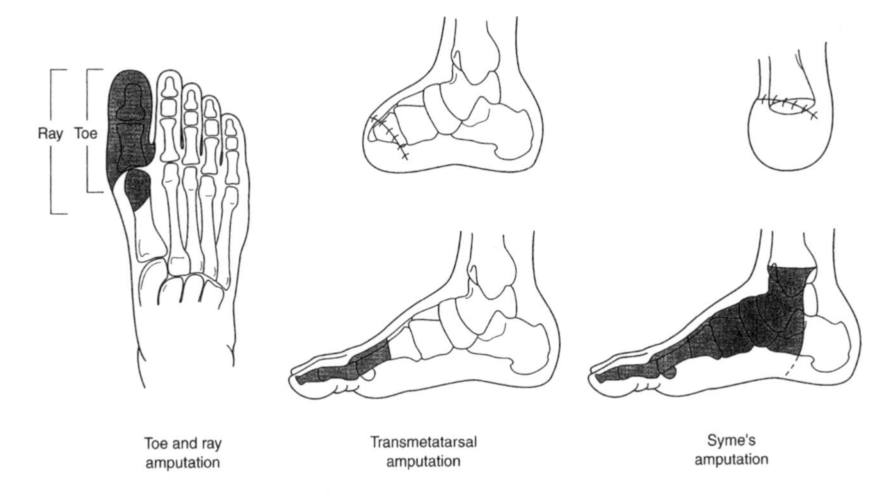

Figure 11.2 Levels of foot amputation.

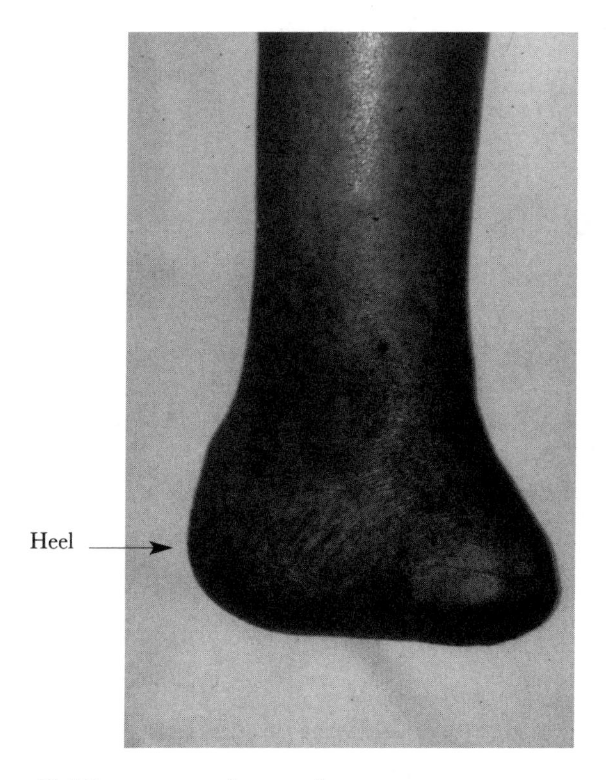

Figure 11.3 Transmetatarsal amputation.

Transtibial or below-knee amputation

The below-knee amputation (BKA) (Figure 11.4) is often favoured, as the preservation of the knee joint allows the amputee to gain as near normal a gait pattern as is possible with a prosthesis. It has been stated that two to three times as many BK amputees achieve full mobility with a prosthesis compared to AK amputees (Dormandy et al., 1999). The effectiveness of a long posterior flap in the BKA was popularised in the 1970s by Burgess (1968). He also highlighted the fact that a poorly designed flap resulted in a deformed stump, and that the ensuing pressure and ulceration caused problems with the prosthesis.

Robinson advocated the skew flap method, which is now predominantly used. By positioning the join of the flap obliquely, the tibial crest is covered by gastrocnemius muscle and the blood supply to the flap is maximised (Robinson et al., 1982). Ideally the BKA stump is fashioned 14 cm distal to the tibial plateau; if the stump is under 8 cm there will be a problem fitting a prosthesis (Naylor, 1995). Other techniques can be used, with some surgeons dividing the tibia into thirds, leaving the upper third, whereas others amputate at the largest diameter of the calf.

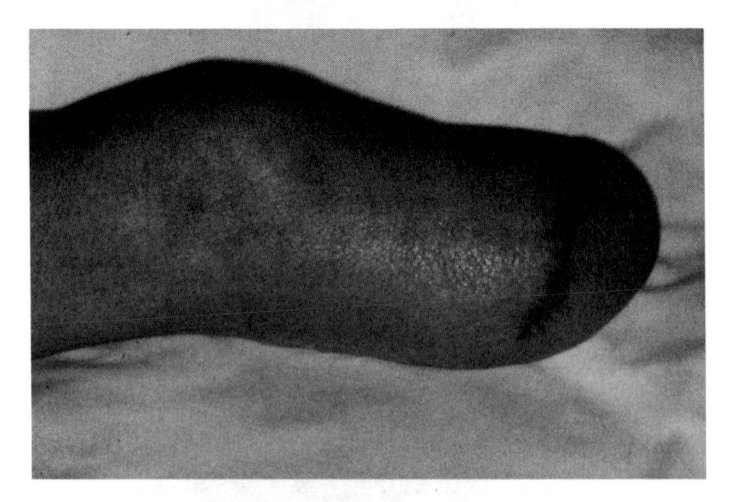

Figure 11.4 Below-knee amputation.

Knee disarticulation or through-knee amputation

A through-knee amputation (TKA) or knee disarticulation, is a rapid and relatively less traumatic amputation, as no bone needs to be cut.

The TKA tends to be used when expectations of postoperative mobility are limited. The patella is preserved, and the patellar tendon is sutured to the hamstring tendons and cruciate ligaments around the end of the femur. The residual limb allows the fitting of a prosthesis, although cosmesis is often unacceptable as the knee joint line appears more distal compared to the other leg, with a short shin. Where mobility is not an option, the long residual limb aids good sitting balance in the wheelchair.

Gritti-Stokes amputation

This amputation involves transecting the femur above the adductor tubercles, and attaching the patella over the end of the cut femur in order to allow weight bearing. However, as the union of the fracture takes a long time and the distal end of the femur often retracts, this level of amputation is now rarely used.

Transfemoral or above-knee amputation

The above-knee amputation (AKA) (Figure 11.5) is often the only option for patients with few viable arteries below the knee joint due to long-term peripheral vascular disease. The thigh is divided into thirds, with the distal third being removed. Ideally the AKA stump should have a gap of 13 cm between the distal end of the stump and the natural knee joint line. This will avoid the prosthetic knee

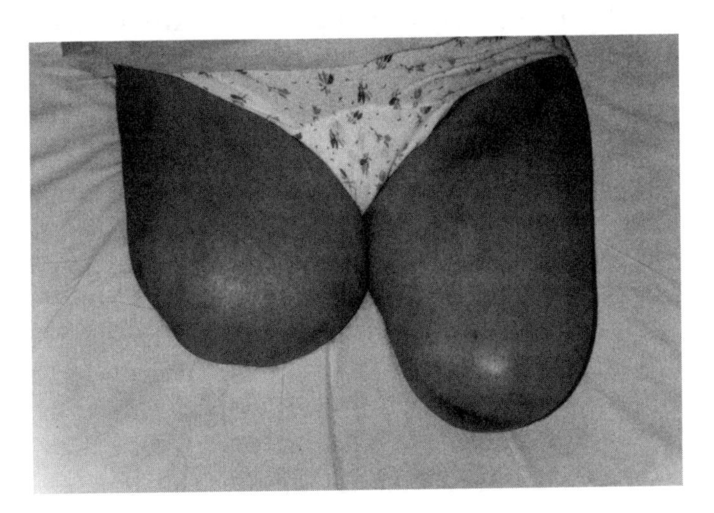

Figure 11.5 Bilateral above-knee amputee.

component protruding when sitting. The stump has anterior and posterior flaps that are equal in length, and the femur is sculptured and smoothed before the muscles are sutured together. The arteries and veins are ligated separately to allow the maximum number of collateral vessels to survive. A suction drain is normally inserted to prevent haematoma formation. Intensive physiotherapy is essential to avoid hip flexion, as greater than 25 degrees of hip flexion seriously limits the provision of a prosthesis.

There is a higher mortality rate for this level of amputation than for more distal levels (Dormandy and Ray, 1994), and even when successful, mobility with an artificial knee joint requires a much higher oxygen consumption than normal (see Table 11.2).

Hip disarticulation (hind quarter)

This amputation is generally only performed for malignant tumours in the lower limb, or as a life-saving operation. The wound is anterior to avoid faecal contamination, and it is essential that the patient be catheterised and given intravenous antibiotic cover both pre- and postoperatively. Mobility using a prosthesis is a possibility but is slow, difficult, and energy consumption is exceptionally high (see Table 11.2). Every effort must be made by the multidisciplinary team to avoid contracture of the hip, infection and breakdown of the wound.

Pre- and postoperative care of the lower limb amputee

Limb amputation is ideally a planned procedure, with the preoperative period allowing the nurse and other members of the multidisciplinary team to carry out a full assessment of the physiological, psychological and social preparation required by the patient. The postoperative period is a time when the multidisciplinary team work together to fulfil these needs. The multidisciplinary teams are interdependent, and communication between the teams is essential to the wellbeing of the amputee (Figure 11.6).

The preoperative role of the nurse

The nurse's role is central to the patient's care and the preoperative nursing assessment is concerned with the physiological and

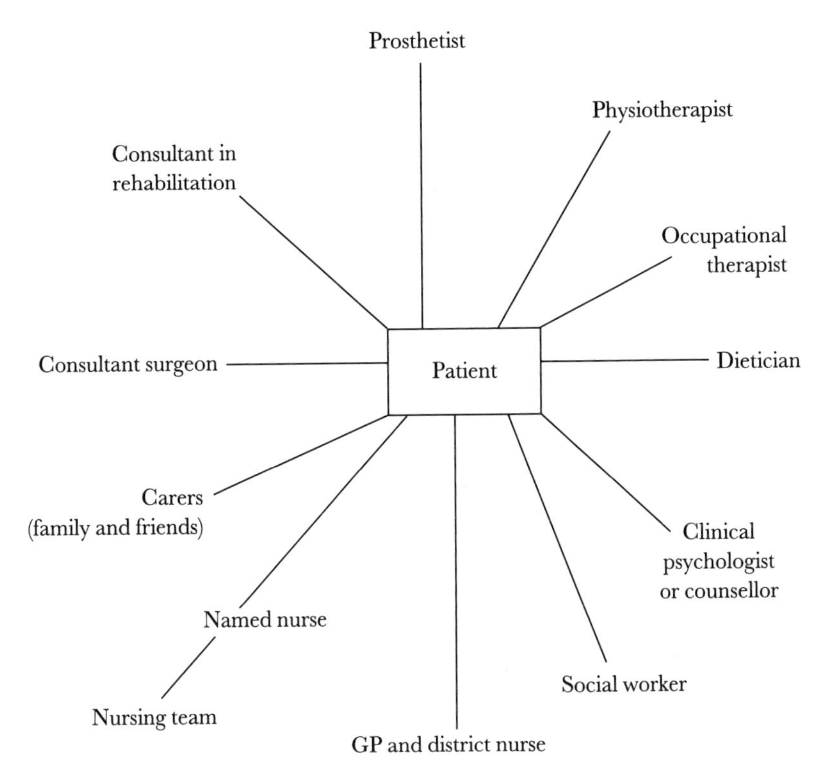

Figure 11.6 Clinical services and support available to the amputee.

psychological status of the patient, their social situation, home environment and available help.

Physiological Assessment

Patients awaiting amputation are usually physiologically unprepared for an operation because of the coexistence of other pathologies. This may be due to generalised cardiovascular and/or respiratory disease, infection, uncontrolled diabetes mellitus, poor nutritional status, pain, and immobility.

Cardiovascular and respiratory stability

The anaesthetist, medical team and physiotherapist will perform a full cardiovascular and respiratory assessment of the patient preoperatively. Hypertension, atrial fibrillation, chronic obstructive pulmonary disease, coronary heart disease and renal failure are common complications in patients awaiting amputation. To ascertain whether any of the complications can be minimised preoperatively, regular and accurate observations of blood pressure, pulse, fluid and electrolyte balance, respiratory rate and oxygen saturation should be recorded by the nurse.

Infection

The level of the amputation will be affected by the extent of infected tissue (Helt, 1994). Infection may be localised to a lesion, diffuse (e.g. cellulitis) or systemic. The nurse can monitor the progression of infection by observing the limb regularly and documenting any changes in appearance, warmth, sensation and movement, as well as monitoring for a pyrexia and hyperglycaemia. Preoperative intravenous antibiotics may be necessary to control infection prior to surgery, as ischaemic gangrene may develop rapidly into a life-threatening condition due to circulating toxins causing septicaemia. It is not unusual for a patient awaiting amputation to become acutely confused secondary to infection, and this indicates the need for immediate surgery.

Diabetic control

Diabetic patients undergoing vascular surgery are likely to have endocrine instability as a result of infection and pain. They also tend to have poor nutritional intake as their appetite has been suppressed by their physical condition (Holmes, 1996). The nurse plays an essential part in assessing the patient's diabetic control and the optimum blood glucose level prior to surgery is between 4 and 10 mmol/l (Marshall, 1996). Fasting times will vary in different centres, but should be determined by research-based practice, and patients should be allowed to drink clear fluids until 2-3 hours prior to surgery (Chapman, 1996). Occasionally surgery will be needed before optimum blood glucose levels are achieved, and a titrated intravenous infusion of insulin and glucose may be needed preoperatively instead of the patient's normal regimen of insulin or oral hypoglycaemic drugs. The nurse should inform the medical and anaesthetic staff of the patient's blood glucose levels prior to theatre so that the levels can be closely monitored perioperatively. Generally, diabetic patients normally controlled on insulin or oral hypoglycaemics will require a dextrose and insulin sliding scale regimen postoperatively until they are able to resume their normal diet.

Nutritional intake

The patient's nutritional intake may be adversely affected by pain, and the nurse, who has a key responsibility in pre-empting malnutrition (UKCC, 1997), should work closely with the dietician, the patient and his/her family in an effort to replete a patient's energy stores prior to surgery. Malnutrition slows down healing, and increases the risk of postoperative infection. The dietician may discuss food preferences with the patient and can provide a high protein diet and recommend suitable supplement drinks.

Pain control

Many patients awaiting an amputation experience uncontrolled pain, and may be prescribed opiates, such as oral morphine (Sevredol) or slow release morphine, in an attempt to control the pain (see Chapter 6). Adequate pain control is often difficult to achieve due to the severity of the pain, yet without it patients will find it extremely difficult to prepare themselves psychologically and socially for the amputation. The sensitivity of the ischaemic limb cannot be overemphasised as even the weight of a sheet can cause unbearable discomfort. Bed cradles should be used to alleviate pressure, and keeping the limb warm will promote reflex vasodilatation.

It has been widely documented that there is a difference in pain perception between the patient and the nurse (Seers, 1987; Field, 1996), and that verbal and non-verbal signals of pain should be used to ascertain the severity of the pain, with many pain assessment tools being available (Schofield, 1995). There is a correlation between the use of preoperative prophylactic pain relief and decreased post-amputation pain (Diamond and Coniam, 1991), and Bach et al. (1988) found that a preoperative epidural block correlated with a reduction in phantom limb pain (Chapter 6).

Immobility

Pressure sores, chest infection, deep vein thrombosis, constipation and sensory deprivation can pose significant problems pre- and post-amputation (Rubin, 1988). An ischaemic limb may render a person more immobile before the amputation than afterwards. The nurse is responsible for assessing the patient's risk of developing pressure sores using scores such as the Waterlow score (Waterlow, 1988), and for selecting a suitable pressure-relieving mattress (see Chapter 5). Some types of alternating pressure mattresses are not suitable for amputees, and the manufacturers' instructions should be consulted.

If the amputation is a planned procedure, the ward physiotherapist will assess the patient's normal and/or current mobility, and discuss the exercise regimen that will start on the first day following the amputation.

Psychological assessment

The nurse should view the psychological preparation of the patient and family as a priority. It is the nurse's responsibility to assess the extent of psychological preparation that is needed and what form it should take. Swindale (1989) documented that postoperative anxiety was reduced by giving preoperative information, and many patients have commented that they feel more able to cope with surgery if they understand what to expect, rather than fearing the 'unknown'.

Each patient will have different psychological needs and the needs themselves will be dynamic and constantly changing. Some patients will appear confident in their decision, anxious only for their partners/family, whereas others will see the amputation as the loss of their autonomy, being viewed as an 'amputee', not as a person. Any person facing an amputation will also face an alteration in their body image. Body image is neither a motionless nor simplistic concept; the external environment alters the way we see ourselves and we often utilise various coping strategies, both consciously and unconsciously, to cope with this alteration (Salter, 1988). Price (1990) developed a body-image care model where the body reality (how the body really exists), the body ideal (how we would prefer our body to look) and the body presentation (how we present our body to the outside world) are three equal components. A satisfactory body image is dependent on the equilibrium of these three components, and when the equilibrium is threatened we use our environment, social networks, and additional coping mechanisms to help facilitate a positive response to circumstances. For example, when our body ideal and body reality are different, we utilise coping mechanisms to find a mean body presentation that we are comfortable with. However, physiological changes such as the amputation of a limb do not allow the body reality and body presentation to be manipulated, and the body-image equilibrium is disrupted.

The attribution of causes of the altered body image plays an important part in the individual's recovery, and the nature and intensity of their grief is seen to depend largely on to whom, or to what, the individual attributes the cause of the physiological changes (Abramson and Martin, 1981). For example, if a patient attributes the amputation to a cause that was 'not their fault', they are likely to be bitter. In contrast, a patient whose amputation is attributed to peripheral vascular disease secondary to a refusal to give up smoking may accept responsibility in causing the amputation (Donohue, 1997c).

Preoperatively, an assessment by the nurse of the person's present body image and self-esteem is important. A patient may already have an altered body image due to uncontrolled pain, non-healing ulcers or a previous limb amputation, but they will still experience further body-image alteration, and should still be assisted in the preparation for the loss of a limb. An assessment by the nurse of a patient's support systems is useful to help predict their ability to cope with the forthcoming operation. If a patient fears the responses of others to their altered body reality, then an empathetic response by close family and friends will be important. If those significant others are included in preoperative discussions concerning the surgery, they are more likely to provide that empathetic response and to assist in the redevelopment of a satisfactory body image (Price, 1990). The presence of other amputees on the ward can often be useful, as they demonstrate established coping strategies. Some people have the confidence to talk to other patients and to share their fears and experiences, others may rely on the nurse to approach the possibility of discussing experiences with other amputees rather than instigate it themselves (Donohue, 1997c). Every person's ability to cope with situations differs, and being able to identify the patient's individual needs helps the nurse to formulate an effective care plan.

Social assessment

Although the social assessment does not stand apart from the physical and psychological assessment, the nurse should ascertain specific facts regarding the patient's home environment, support from relatives/carers/social services, place and type of work, and leisure activities in order to formulate a care pathway and discharge plan. A successful discharge is one that allows the patient to return to a life that is as near as, or better than, pre-admission. As a large number of lower limb amputations are due to peripheral vascular disease, many patients have an extremely poor life expectancy (Dormandy and Ray, 1994), and it is unacceptable to waste any time due to a poorly planned discharge. Communication with the occupational therapist and physiotherapist to ascertain how they feel the patient will cope following the amputation is integral to the discharge plan. Many homes will need alterations to allow wheelchair access, and if the person lives alone or their home is not wheelchair accessible, then the social work team will need to be involved. The social work team will also be able to give financial advice concerning social security benefits and allowances that may be available.

Postoperative role of the nurse

After the amputation, the nurse's care plan should identify and address the physical, psychological, and social needs of the patient, and as part of the multidisciplinary team, the nurse will help address these in the discharge plan.

Physiological needs

During the initial postoperative period, the nursing needs of an amputee are similar to any other patient. Haemodynamic stability including respiratory and renal function, diabetic control, pain control, wound and pressure area care remain the postoperative concerns of the nurse. The nurse should also communicate with the physiotherapist and occupational therapist concerning any mobility or personal activities that they are practising with the patient, in order to carry over the practice in the ward setting.

Haemodynamic stability

The amount of blood lost during the operation differs according to the level of the amputation. A through-knee amputation is a relatively bloodless amputation, whereas a below- or above-knee amputation will have more effect on haemodynamic stability. Regular monitoring of the patient's blood pressure, pulse, respiratory rate, oxygen saturation and urinary output should occur, with the parameters being similar to any other postoperative condition. Intravenous hydration will continue until the patient is tolerating fluid and diet adequately. Below- and above-knee amputees usually return from theatre with a suction drain in the wound to avoid haematoma formation in the stump. The drain is normally sited, but not sutured, in a place that allows it to be removed without disturbing the bandages.

Diabetic control

Once the patient can tolerate an adequate diet they should return to their normal regimen of insulin or oral hypoglycaemic tablets. However, the nurse should continue to monitor the blood glucose levels closely, as the patient may still become hypoglycaemic following trauma of surgery, and hyperglycaemia delays wound healing.

Pain control

The pain experienced following an amputation may scare and confuse patients, with the altered sensations being attributed to a loss of sanity, and therefore constant explanation and reassurance is essential. It is important that patients are alerted to the possibility of experiencing phantom limb pain and sensation (Wilson, 1994). In order to help control the pain and support those experiencing it, all healthcare professionals caring for people undergoing lower limb amputation should understand the various pain responses to surgery (see Chapter 6).

The initial pain experienced post-amputation differs from the ischaemic pain experienced prior to surgery. Because of tissue damage and neurological disturbance during surgery, the pain is acute and is often termed *stump pain*. Stump pain can often be successfully relieved by the use of opiates, non-steroidal anti-inflammatory agents and local anaesthetics. The current treatment choices for phantom limb pain and sensation tend to combine tricyclic antidepressants such as carbamazepine, and anticonvulsant drugs such as sodium valproate, with non-invasive stimulatory techniques such as TENS (transcutaneous electrical nerve stimulation). *Phantom limb pain* is literally pain experienced in the limb that has been amputated, and is often described as a crushing, tearing pain. It has been described as one of the worst clinical pain syndromes (Melzack and Wall, 1995) and its true cause is poorly understood. The episodes of pain may differ in intensity and frequency and may cease after a short period or continue indefinitely (Diamond and Coniam, 1991). In one study, 60% of amputees were still experiencing phantom limb pain 7 years after their amputation (Krebs et al., 1984). *Phantom limb sensation* is not pain, but a sensation that is experienced. Jensen and Rasmussen (1994) have divided the clinical characteristics of phantom limb sensation into three categories: simple sensations (touch, itching and heat); more complex sensations (limb length, posture and size); and limb movement (spontaneous or willed movements). Initially, the illusory limb may appear identical to the amputated limb, and then gradually shrink or become distorted and grotesque (Chapman, 1986).

In order to distinguish between stump pain, phantom limb pain and phantom limb sensation, the nurse can use pain assessment charts to obtain comprehensive information concerning the type, location and intensity of the pain, not simply quantitative symptomatic information, i.e. blood pressure, pulse and respiratory rate. However, pain assessment charts rely on the individual's ability to verbalise their pain (Mackintosh, 1994), and culture, gender and age all affect expression of pain (Seers, 1987).

Inadequate pain control correlates with poor postoperative pain relief, respiratory and cardiovascular complications, and restricted postoperative mobilisation (Hollinworth, 1994), and if the pain persists for longer than 6 months, it is generally difficult to treat (Davis, 1993). Chapter 6 may be referred to for a more detailed description of pain control methods.

The wound

The flap of the stump is normally sutured using a continuous suture, which should not be removed until at least 12-14 days postoperatively. Some surgeons prefer to use clips but Galvani (1997) states that using clips has been correlated with a higher incidence of wound pain. The bandages surrounding the stump help to shape the stump and reduce oedema. Some vascular units leave the bandages intact for up to 5 days unless there is significant rationale for their removal, i.e. haemorrhage, odour or staining; others change them for a tubular retention bandage, e.g. Tubifast™ once the wound drain is removed. Usually, the blue-line Tubifast™ is applied to a below-knee stump, and the yellow-line Tubifast™ is applied to an above-knee amputation. However, if the patient has a below-knee stump with a very wide girth, the blue-line Tubifast™ may cause too much compression with subsequent ischaemia or mis-shaping of the stump. The nurse should therefore assess the patient's stump before applying the Tubifast™. Transmetatarsal amputations tend to have individual sutures/clips along the wound, or they may be left open to heal by secondary intention, or have a skin graft applied at a later date to aid healing (see Chapter 14).

Hypovolaemia and malnutrition can prevent the wound from healing and may necessitate revision of the stump to a higher level. This is yet another indication of the importance of the nurse's role in assessing and addressing any nutritional and fluid imbalance.

Psychological needs

Postoperatively, the amputee may wish to conceal the stump with bedding or clothing until they feel that they can cope with viewing the limb. The altered body part should be referred to as the 'residual limb' and not as 'your bad leg'. The patient should be given privacy to investigate the limb and to express their feelings, and only when they are ready will they begin to acknowledge the changes that have occurred and become more inquiring about the future (Donohue, 1997c). Price (1990) suggests that body-image sustenance and development is best achieved within a supportive social support framework. A 'normal body' is first formed in such networks, and these allow an altered body image to be integrated into society.

One of the roles of the nurse is to encourage both the patient and their family to express their true feelings (Helt, 1994). All healthcare professionals need to be truthful and non-judgemental, yet help facilitate rehabilitation goals by guiding the person through recovery. A trusting, truthful relationship that involves realistic appraisal and ongoing evaluation of progress is essential, and the integration with other amputees, and engaging in activities where others are present, is an important step. A person who has undergone such a major alteration in their body image is not going to possess a fully constructed body image by the time they leave hospital.

Social needs

Ideally, the discharge process should have commenced prior to surgery and the nurse should have already liaised with the patient, carer and professionals both within the hospital and community. The occupational therapist will assess the patient's ability to perform activities of daily living (ADLs) such as cooking, and personal ADLs such as washing and dressing. They will practise wheelchair mobility, and visit the patient's home (often without the patient) to identify any particular problems such as inaccessible rooms, and any equipment required before discharge. Family and carers may approach the nurse with questions concerning discharge home and the future. Documenting discussions, information given and unmet needs will allow the nursing team to achieve continuity in their care.

Mobility

The physiotherapist will see the amputee the day after surgery to prevent postoperative respiratory complications, and will normally begin an exercise programme to prevent the development of joint contractures and other complications associated with immobility. The physiotherapist will work with the amputee to teach them how to develop the strength in the amputated limb, their remaining limb and their upper body. If the amputee is not physically able to begin gentle exercise, then the physiotherapist will initially help the patient to perform the activities, then progress to the patient doing it themselves, and finally to the patient exercising against resistance to increase their strength.

Sitting out in a wheelchair on the first or second day postoperatively will help to improve the person's confidence in their independence and their future, but the first time they get out of bed will be traumatic unless they receive adequate explanations and reassurance (Andrews, 1996). Many amputees are nursed on an alternating cell mattress to avoid the development of pressure sores, which often makes independent movement from bed to wheelchair difficult. Deflating the mattress enables the person to move across the mattress with minimum energy expenditure, as can the use of a 'transfer' or 'sliding-board'. Standing and hopping are not recommended, as the remaining foot may have fragile tissue viability and break down. Transmetatarsal amputees will require a soft-infill in their shoes, which may be measured and supplied by the orthotics department of the hospital, or by the local limb-fitting centre. For other amputees, a temporary wheelchair is provided on the first day after the amputation to allow the patient to be mobile until a permanent wheelchair has been delivered. A pressure-relieving cushion will be provided, and the patient will be taught how to 'hip-hitch' whilst seated to help relieve pressure on their ischial tuberosities. All amputees who have a below- or through-knee amputation must have a stump board fitted to their wheelchair, so that the stump is supported at all times. This prevents dependent oedema of the residual limb, which may cause the wound to break down, or form a stump shape that is difficult to fit with a prosthesis. If an above-knee stump is very short, and is fully supported by the seat cushion, the occupational therapist may decide that a stump board is not necessary. The position of the wheels differs according to the level of the amputation, with bilateral above-knee amputees having set-back wheels to compensate for the change in their centre of gravity and prevent the wheelchair from tipping backwards.

In the early stages of rehabilitation, the wheelchair will be the only method of mobility, but from day 5 to 7 postoperatively, provided the surgeon has given permission, the physiotherapist may start the patient walking with an early walking aid such as the Ppam aid™ (Pneumatic post-amputation mobility aid; Vessa Limited). This can be used with the sutures/clips still in place, but is only a partial weight-bearing device, and should only be used with supervision, usually with the physiotherapist (Figure 11.7).

Transmetatarsal amputations will require the person to be non-weight-bearing for up to 5 days. They can move from bed to chair, but will only be able to use their heel to weight-bear through. The physiotherapist may give a walking frame to enable the patient to 'heel walk' and remain mobile, but the patient must be mentally alert enough to remember not to fully weight-bear.

Assessment for lower limb prosthesis

Early referral to the Prosthetic Rehabilitation Service (which may be a satellite clinic within the hospital, or a regional specialist prosthetic service) is essential for amputees that are anticipated to make an uneventful recovery from surgery. Written referral can be made using a form AOF3 or a local referral form, and should be sent before the sutures are removed. By the time the first appointment

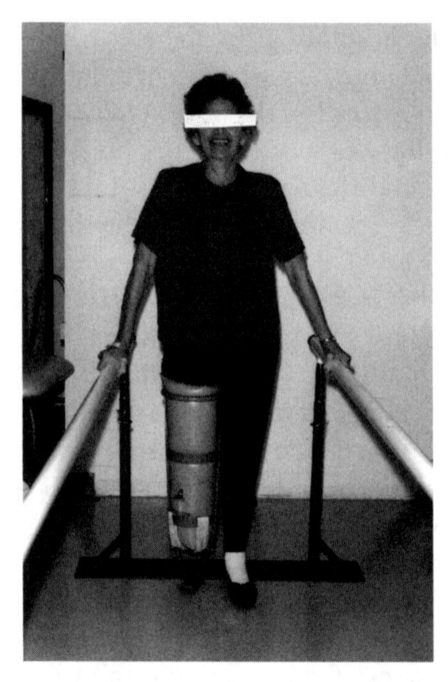

Figure 11.7 Below-knee amputee using Ppam aid for early mobility.

date arrives, the patient should be independent in dressing and transferring, and able to tolerate a full day's activity.

Before referring a patient for prosthetic fitting, the nurse should ensure that it is appropriate. Due to the high energy-expenditure of walking with a prosthesis (Table 11.2) it is inappropriate to refer a patient with severe cardiac or respiratory dysfunction, or frailty. The patient must be able to remember and carry out instructions, *want* to walk, be *able* to walk, and show that quality of life will be improved by having a walking prosthesis. Another option, for psychological benefit, is a 'cosmetic' prosthesis that is fixed to the wheelchair footrest in order to present a 'whole body' image.

Blindness and stroke, pre-existing or postoperatively, are not absolute contraindications to a prosthesis, but the patient must be assessed by the physiotherapist and the prosthetic rehabilitation service.

Discharge advice

The patient should be given information and advice on care of the remaining limb/foot and care of the stump, and how to reduce their risk factors of developing or exacerbating peripheral vascular disease. Patients should be advised to stop smoking although some amputees will continue to smoke despite their future health risks. Diabetics or those who have difficulty caring for their feet, should be referred to a chiropodist because of the increased risk of peripheral lacerations. Relatives/carers should also be given information on how to care for the stump and the remaining limb. Information such as the addresses of the local prosthetic service, the local Limbless Association, and the name and contact number of the therapists should be given prior to discharge. Although any member of the multidisciplinary team may carry out these tasks, the nurse should check that it has been given, and document it in the discharge checklist.

Ethical considerations

To many people an amputation offers an escape from the pain, infection and disability that has been affecting their quality of life for many years, and for them the advantages far outweigh the disadvantages. However, what if someone decides that their quality of life is so poor that they prefer the thought of death to continuing life as an amputee? A person refusing treatment when the alternative prognosis is death generates conflicting attitudes and beliefs between their family, carers and the healthcare professionals (Donohue, 1997d). The ethical principles are outlined briefly below, but have been discussed in depth by Donohue, (1997d), to which the reader is directed.

The sanctity of life

For many people the basic law of ethics is that 'human beings should revere life and accept death' (Tschudin, 1986), and all other ethical principles should be considered in relation to the preservation of life. The Suicide Act 1961 (UK) concedes that although a person may take their own life, others are not allowed to withhold treatment or otherwise assist in order to end their life.

Lowe (1997) states that it is important to differentiate between 'killing' and 'allowing to die', and says that according to current legal opinion 'a medically competent patient, fully understanding the consequences of refusing life-preserving drugs may refuse to take them even though his death must be the natural outcome'. An example of this could be a person with an ischaemic, infected limb refusing an amputation.

Autonomy

Autonomy implies the ability to think and act for oneself, and involves rational thought. It has been described as 'a form of personal liberty of action where the individual determines his or her own course of action in accordance with a plan chosen by himself or herself' (Beauchamp and Childress, 1983), or 'a subclass of freedom' (Gillon, 1986). An individual's autonomy is viewed in terms of their autonomy of thought, will and action; the ability to consider variables, to choose which variable best fulfils their needs and then to act according to that decision. 'The obligation to respect the autonomy of thought and will is not impaired or even removed by disease' (Weale, 1988).

An individual with an ischaemic limb who has deliberated on the consequences of not having an amputation, and who as a sentient person has made a rational choice to accept those consequences, should have his/her autonomous choice accepted.

Beneficence and non-maleficence

Beneficence (doing good for others), and non-maleficence (doing no harm), could be viewed as moral goals in health care. The active pursuit of goodness and the avoidance of harm are fundamental philosophies in both nursing and medical codes of conduct, with the Hippocratic Oath stating 'I will follow that system or regimen which, according to my ability and judgement, I consider for the benefit of my patients' (cited in Gillon, 1986).

Many clinical situations arise where acting in a beneficent manner is a complex process. A person may decide that they wish to die rather than have an amputation, yet their family and friends are urging them to have the surgery in order to prolong the life of their loved one. In this scenario a beneficent act would be to go against the wishes of the patient, as the greatest benefit would be to listen to the wishes of the majority, i.e. the family. However, people should be seen as an end, not as a means to an end, and a beneficent action should be one that respects the wishes of the person involved, i.e. the patient, rather than the value that the healthcare professional places on the patient's life (Donohue, 1997d).

Veracity

The principle of veracity or honesty is often fundamental to ethical dilemmas, but telling the truth is often painful and time-consuming. It requires an effective communicator who approaches the situation with empathy and skill. The fear of not upsetting a person with the truth may also be disguising a fear by the health professional to discuss death (Donohue, 1997d). As Henderson (1964) states, harm can be done both by telling the truth and by lying – there are no easy solutions in this situation.

Justice

In any healthcare setting each professional must act justly by treating each individual as an equal, and by respecting their individual worth and human rights. The patient and the professional have jointly entered into a relationship where both parties have equal footing and therefore should treat each other as equals. Nurses may be involved in situations where the medical staff, nursing staff or family are objecting to the patient's choice to refuse treatment, and this may necessitate the involvement of an impartial third party, such as a counsellor, to define the wishes of the patient and to assist the others involved in accepting those wishes. The nurse should then ensure that their decision to refuse treatment does not cause the patient to feel that they will be left to die without support. Adequate analgesia, social support and counselling should be offered. In the case of the person with the ischaemic limb, confusion due to septicaemia may soon follow, thus the nurse can ensure that time is allowed for them to spend time with their family and significant others (Donohue, 1997d).

In any ethical dilemma it may be impossible to satisfy the different ethical views of the people involved in the situation. People will always possess varying moral attitudes and beliefs when someone has made the decision to die. All that can be done is to remember that on entering a healthcare setting an individual does not lose the right for his autonomy of thought and will to be respected. The value of the patient's life can only be judged by the person experiencing it.

'Autonomy has a very special and central role in the value of life ... to deny people the power of choice over their own destiny is therefore to offer them the most profound of insults' (Harris, 1985).

Summary

Although the incidence of lower limb amputation is decreasing in the Western world, it is still a distressing operation for those who need it. Dealing with lower limb amputation requires a wide-ranging multidisciplinary team, of which the nurse is an important member. The nurse is in the position of being able to help the patient awaiting an amputation to prepare physically and psychologically, and where the patient has not had the time to prepare for the amputation, can address these needs and social needs postoperatively.

Whilst the nurse does not have the expertise to deal with all aspects of the patient's care, he/she should know which member of the team to refer to, and have an understanding of pain control and ethical issues. By working closely with other team members, the nurse can ensure that the patient is rehabilitated to maximal functional independence.

References

Abramson LY, Martin DJ (1981) Depression and the causal inference process. In: Gross RD (ed.) (1990) Key Studies in Psychology. London. Hodder and Stoughton.

Andrews KL (1996) Rehabilitation in limb deficiency: the geriatric amputee. Archives of Physical and Medical Rehabilitation 77: 14–17.

Bach S, Noreng MF, Tjellden NU (1988) Phantom limb pain in amputees during the first 12 months following limb amputation, after pre-operative lumbar epidural blockade. Pain 33(3): 297–301.

Beauchamp TL, Childress JF (1983) Principles of Biomedical Ethics. Oxford: Oxford University Press.

Burgess EM (1968) The below knee amputation. Bulletin of Prosthetics Research 19–25.

Campbell WE (1982) The ischaemic lower limb (2). Hospital Update May: 549–560.

Chapman A (1996) Current theory and practice: a study of pre-operative fasting. Nursing Standard 10(18): 33–36.

Chapman R (1986) Pain, perception and illusion. In: Sternbach RA (1986) The Psychology of Pain, 2nd edn, pp 153–179. New York: Raven Press.

Davis RW (1993) Phantom sensation, phantom pain, and stump pain. Archives of Physical and Medical Rehabilitation 74: 79–86.

Diamond AW, Coniam SW (1991) The Management of Chronic Pain. Oxford: OUP.

Donohue SJ (1997a) Lower limb amputation 1: Indications and treatment. British Journal of Nursing 6 (17): 970–977.

Donohue SJ (1997b) Lower limb amputation 2: Once the decision has been made. British Journal of Nursing 6(18): 1048–1052.
Donohue SJ (1997c) Lower limb amputation 3: The role of the nurse. British Journal of Nursing 6(20): 1171–1190.
Donohue SJ (1997d) Lower limb amputation 4: Some ethical considerations. British Journal of Nursing 6(22): 1311–1314.
Dormandy JA, Ray SA (1994) The fate of amputees. Vascular Medicine Review 5: 331–346.
Dormandy J, Heeck L, Vig S (1999) Major amputations: Clinical patterns and predictors. Seminars in Vascular Surgery 12(2): 154–161.
Faris I (1991) The Management of the Diabetic Foot. Edinburgh: Churchill Livingstone.
Field L (1996) Are nurses still underestimating patient's pain postoperatively? British Journal of Nursing 5(13): 778–784.
Galvani J (1997) Not yet cut and dried. Nursing Times 93(16): 87–89.
Gillon R (1986) Philosophical Medical Ethics. Chichester: John Wiley.
Graham LM, Ford MB (1994) Arterial disease. In: Fahey VA (ed.) Vascular Nursing, 2nd edn. Philadelphia: WB Saunders.
Ham R, Cotton L (1991) Limb Amputation. London: Chapman and Hall.
Harris J (1985) The Value of Life. London: Routledge & Kegan Paul.
Helt J (1994) Amputation in the vascular patient. In: Fahey VA (ed.) Vascular Nursing, 2nd edn. Philadelphia: WB Saunders.
Henderson N (1964) The Nature of Nursing. New York: Macmillan.
Herbert LM (1997) Caring for the Vascular Patient. New York: Churchill Livingstone.
Hollinworth H (1994) No gain? Nursing Times 90(1): 24–27.
Holmes S (1996) The incidence of malnutrition in hospitals. Nursing Times 92(12): 43–47.
Huang CT, Jackson JR, Moore NB et al. (1979) Amputation: energy cost of ambulation. Archives of Physical Medicine and Rehabilitation 60: 18–24.
Jensen TS, Rasmussen P (1994) Phantom pain and other phenomena after amputation. In: Melzack R, Wall PD (1995) Textbook of Pain, 3rd edn. London. Churchill Livingstone.
Krebs B, Jenson TS, Kroner K et al. (1984) Phantom limb phenomenon in amputees seven years after limb amputation. Pain Supplement 2: 585.
Lowe SL (1997) The right to refuse treatment is not a right to be killed. Journal of Medical Ethics 23(3): 154–158.
Mackintosh C (1994) Do nurses provide adequate pain relief? British Journal of Nursing 3(7): 342–347.
Macleod J (1986) Davidson's Principles and Practice of Medicine, 14th edn. New York: Churchill Livingstone.
Marshall SM (1996) The peri-operative management of diabetes. Care of the Critically Ill 12(2): 64–67.
Melzack R, Wall PD (1995) Textbook of Pain, 3rd edn. London: Churchill Livingstone.
Murray D, Fisher FR (1982) Normal gait. In: Handbook of Amputations and Prostheses, pp 28–31. Ottowa: University of Ottowa.
Naylor AR (1995) Amputation: when and where. Unpublished lecture, Leicester Royal Infirmary.

Price B (1990) A model for body-image care. Journal of Advanced Nursing 15: 585–593.
Robinson KP, Hoile R, Coddington T (1982) Skew flap myoplastic below knee amputation: a preliminary report. British Journal of Surgery 69(9): 554–557.
Rubin M (1988) The physiology of bed-rest. American Journal of Nursing 1: 50–55.
Salter M (1988) Altered Body Image: The Nurse's Role. Chichester: John Wiley.
Schofield P (1995) Using assessment tools to help patients in pain. Professional Nurse 10(11): 703–706.
Seers K (1987) Perceptions of pain. Nursing Times 33(48): 37–-39.
Swindale J (1989) The nurse's role in giving pre-operative information to reduce anxiety in patients admitted to hospital for elective minor surgery. Journal of Advanced Nursing 14: 899–905.
Tschudin V (1986) Ethics in Nursing: The Caring Relationship. London: Heinemann Nursing.
UKCC (1997) Nurses are responsible for feeding patients. Register (20): 5.
Vitali M, Robinson KP, Andrews BG, Harris EE, Readhead R (1986) Amputations and Prostheses, 2nd edn. London: Baillière Tindall.
Waterlow J (1988) Calculating the risk. Nursing Times 83(39): 58–60.
Weale A (1988) The Cost and Choice in Health Care; the Ethical Dimension. London: King's Fund.
Wilson PG (1994) Phantom pain. In: Tollison CD (ed.) Handbook of Pain Management, 2nd edn. Baltimore: Williams & Wilkins.

Further reading

Engstrom B, Van de Ven C (eds) (1999) Therapy for Amputees, 3rd edn. London: Churchill Livingstone.

CHAPTER 12

Abdominal Aortic Aneurysm Repair

FRANCES COLLINS

Introduction

In 1951 Charles Dubost and colleagues performed the first successful aortic aneurysm repair by substituting an aortic aneurysm with a cadaver homograft (Dubost et al., 1952). Since this time much progress has been made. Abdominal aortic aneurysms (AAAs) are responsible for approximately 1–2% of all deaths within the United Kingdom (OPCS, 1993) and there is still around 80% mortality associated with ruptured aneurysms (Anidjar, 1992). A significantly large proportion of deaths caused by a ruptured aortic aneurysm go unrecorded resulting in the exact figure being unknown (Collin, 1996). The diagnosis of AAA has increased over the last decade due to greater diligence by the medical profession and a larger ageing population (Shealy and Elliott, 1997).

Although there is no uniform definition available, the consensus is that an abdominal aortic aneurysm is a localised, permanent dilatation within the artery. The increase of diameter must be greater than 1.5 times or 50% of the 'normal' (Santilli and Santilli, 1997). Age, gender, body weight and blood pressure can influence normal diameter size (Graham and Ford, 1999).

Caring for patients with aneurysmal disease requires all practitioners to be aware of the individual's health needs in order to deliver safe and effective care. The nurse is in a prime position to assist in identifying and modifying the risk factors by giving pre- and postoperative health promotion advice to patients and their families. The nurse must also play a key role in providing exemplary care and continuous support to the patient and family throughout the period when major surgery is required.

This chapter will briefly examine the aetiology and the prevalence of AAA, and the risk factors associated with its development. Screening and diagnostic methods will be discussed and the types of AAA will be described. A detailed explanation of the investigations required prior to surgery will be given and the factors that contribute to the decision whether to operate or observe. Guidelines for pre- and postoperative care will be presented using an integrated care pathway (ICP) format to help illustrate patient management. Finally, new developments and advances in the management of abdominal aortic aneurysms are highlighted.

Aetiology and pathogenesis

Evidence from animal models suggests that inflammatory cells releasing cytokines and proteases that digest proteins such as elastin within the blood vessel wall may play an early role in pathogenesis of aneurysm formation. Elastin allows the aortic wall to stretch and accommodate the increased blood flow and pressure and then return to a normal diameter during each cardiac cycle. Once destruction of elastin has taken place it cannot be replaced and places further demands on collagen fibres. Increased mechanical load and shear stresses cause the breakdown and the destruction of the collagen and result in aortic dilatation (Rehm et al., 1998). Amongst others, Campa et al. (1987) have reported that elastin loss is a key step in the development of AAA and stated that elastin identified within the walls of an AAA is greatly reduced from that of a normal aortic wall. Though aortic atherosclerosis is a common association in patients with AAA it remains unclear why some atheromatous vessels dilate when others do not (Rehm et al., 1998).

Clifton (1977) recognised that there is an increased risk of developing an AAA if a first-degree relative is affected and suggest this may be associated with elastin and collagen defects or gene variants. Mutation in a fibrillin-1 gene, thought to be responsible for the congenital disorder Marfan's syndrome, causes premature degenerative disease of connective tissue which can result in aortic aneurysm, aortic dissection, mitral valve regurgitation and early death (Graham and Ford, 1999). In the inherited disorder Ehlers–Danlos syndrome (type IV), patients are found to have defects in certain collagen genes which result in a weakening of the vessel wall and eventual rupture of the large arteries (Krupski, 1995). Other causes of AAA are trauma, arteritis, syphilis and mycotic aneurysms that can occur at the site of infection.

Although the aetiology of aneurysm formation is multifactorial, the central pathophysiological mechanisms are atheroma formation and elastin and collagen loss in the vascular wall.

Incidence

Men are three times more likely than women to develop an AAA (Tennant, 1994; Cheatle, 1997). Incidence increases with age and the gap between men and women narrows when women reach their 70s. Recent studies (Hallett et al., 1994; Vardulaki et al., 1998) suggest an increase in incidence attributable to a number of factors: primarily longevity as AAAs are more prevalent in the elderly. It would be considered rare for a patient to develop an AAA before the age of 60 years (unless congenital) (Collin, 1996). Other main causes for an increase in prevalence can be attributed to increased technology and screening programmes.

Risk factors

Of the many factors that play a part in the development of an AAA, atherosclerosis appears to be important (Rehm et al., 1998), though the causal relationship is still not fully understood (Shealy and Elliott, 1997). Risk factors include smoking, hypertension, hyperlipidaemia and diabetes (Table 12.1) and are also implicated in the aetiology of atherosclerosis (see Chapters 2 and 3). Approximately 50% of patients who present with an AAA have evidence of coronary heart disease, 10–15% suffer from a degree of pulmonary disease and approximately 10% show evidence of carotid artery disease (Hallett, 1992). Around 50% of patients presenting with a femoral or popliteal aneurysm have also been found to have an abdominal aortic aneurysm (Nehler et al., 1995).

Table 12.1 Risk factors

Age
Smoking
Hypertension
Diabetes
Sex
Hyperlipidaemia
Connective tissue disorder

Screening

Approximately 75% of AAAs are asymptomatic (Datta, 1989). Detection is made during routine check-ups or the aneurysm is discovered during other procedures or investigations. For many patients the first sign of trouble is excruciating lower back pain, or they may present in an accident and emergency department in a clinically shocked state.

It has been demonstrated that screening for an AAA can be beneficial by effectively identifying aortic aneurysms early enough to offer treatment, reducing the mortality rate from ruptured aortic aneurysm (Lucarotti et al., 1993; Scott et al., 1995). Information gathered from earlier smaller local studies suggested that a national screening programme should be established (Harris, 1992) and aimed at men between the ages of 65 and 80 years. Acting upon this recommendation, a large screening programme was launched, the United Kingdom Small Aneurysm Trial, which was completed in 1995 (UK Small Aneurysm Trial Participants, 1998). The UK trial enrolled 1090 patients between the ages of 60–76 years and attempted to identify the ideal management of small abdominal aortic aneurysm (4.0–5.5 cm). They concluded that elective AAA repair for those with small, non-tender aneurysms was not always the appropriate management. Supervision and follow-up scanning of these patients was recommended. Those with 4.0–4.9 cm AAA underwent an ultrasound scan every 6 months and those found to have a 5–5.5 cm abdominal aortic aneurysm had a scan performed every 3 months. Recently, a multicentre aneurysm screening trial (MASS) was conducted to assess the benefits of using ultrasound for screening abdominal aortic aneurysms (Vardulaki et al., 1998). By providing a national screening programme it has been estimated that as many as 2000 deaths per year from ruptured aneurysm could be prevented in the UK, despite many of the aneurysms identified being less than 4.5 cm in diameter (Law, 1998). By ensuring the screening programme is worthwhile and beneficial, an attempt would have to be made to establish the number of lives saved and the cost effectiveness of screening. Scott et al. (1995) conducted an in-depth study in order to demonstrate this and the cost of early detection. Their results equated to 7 out of 3205 lives being saved, an increase of elective AAA repair by 34 per year within a population of 250 000. They also predicted large additional costs such as operation, prolonged stay and failure to return to former quality of life, perhaps demonstrating that a national screening programme cannot be recommended.

Often the first description of the aneurysm can be very frightening for patients and few are able to return to normal life for fear of causing the AAA to rupture. Patients tend to limit activities and choose a sedentary way of life. Following diagnosis, the vascular team will then offer the type of management that is appropriate. If it is to operate, patients are asked to agree to a major operation, with a mortality rate of between 3% and 10% depending on where the operation is performed (Campbell, 1991). Even if the patient survives the operation, their quality of life or their life expectancy may be reduced (Cheatle, 1997). With conservative management, the patient may be required to attend a hospital on a regular basis for ultrasound scans to detect any change in the size of the aneurysm. Small aneurysms, less than 4 cm in diameter, have an expansion rate of around 2–4 mm per year and a far smaller chance of rupture than the AAA greater than 5.5 cm (Nevitt et al., 1989; Bengtsson et al., 1993).

Location and types

The location of an AAA influences perioperative complications. Anatomically the abdominal aorta can be divided into three sections and traditionally 90% of abdominal aortic aneurysms are infrarenal (Phillips, 1998).

- An *infrarenal aneurysm* occurs when the upper end of the aneurysm is below the origins of the level of the renal artery.

- A *juxtarenal aneurysm* is the second level. This is when the upper end of the aneurysm borders on the renal artery origins.
- A *suprarenal aneurysm* involves visceral vessels, such as the superior mesenteric artery and renal arteries and the lower aorta (Tennant, 1994).

There are several different types of aneurysm (see Chapter 2, Figure 2.2):

- The commonest aortic aneurysm is the *fusiform*. This takes the shape of an enlargement of the entire circumference.
- A *saccular* aneurysm is a localised swelling.
- A *dissecting* aneurysm occurs when there is a tear in the aortic intima; this causes blood to escape into the vessel wall and results in the media being stripped from the adventitia.
- A *pseudoaneurysm* develops when an entire tear occurs in all the layers of the vessel and allows blood to flow from the artery into the periarterial tissues. This results in a collection or haematoma (Hatswell, 1994a).

Diagnosis and investigations

For patients who have asymptomatic AAA, a physical examination is not the most reliable method of diagnosing and detecting an aortic aneurysm (Hallett, 1992). Clinical examinations have been found to miss approximately 50% of aneurysms that have later been identified by ultrasonography (Hatswell, 1994a). Abdominal B-mode ultrasonography is a highly sensitive technique and can detect most aortic aneurysms. Unfortunately there is discrepancy in size and precise location of the AAA and the technique should not be relied upon solely when making management decisions (Ellis et al., 1991; Lederle et al., 1995). Ultrasonography can be recommended as a screening tool as it can give a clear picture, is non-invasive and inexpensive (Figure 12.1). When planning surgery or in initial diagnosis of suprarenal or juxtarenal aneurysms, spiral computerised tomography (CT) with overlapping axial reconstruction is more useful for sizing the aneurysm (Albrecht et al., 1997). Magnetic resonance imaging (MRI) is also able to identify size and location but is costly, timely to conduct the test and not always available or necessary as CT provides adequate views.

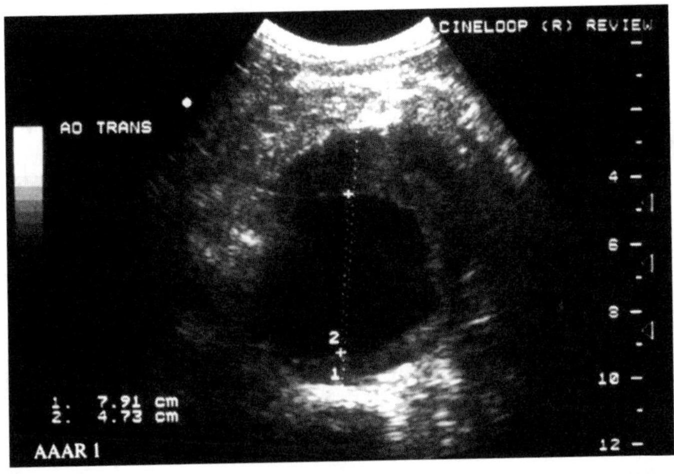

Figure 12.1 Ultrasound scan of an abdominal aortic aneurysm. (Courtesy of Sulzer Vascutek Ltd.)

Once a diagnosis has been made, a detailed history must be taken from the patient. This must include a past medical history, paying particular attention to any other concomitant diseases such as cardiac or cerebrovascular disease and family history. A full physical examination will be undertaken and should include a thorough vascular assessment ensuring that the ankle brachial index pressures (ABPI) are documented, and all peripheral pulses are identified either by palpating or by portable Doppler machine. If any of the pulses are absent or the ABPI is less than 0.7 this indicates some occlusion that may require further investigation by arteriography (see Chapter 4). Patients with carotid bruits or those who show evidence of carotid artery disease, such as transient ischaemic attacks or a history of stroke, should have a carotid duplex. If more than 80% stenosis is identified bilaterally, carotid endarterectomy should be considered before the aneurysm repair (Hallett, 1992).

A full blood screen should be taken to obtain baseline values and identify any possible problems such as anaemia or renal damage. This should include:

- full blood count
- clotting studies
- liver function
- urea, electrolytes and creatinine

- fasting lipids (to enable treatment to commence at the earliest point).

Several days prior to surgery the patient's blood should be cross-matched. Between 6 and 12 units of blood should be requested depending on the location of the aneurysm.

Preoperative evaluation should also include a chest X-ray. The chest X-ray will show any underlying pathology or if the patient suffers from chronic obstructive pulmonary disease. A pulmonary function test should be performed and from these baseline readings an assessment can be made about appropriate treatment. It is possible that bronchodilators and chest physiotherapy can be administered preoperatively to enhance recovery postoperatively (Phillips, 1998). An electrocardiogram (ECG) is performed routinely to detect cardiac ischaemia or previous myocardial infarctions and establish a baseline trace. In the event of an abnormal ECG or if there is evidence of angina pectoris, a cardiologist's opinion should be sought. A recommendation may be made for the patient to undergo a dipyridamole-thallium scan or a dobutamine stress echocardiogram. The first assesses cardiac perfusion and the latter enables ventricular function to be assessed under pharmacologically induced stress. If either of these studies identify abnormal findings, more invasive tests such as coronary arteriography will be performed and coronary revascularisation may be considered in advance of the aneurysm surgery, or in rare cases a combined procedure may be indicated (Hertzer et al., 1984). In juxtarenal and suprarenal AAA repairs a renal scan may provide valuable information about renal blood supply, functional abilities and rate of excretion prior to surgery. A summary of preoperative investigations can be seen in Table 12.2.

Table 12.2 Preoperative investigations

Computed tomography or B-mode ultrasound
Clinical history and physical examination
Chest X-ray
Blood tests
ABPI
ECG +/– stress echo
Lung function
+/– Arteriography

Indications for surgery

Lower back pain, a pulsating mass and abdominal tenderness when examined suggest a symptomatic AAA. Other symptoms include painful toes due to microemboli obstructing blood supply to peripheries, scrotal pain and abdominal pain. The patient with a ruptured aneurysm may present via an accident and emergency department or following routine admission to a vascular ward. The patient appears clinically shocked or very agitated and complaining of excruciating back pain. Aggressive resuscitation should be carried out with the administration of oxygen and intravenous plasma substitutes if blood is not available, followed by immediate surgery; without this death will follow rapidly (Table 12.3). The mortality rate still remains high when surgery is performed following rupture (Shealy and Elliott, 1997). The nurse needs to be available at all times to provide vital emotional support to the patient and their family and reinforce the gravity of the situation.

Table12.3 Indications for surgery

Ruptured AAA
AAA >5.5 cm
Symptomatic AAA
< 5.5 cm but increasing >5 mm per 6 months
Peripheral emboli

For the remaining 75% of patients, who are not under surveillance and present with asymptomatic abdominal aortic aneurysm, guidance should be taken from the results of the UK trial (UK Small Aneurysm Trial Participants, 1998). When a patient presents with an AAA greater than 5.5 cm the surgeon has to assess the patient and make an informed decision with the patient and family about the operative risk for the patient. Surgery should be considered if perioperative death is considered to be less than 5% unless contraindicated (Table 12.4). However, it must always be remembered that the main goal of aortic surgery is to prevent rupture and premature death.

Patients may also present with *mycotic* AAA. The principal symptoms and signs of infected AAAs are abdominal pain, fever, palpable mass and positive blood cultures, although up to 40% of these may

Table 12.4 Contraindications for surgery

Terminal illness
Recent myocardial infarction or unstable angina
Severe pulmonary disease
Chronic renal failure
Poor quality of life, which will increase the operative risk to 5–10%

not be palpable and may go unrecognised until rupture occurs (Reddy and Ernst, 1995). The timing and type of surgery required for infected AAAs remains controversial with some studies advocating 'in situ' aortic grafts (Chan et al., 1989), and others recommending extra-anatomical reconstruction (Taylor et al., 1988). All patients with mycotic AAA will require long-term antibiotic therapy (Reddy and Ernst, 1995).

Pre-admission care and health promotion

After the initial decision for surgery has been taken, patients will be admitted electively, although a short delay should be expected. Within this time, patients should be encouraged to optimise their health through smoking cessation and gentle exercise in an attempt to reduce perioperative complications. Correct medication must be administered to control high blood pressure and maintain a good diabetic control. If the patient is overweight, a reducing diet is advisable as excess weight may influence the patient's recovery (see Chapter 3). During this waiting period the patient and their family feel most vulnerable to a catastrophic event and they will benefit from the support of a vascular nurse specialist or a nurse on the ward. By providing a contact telephone number, the patient and their family will be able to speak to someone who can answer their questions and alleviate any concerns relating to the impending surgery. Information leaflets detailing the surgery and investigations required, as well as outlining milestones throughout the patient's stay in hospital, should be provided in the outpatient department.

Preoperative care

The patient is admitted a couple of days prior to surgery, and the standard preoperative preparations and a full nursing assessment should be undertaken before surgery, placing a strong emphasis on the psychological wellbeing of the patient (see Chapter 4). Providing accurate information to patients will help them to feel more at ease with the environment and procedure and to understand the nature of the multidisciplinary team involved in their care. Following recent recommendations by the Royal College of Surgeons (1997), only a doctor who is competent and technically able to perform the operation should obtain written informed consent from the patient. The consultant or the vascular registrar will usually undertake this task.

Prior to surgery, long-acting anticoagulants such as warfarin should be replaced by intravenous heparin, which is a shorter-acting agent. Heparin is more easily titrated to the required anticoagulant effect, which helps to avoid haemorrhagic complications. Patients will be nil by mouth for several hours prior to surgery, as per local guidelines (normally 6 hours for food and 2 hours for water), and diabetic patients will require regular recordings of blood sugar to prevent any hypoglycaemic episodes. Patients who usually require subcutaneous insulin or oral hypoglycaemic medication will be commenced on a sliding scale regimen of intravenous insulin and glucose 5% on the morning of surgery. This allows control of their blood sugar throughout surgery and the postoperative period.

On the morning of surgery the patient should be advised to shower in a skin cleansing preparation according to local policy, to reduce risk of cross-infection. The physiotherapist will review the patient and provide advice on breathing exercises that should be repeated postoperatively. The ward nurse should ensure all investigations and test results are available and with the case notes. The abdominal area will be shaved in theatre immediately before the skin incision.

The anaesthetist will review the patient and discuss perioperative risks with the surgeon. If the anaesthetist shows concern over the cardiac, respiratory or renal function further investigations or treatment may be required, possibly delaying surgery. The anaesthetist will decide on the appropriate preoperative sedative and request that all cardiac related drugs and diuretics are administered at 6 a.m. for the patients scheduled for surgery that day. The anaesthetist will also discuss analgesia with the patient as it has been demonstrated that this can reduce the amount of pain experienced and the amount of analgesia the patient will require following surgery. The current trend is for use of an epidural for perioperative and postoperative analgesia. Excellent analgesia is provided by epidural infusion while avoiding the side effects of systemically administered opiates. The major advantage is in reducing postoperative respiratory complications and pain, which enables early mobilisation. Epidurals also help increase peripheral blood flow, which may assist in preventing graft failure (Tuman et al., 1991). The disadvantages include possible hypotension (systolic blood pressure <100 mmHg), followed by nausea and vomiting, and if the block is complete, some complications such as haemorrhage may be masked. Depending on the location of the incision, the epidural block may have to be as high as the T4 dermatome to provide effective analgesia and that may result in respiratory function being compromised. There are different combinations available, bupivacaine and fentanyl being one common combination that acts synergistically. Some patients are adverse to the idea of an epidural causing numbness in the lower body and may choose other forms of analgesia such as intravenous patient-controlled analgesia or intramuscular opiates (see Chapter 6).

To optimise the condition of some patients, they may be required to spend 24–48 hours in a high dependency unit to receive respiratory support or pharmacological assistance in controlling blood pressure. This may result in regular arterial blood gases being obtained, frequent physiotherapy, nebulisers and oral or intravenous medication being administered.

The operative procedure

An AAA repair requires either a midline incision for a retroperitoneal approach or a transverse approach above the umbilicus for renal vessel involvement (Lamont et al., 1999). Fewer complications are associated with a midline retroperitoneal approach (Sicard et al., 1995). The aneurysm is exposed and clamps are placed proximally and distally to stem bleeding and allow the surgeon to operate (Figure 12.2). Following this, the aneurysmal sac is incised and any clots or thrombus are removed. To reduce the risk of further clotting and distal thrombosis, 5000 units of heparin are administered intravenously (Phillips, 1998). Prophylactic intravenous antibiotics are administered during the procedure to minimise the risk of a graft

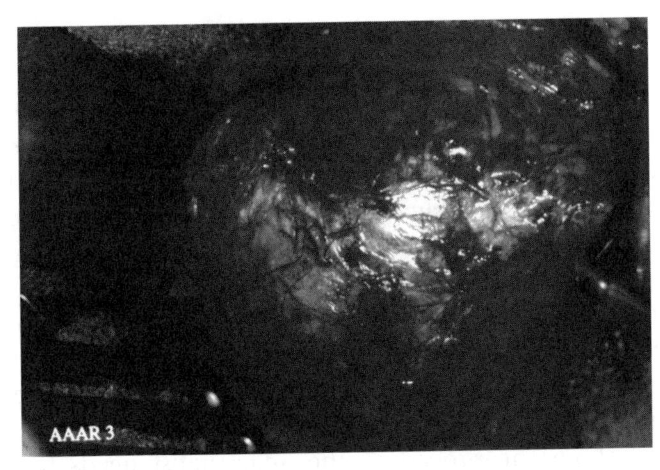

Figure 12.2 The proximal aortic clamp is shown on the left side of the aneurysm. (Courtesy of Sulzer Vascutek Ltd.)

infection. The sac is laid open and any lumbar vessel apertures are sutured. The prosthetic graft is then sewn in place and the walls of the aneurysm are closed over the graft before the clamps are removed (Figure 12.3) (Hatswell, 1994b). The abdomen is then closed. An embolectomy may be performed via the femoral artery to remove any debris from the aneurysm floating down towards the feet and causing occlusions (Lamont et al., 1999).

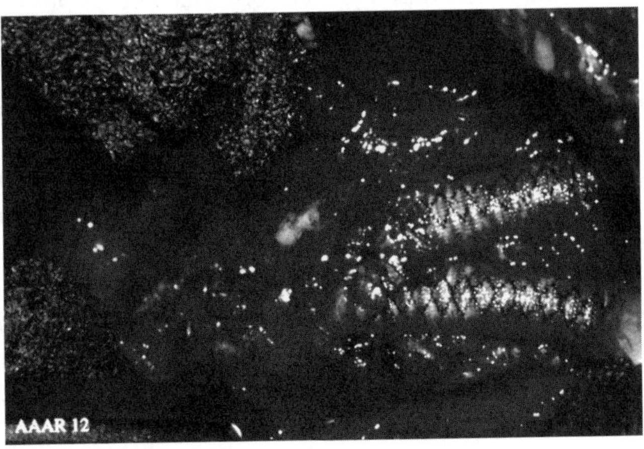

Figure 12.3 A bifurcated graft is in situ with the original aortic aneurysm sac in place over the top of the graft. (Courtesy of Sulzer Vascutek Ltd.)

Depending on the site of the aneurysm either a straight tube graft (Figure 12.4a) or a bifurcated graft can be used (Figure 12.4b). The grafts are constructed from either polyethylene terephthalate (Dacron), which is either a knitted or woven polyester fibre, or polytetrafluoroethylene (PTFE). The surgeon, based on preference, availability and previous surgery, makes the choice of graft material. One of the main advantages of PTFE is its easy handling and it does not require pre-clotting. Unlike PTFE, the Dacron graft requires pre-clotting prior to insertion which requires the surgeon to soak the graft in non-heparinised blood before use. Some manufacturers are attempting to line the prosthetic graft with cultured endothelial cells in an attempt to promote resistance and reduce graft infections (Lamont et al., 1999).

Throughout the procedure the anaesthetist needs to ensure adequate fluid replacement is made with both crystalloid and colloid intravenous fluids. It is now common practice in larger centres to use some form of cell saver autotransfusion device, which reduces the amount of stored blood required. Widespread use of this device is limited due to the cost. Large fluctuations in haemodynamics occur when clamping or unclamping of the aorta is performed. Cross-clamping causes a dramatic rise in the afterload seen by the left ventricle and the left ventricular end-diastolic volume and pressure may increase. This in turn can cause a fall in coronary perfusion with the risk of myocardial ischaemia. At unclamping, the large fall in systemic vascular resistance can cause hypotension, which needs prompt treatment with intravascular fluids and vasoactive drugs. During repair of juxtarenal or suprarenal aneurysm the cross-clamp is located above the renal arteries. This reduces renal blood flow and puts the patient at risk of acute renal failure (Hatswell, 1994b). In an attempt to reduce long-term damage, mannitol, an osmotic diuretic, may be given intravenously to help increase glomerular filtration. A continuous infusion of renal dose dopamine may also be given if preferred. Following surgery patients will either return to the intensive care unit (ICU) or a high dependency unit (HDU) where they will be closely monitored. The patient should not require prolonged ventilation unless they have pre-existing pulmonary disease or arterial blood gases are poor.

Postoperative care

Before collecting the patient from the theatre recovery room, the nurse must ensure the bed space is ready to receive the patient. The

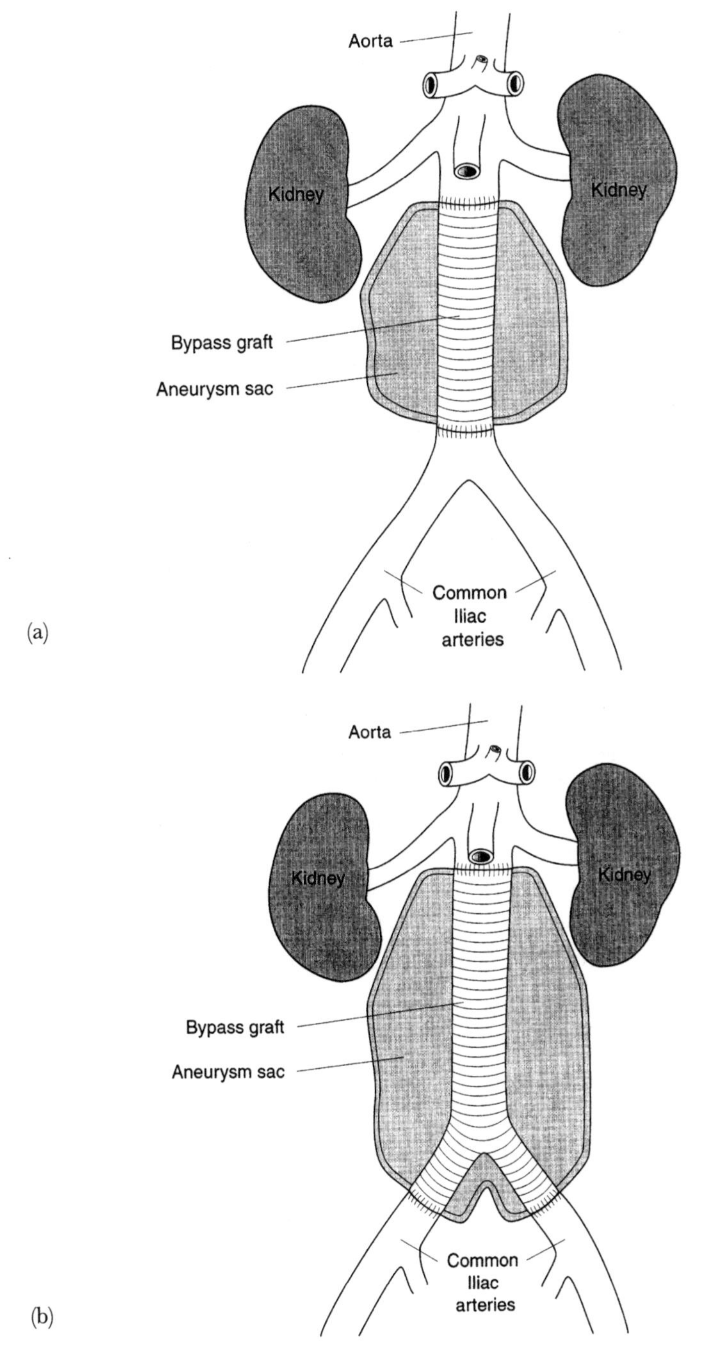

Figure 12.4 (a) An abdominal aortic aneurysm repair using a straight tube graft. (b) An abdominal aortic aneurysm repair using a bifurcated graft.

bed area must have a cardiac monitor, a working suction unit, an oxygen point with a facemask and a range of airways. In addition, a drip stand with several infusion pumps should be in close proximity and a specific nurse should be identified to provide additional care to the patient. The main priorities of care are as described below.

Cardiovascular system

Blood pressure (BP) will be recorded continuously via an arterial line and should be documented every 15 minutes for a minimum of 1 hour. The nurse must aim to keep the blood pressure within the set range, typically 120–160 mmHg systolic, to prevent complications. High blood pressure can cause bleeding around the graft site. The blood pressure should be controlled by intravenous glyceryl trinitrate, which should be titrated against the current blood pressure. Hypovolaemia or rapid re-warming of the patient may cause hypotension. Treatment priority is to normalise intravascular volume as quickly as possible and identify the cause of the hypotension. Intravenous fluids of colloid and crystalloids should be administered followed by inotropic support if fluid alone is unsuccessful (Sielenkamper and Sibbald, 1999). As a result of prolonged low blood pressure inadequate amounts of oxygen will be delivered to the tissues and multiple organ failure may eventually occur. The patient's heart rate will be continuously monitored to detect any arrhythmias, the commonest being sinus tachycardia and atrial fibrillation (Sayers and Gasperetti, 1999). It is important to treat the patient rather than the monitor as artefacts can often appear on the monitor and interfere with the patient's true rhythm. When the patient is adequately warmed, passing a good quantity of urine and in a sinus rhythm, the frequency of the observations can be reduced.

Respiratory

Between 40% and 60% of warmed, humidified oxygen should be administered via a facemask to maintain oxygen saturation of 95% or higher. Oxygen saturation must be monitored regularly by either oximetry or arterial blood gases, and respiratory rate must be recorded hourly. Deep breathing exercises should be encouraged regularly to ensure bilateral lung expansion is maintained and secretions are removed. The physiotherapist will treat the patient morning and afternoon.

Renal

The kidneys can survive for approximately one hour without adequate perfusion (Phillips, 1998). This patient population is often elderly and some narrowing of the renal artery and reduced renal perfusion should be expected. It may be enough to cause oliguria (<20 ml per hour). Urine output should be recorded hourly via a urinary catheter (inserted perioperatively) and if the patient becomes oliguric the nurse should perform a bladder washout to ensure patency of the catheter, record central venous pressure (CVP) and BP and inform the doctor. The CVP should be recorded 1–4-hourly from a fixed site, either sternum or mid-axilla and the range should be set accordingly. Depending on these recordings a fluid regimen will be prescribed, usually 1 litre every 6–8 hours. The CVP will reflect the intravascular volume status. If urine output is low, dopamine can be administered intravenously at a starting dose of 1–4 μg/kg/min to increase cardiac output and blood flow (Cordingley and Palazzo, 1999). By increasing renal vascular dilatation, it is hoped that renal blood flow will increase, causing an increase in glomerular filtration rate and urine output. No prospective randomised controlled trial has shown the benefits of using dopamine in preventing acute renal failure, hence leaving the decision to use dopamine to the discretion of the lead doctor (Cordingley and Palazzo, 1999).

Eating and drinking

A nasogastric (NG) tube will be in situ and left on free drainage. It should be aspirated every 4 hours until the paralytic ileus has resolved. The NG tube will remain in place for approximately 3–4 days and during this time oral fluid will be introduced gradually according to bowel sounds, commencing on day 1 with 30 ml of water hourly. If a patient's appetite does not return immediately, high protein fluid supplements should be encouraged. Mouth care should be offered regularly to alleviate dryness and discomfort.

Mobility

Vascular limb perfusion observations should be recorded hourly. This must include identifying all peripheral pulses, limb colour, sensation, movement, temperature and capillary refill time (Chapter 4). The nurse should take into consideration the reduced sensation and movement if an epidural is in situ. A pressure sore assessment tool should be completed preoperatively and immediately postoperatively to assess the patient's risk of developing pressure sores (Chapter 5). It is recommended that all patients have the use of an appropriate pressure-relieving mattress until their mobility increases. Position change and deep breathing exercises should be encouraged to reduce the risk of chest infection. Subcutaneous heparin should be prescribed to prevent development of deep vein thrombosis, and if indicated anti-embolic stockings can be worn if the ABPI is greater than 1.0 (Fahey, 1999).

Analgesia

This was discussed earlier with preoperative care and is reviewed in more detail in Chapter 6. When an epidural is used to provide postoperative pain relief, the nurse must be aware of possible complications being masked such as haemorrhage or paralysis. If the nurse has any concerns the anaesthetist should be contacted. Reduced mobility and sensations in the lower limbs due to an effective epidural can lead to prolonged pressure on vulnerable areas such as heels and sacrum. It is the nurse's role to alleviate pressure regularly and inspect areas for tissue ischaemia and serious damage.

Wound care

The dressing should be checked on an hourly basis. The nurse should observe the size of the patient's abdomen for possible swelling due to haemorrhage. If there is any doubt the abdomen should be measured. In some cases vacuum drains may be used. These should be removed as soon as possible, usually within 24–48 hours postoperatively.

Anxiety

Patients can feel extremely vulnerable at this time. The nurse should ensure that the patient and family are given all the relevant information and support required, and that all their concerns are addressed and answered. The patient must be encouraged to have adequate rest, as this will assist the healing process. Guidelines on postoperative care can be seen in the form of an integrated care pathway (ICP) in Table 12.5.

Table 12.5 Integrated care pathway for postoperative care following repair of AAA (days 1–7)

	Day 1	Day 2	Day 3	Day 4	Day 5	Day 6	Day 7
CVS and limb circulation	BP, T and P 1–2 h Doppler 2 h	BP 2–4 h; T and P 4 h Doppler 4 h	BP, T and P 4 h Doppler 4 h	BP, T and P 4 h Doppler 8 h	BP, T and P 6 h Doppler 8 h	BP, T and P 12 h Doppler OD	BP, T and P 12 h Doppler OD
Chest	Resp 1 h 40–60% O_2 Physio BD	Resp 1 h 40–60% O_2 Physio BD	Resp 1 h 35–40% O_2 Physio BD	Resp 1 h 28–35% O_2 Physio BD	Resp 4 h Discontinue O_2 Physio OD	Resp 4 h Physio OD	Resp 4 h Physio OD
Renal	Urine 1 h CVP 2 h IVI 6–8 h	Urine 2 h CVP 4 h IVI 6–8 h	Urine 4 h CVP 4 h IVI 8–10 h	Urine 4 h CVP BD Discontinue IVI	prn N/A N/A	N/A N/A N/A	N/A N/A N/A
Medication	IVAB IV ranitidine Epidural	IV ranitidine Epidural	IV ranitidine Reduce epidural	IV ranitidine Discontinue epidural	Oral drugs	Oral drugs	Oral drugs
Diet and oral fluids	30 ml H_2O/h NG 2–4-hourly	30–60 ml/h NG 4-hourly	60–90 ml/h NG 4-hourly	Free fluids	Light diet supplements	Normal diet	Normal diet supplements
Hygiene	M/C prn Bedbath	M/C prn Bedbath	M/C prn Assisted	M/C prn Assisted	Bathroom	Bathroom	Shower

(contd)

Table 12.5 (contd)

	Day 1	Day 2	Day 3	Day 4	Day 5	Day 6	Day 7
Psychosocial	Relieve anxiety and liaise with family Plan discharge	Relieve anxiety and liaise with family Review plan	Relieve anxiety and liaise with family	Relieve anxiety and liaise with family Set date for discharge	Relieve anxiety and liaise with family	Liaise with services Arrange transport	Liaise with services
Day plan	Sit out × 1 FBC, U&Es CXR ABPI	Sit out × 1 Reduce O_2 Dress wound Remove arterial line FBC, U&Es	Sit out × 2 Reduce O_2 Increase oral fluids Move to ward Remove NG tube Remove CVP	Walk Reduce O_2 Increase oral fluids Wound dressing Check bowels Remove epidural Remove catheter FBC, U&Es	Walk × 2 ?Discontinue O_2	Stairs Discontinue O_2 Dress wound Check bowels	Walk and stairs FBC, U&Es

BP, blood pressure. T, temperature. P, pulse. Resp, respiration. O_2, oxygen. Urine, urine output. IVAB, intravenous antibiotics. M/C, mouth care. CVP, central venous pressure. FBC, full blood count. U&E, urea and electrolytes. ABPI, Ankle brachial index pressure. CXR, chest X-ray. NG, nasogastric. IVI, intravenous infusion. BD, twice a day; OD, once a day. prn, As required.

Discharge planning

The speed of recovery and lack of potential complications (Table 12.6) guide the length of inpatient stay. To ensure a smooth transition from inpatient to outpatient status, discharge planning should begin on admission following the initial assessment. AAAs affect the elderly and many live alone and it may take up to 6 months before a full recovery is made following major surgery. Social services need to be involved and a care manager should be selected. Family/carers should be involved in discharge discussions as this provides the family with information, and allows partners or loved ones to ask questions regarding their concerns. Health promotion advice must be given (see Chapter 3).

A ward nurse or GP practice nurse will remove the sutures between 10 and 14 days postoperatively. If the wound becomes swollen, inflamed or starts leaking after discharge, the patient should be advised to visit their GP. Other advice should include undertaking gentle exercise, perhaps a short walk each day, limiting the amount of lifting done, and to elevate the legs when sitting to increase venous return and reduce swelling. Depending on their occupation, patients can return to work when they feel able which can be between 6 and 12 weeks following operation.

A discharge checklist should incorporate the following advice:

- Health promotion advice and risk factor modification; smoking cessation, diet, medication compliance.
- Exercise.
- Avoid heavy lifting for 12 weeks.
- Wound care and removal of sutures.
- Medication (this may have changed during admission).
- Driving may be resumed when an emergency stop can be performed.
- Returning to work within 6–12 weeks (discuss with GP).
- Follow-up appointment and contact number.

New developments

Future management of patients with AAA now lies in the improvement of recently developed techniques such as *endoluminal repair*. The first successful endovascular stent was performed in 1991 (Parodi et al.,

Table 12.6 Potential complications following repair of AAA

Problem	Cause	Action
Myocardial infarction	Pre-existing ischaemia. Hypertension or anaemia. Increased oxygen required by myocardium	Continuous monitoring. Prompt treatment of arrhythmias and hypertension. Maintenance of circulatory volume. Keep electrolytes within normal range. Administer oxygen
Respiratory disorders	Anaesthesia, surgery and postoperative pain impairs lung function. Exacerbation of pre-existing disease	Administer oxygen, nebulisers and chest physiotherapy. Ensure analgesia is effective. Monitor with oximetry, blood gases and chest X-ray
Limb ischaemia or 'trash' foot	Reduced blood flow due to embolisation or thrombosis	Anticoagulation, regular vascular observations. May need embolectomy or revascularisation and analgesia
Acute renal failure	Hypotension, prolonged clamping, dehydration or embolisation	Monitor CVP, blood pressure and urine output. Check U&Es. Consider IV dopamine, frusemide or dialysis
Ischaemic colitis	Inferior mesenteric artery occlusion	Maintain hydration, record white cell count and drainage from NG tube. Observe bowel movement, colour, smell, consistency
Haemorrhage	Suture line failure exacerbated by hypertension and coagulopathy	Observe wound and abdomen for swelling or oozing of blood. Monitor haemodynamics, FBC and clotting profile. Correct if abnormal. Inform surgeon, may require re-exploring
Sexual impotency	Due to division of nervi erigentes.	Assess level; unable to obtain an erection or inability to ejaculate. Perform urological evaluation and referral. Counselling should be offered

Table 12.6 (contd)

Problem	Cause	Action
Graft infection	Due to presence of bacterial colonisation at the graft site during or after surgery	Monitor vital signs and white cell count. Administer IVAB. White blood cell scan to locate area of infection. Graft may need replacing
Spinal cord ischaemia	Due to prolonged clamping, hypotension or division of blood vessels supplying the spinal cord. Cord swelling may worsen ischaemia	Assess sensory and motor impairment. Monitor neurological changes. Refer to a neurologist
Lymph leak	Due to damage of para-aortic lymphatics	Monitor output, reduce mobility. If persistent apply light pressure. Rarely a problem and normally lymph gets reabsorbed
Aortic-enteric fistula	Due to infection or trauma around the suture line or a false aneurysm	Monitor vital signs and maintain circulating volume. Monitor gastric drainage. Treat fever and infection. Provide adequate analgesia. Endoscopy or surgical exploration may be required

IVAB, intravenous antibiotics. FBC, full blood count. U&E, urea and electrolytes. NG, nasogastric.

1991). Since then a number of devices have been produced with many centres undertaking endoluminal repairs. The procedure involves intraluminal insertion via the femoral artery of a 'stent graft' that is delivered by a deployment device with the assistance of fluoroscopic imaging. An expandable anchoring feature secures the graft proximal to the neck of the aortic aneurysm. The aim is to exclude the aneurysm and restore normal blood flow. Endoluminal repair remains controversial and complications include suture breakage, graft erosion, stent migration, graft kinking or failure (Zarins, 1999). Endoluminal repair of infrarenal aortic aneurysm undertaken by experienced surgeons and interventional radiologists is reducing mortality rates and length of stay as it is less invasive than conventional surgery and may be favourable for those patients who are considered to be high risk (Zarins, 1999). In some cases, general anaesthetic can be avoided by the use of an epidural for the endoluminal repair (Cao et al., 1999). When deciding on the method of treatment, the surgeon must use their judgement and consider other factors such as position, size and risk of rupture. However, the anatomy of some AAAs prevents endoluminal repair being the first line of treatment.

We are now also getting closer to identifying the pathogenesis associated with aneurysm development and it may not be too long before drug treatment is available to inhibit the growth of smaller aneurysms (Rehm et al., 1998).

References

Albrecht T, Jager HR, Blomley MJ, Lopez A, Hossain J, Standfield N (1997) Pre-operative classification of abdominal aortic aneurysms with spiral CT: the axial source images revisited. Clinical Radiology 52(9): 659–665.

Anidjar SAKE (1992) Pathogenesis of acquired aneurysm of the abdominal aorta. Annals of Vascular Surgery 6(3): 298–305.

Bengtsson H, Nilsson P, Bergqvist D (1993) Natural history of abdominal aortic aneurysm detected by screening. British Journal of Surgery 80(6): 718–720.

Campa JS, Greenhalgh RM, Powell JT (1987) Elastin degradation in abdominal aortic aneurysms. Atherosclerosis 65: 13–21.

Campbell WB (1991) Mortality statistics for elective aortic aneurysms. European Journal of Vascular Surgery 5: 111–113.

Cao P, Zannett MD, Parlani G, Verzini F, Caporali S, Spaccatini A, Barzi F (1999) Epidural for endoluminal repair is feasible in some patients. Journal of Vascular Surgery 30: 651–657.

Chan FY, Crawford ES, Coselli JS et al. (1989) In situ prosthetic graft replacement for mycotic aneurysms of the aorta. Annals of Thoracic Surgery 47: 193–203.

Cheatle TR (1997) The case against a national screening programme for aortic aneurysms. Annals of the Royal College of Surgeons of England 79(2): 90–95.

Clifton MA (1977) Familial abdominal aortic aneurysms. British Journal of Surgery 64: 765–766.

Collin J (1996) The Oxford Screening Program for aortic aneurysm and screening first-order male siblings of probands with abdominal aortic aneurysm. Annals of the New York Academy of Sciences 800: 36–43.

Cordingley JJ, Palazzo MGA (1999) Management. In: Webb AB, Shapiro MJ, Singer M and Suter PM (eds) Oxford Textbook of Critical Care, pp 409–412. Oxford: Oxford University Press.

Datta P (1989) The pulsating mass. Nursing Mirror 8: 46–49.

Dubost C, Allary M, Deconomos N (1952) Resection of an aneurysm of the abdominal aorta. Re-establishment of the continuity by a preserved human arterial graft, with a result after five months. Archives of Surgery 64: 405–409.

Ellis M, Powell JT, Greenhalgh RM (1991) Limitations of ultrasonography in surveillance of small abdominal aortic aneurysms. British Journal of Surgery 78: 614–616.

Fahey VA (1999) Clinical assessment of the vascular system. In: Fahey VA (ed.) Vascular Nursing, pp 50–73. Philadelphia: WB Saunders.

Graham LM, Ford MB (1999) Arterial Disease. In: Fahey VA (ed.) Vascular Nursing, pp 2–20. Philadelphia: WB Saunders.

Hallett JW, Jr (1992) Abdominal aortic aneurysm: natural history and treatment. Heart Disease and Stroke 1(5): 303–308.

Hallett JW, Jr, Bower TC, Cherry KJ, Gloviczki P, Joyce JW, Pairolero PC (1994) Selection and preparation of high-risk patients for repair of abdominal aortic aneurysms. Mayo Clinic Proceedings 69(8): 763–768.

Harris PL (1992) Reducing the mortality from abdominal aortic aneurysms: need for a national screening programme. British Medical Journal 305: 697–699.

Hatswell EM (1994a) Abdominal aortic aneurysm surgery, Part I: An overview and discussion of immediate perioperative complications. Heart and Lung 23(3): 228–239.

Hatswell EM (1994b) Abdominal aortic aneurysm surgery, Part II: Major complications and nursing implications. Heart and Lung 23(4): 337–341.

Hertzer NR, Beven EG, Young JR, O'Hara PJ, Ruschhaupt WFI, Graror RA, Dewolfe VG, Malijovec LC (1984) Coronary artery disease in peripheral vascular patients: A classification of 1000 coronary angiograms and results of surgical management. Annals of Surgery 200: 255–263.

Krupski WC (1995) Abdominal aortic aneurysm: defining the dilemma. Seminars in Vascular Surgery 8(2): 115–123.

Lamont PM, Shearman CP, Scott JA (1999) Aneurysm disease. In: Lamont PM, Shearman CP, Scott JA (eds) Vascular Surgery, pp 57–74. Oxford: Oxford University Press.

Law M (1998) Screening for abdominal aortic aneurysms. British Medical Bulletin 54(4): 903–913.

Lederle FA, Wilson SE, Johnson GR (1995) Variability in measurement of abdominal aortic aneurysms. Journal of Vascular Surgery 21: 945–952.

Lucarotti M, Shaw E, Poskitt K, Heather B (1993) The Gloucestershire aneurysm screening programme: the first 2 years' experience. European Journal of Vascular Surgery 8: 741–746.

Nehler MR, Taylor LM, Jr, Moneta GL, Porter JM (1995) Indications for operation for infrarenal abdominal aortic aneurysms: current guidelines. Seminars in Vascular Surgery 8(2): 108–114.

Nevitt MP, Ballard DJ, Hallett JW (1989) Prognosis of abdominal aortic aneurysms. New England Journal of Medicine 321: 481–483.

OPCS (1993) 1991 Mortality Statistics: Cause. England and Wales. Series DH2 18(Table 2): London: HMSO.

Parodi JC, Palmaz JC, Barone HD (1991) Transfemoral intraluminal graft implantation for abdominal aortic aneurysm. Annals of Vascular Surgery 5: 491–499.

Phillips JK (1998) Abdominal aortic aneurysm. Nursing 28(5): 34–39.

Reddy DJ, Ernst CB (1995) Infected aneurysms. In: Rutherford RB (ed.) Vascular Surgery, 4th edn, vol. 2, pp 1139–1152. Philadelphia: WB Saunders.

Rehm JP, Grange JJ, Baxter BT (1998) The formation of aneurysms. Seminars in Vascular Surgery 11(3): 193–202.

Royal College of Surgeons (1997) The Surgeon's Duty of Care: Guidance for Surgeons on Ethical and Legal issues: Royal College of Surgeons. London: Senate of Surgery of Great Britain and Ireland.

Santilli JD, Santilli SM (1997) Diagnosis and treatment of abdominal aortic aneurysms. American Family Physician 56(4): 1081–1090.

Sayers MC, Gasperetti CM (1999) Therapeutic strategy. In: Webb AR, Shapiro MJ, Singer M, Suter PM (eds) Oxford Textbook of Critical Care, pp 240–242. New York, Oxford University Press.

Scott RAP, Wilson NM, Ashton HA, Kay DN (1995) Influence of screening on the incidence of ruptured abdominal aortic aneurysm: 5-year results of a randomized controlled study. British Journal of Surgery 82: 1066–1070.

Shealy CB, Elliott BM (1997) Abdominal aortic aneurysms, what's changing? Journal – South Carolina Medical Association 93(1): 13–16.

Sicard GA, Reilly JM, Rubin BG (1995) Transabdominal versus retroperitoneal incision for abdominal aortic surgery: Report of a prospective randomized trial. Journal of Vascular Surgery 21: 174–183.

Sielenkamper A, Sibbald WJ (1999) Therapeutic strategy. In: Webb AR, Shapiro MJ, Singer M, Suter PM (eds) Oxford Textbook of Critical Care, pp 221–228. New York: Oxford University Press.

Taylor LM Jr, Deitz DM, McConnell DB, Porter JM (1988) Treatment of infected abdominal aneurysms by extraanatomic bypass, aneurysm excision, and drainage. American Journal of Surgery 155: 655–658.

Tennant WG (1994) Aneurysms of the abdominal aorta. Surgery 12(10): 235–238.

Tuman KJ, McCarthy RJ, March RJ, Delaria GA, Patel R, Ivankovich AD (1991) Effects of epidural anaesthesia and analgesia on coagulation and outcome after major vascular surgery. Anesthesia and Analgesia 73: 696–704.

UK Small Aneurysm Trial Participants (1998) Mortality results of randomised control trial for early elective surgery or ultrasonographic surveillance for small abdominal aortic aneurysms. Lancet 352: 1649–1655.

Vardulaki KA, Prevost TC, Walker NM, Day NE, Wilmink AB, Quick CR, Ashton HA, Scott RA (1998) Growth rates and risk of rupture of abdominal aortic aneurysms. British Journal of Surgery 85(12): 1674–1680.

Zarins CK (1999) The limits of endovascular aortic repairs. Journal of Vascular Surgery 29(6): 1164–1166.

Chapter 13

Carotid Disease

JILL ARTHUR

Cerebrovascular event (stroke), previously called cerebrovascular accident, is the third commonest cause of death after cancer and ischaemic heart disease and the commonest cause of disability in developed countries (Donayre et al., 1994). Most strokes are caused by cerebral ischaemia due to diseased carotid arteries and the incidence of this is increasing with the ageing of the population.

Until recently nursing input has been directed at caring for patients who have already had a stroke. This is an area of care familiar to nurses working in both acute and community settings, as a stroke often leaves the patient both mentally and physically dependent on others, and a socio-economic burden on both family and society.

Now the role of nurses is widening and they can be increasingly involved in the prevention of stroke by offering health promotion, identifying and modifying risk factors and caring for patients undergoing surgical intervention. This chapter looks at these issues in particular, and discusses features of carotid disease, choice of management, assessment prior to surgery and the surgical technique of carotid endarterectomy.

Incidence of stroke

In developed countries, 12% of all deaths are due to stroke and the incidence of stroke in the UK is 2 per 1000 population. Each year in the UK, 100 000 patients have a first ever stroke, or one every 5 minutes (Bamford et al., 1988).

Stroke is a major cause of disability and institutionalisation among elderly people. It is estimated that stroke-related illness takes up almost 16 000 NHS beds every day and accounts for about 7.7 million lost working days each year (DOH, 1992). Approximately 50% of patients are dependent on carers after a first in a lifetime stroke.

One of the Health of the Nation targets was to reduce the occurrence of stroke and associated death as well as to ensure the maximum quality of life for survivors (Table 13.1).

The mortality of stroke has declined over the last thirty years, more so in women than men. This may be attributed to improved detection and treatment of hypertension, which is the main risk factor for stroke.

Table 13.1 Health of the Nation targets for stroke prevention

Objective: To reduce occurrence of stroke and associated death and to ensure the maximum quality of life for survivors.

Possible targets:
- 30% reduction nationally in death below 65 between 1988 and 2000
- 25% reduction nationally in death in the 65–74-year age group, between 1988 and 2000
- Early detection and treatment of raised blood pressure

Causes of stroke

Stroke is a clinical term used to describe the symptoms and signs of interrupted blood flow to the brain. Strokes are now frequently called cerebrovascular events as the cause is either infarction (80%) or haemorrhage (20%).

Those strokes caused by cerebral infarct are usually related to atherosclerosis of the extracranial carotid arteries (American Heart Association, 1991).

A layer of atherosclerosis (plaque) usually develops at the carotid bifurcation and extends along the internal carotid artery (Figure 13.1). Symptoms are most commonly produced by atheroembolus. Embolus occurs when the endothelial lining of the plaque ruptures and atheromatous debris is discharged into the circulation. This may lead to cell death in the cerebral hemispheres although adequate blood flow via the circle of Willis may be sufficient to support the brain tissue during the acute stage, preventing chronic damage (Figure 13.2).

Alternatively the plaque may ulcerate and attract local thrombus or platelet aggregation, which if loosely attached can also produce emboli (Figure 13.3). Ulceration or haemorrhage within the plaque may be likely if the plaque is soft and unstable, rather than calcified and stable. More rarely, enlargement of the carotid plaque by progression of the atheromatous process produces thrombosis and occlusion of the internal carotid artery and this can also cause a stroke.

Infarcts may also be due to cardiac emboli from atrial thrombus in patients with atrial fibrillation. Primary intracranial haemorrhage is responsible for 20% of strokes. Other rare causes include subdural haematoma, brain tumour, Takayasu's arteritis, carotid aneurysm, fibromuscular dysplasia and cervical radiation of malignant tumours of the neck.

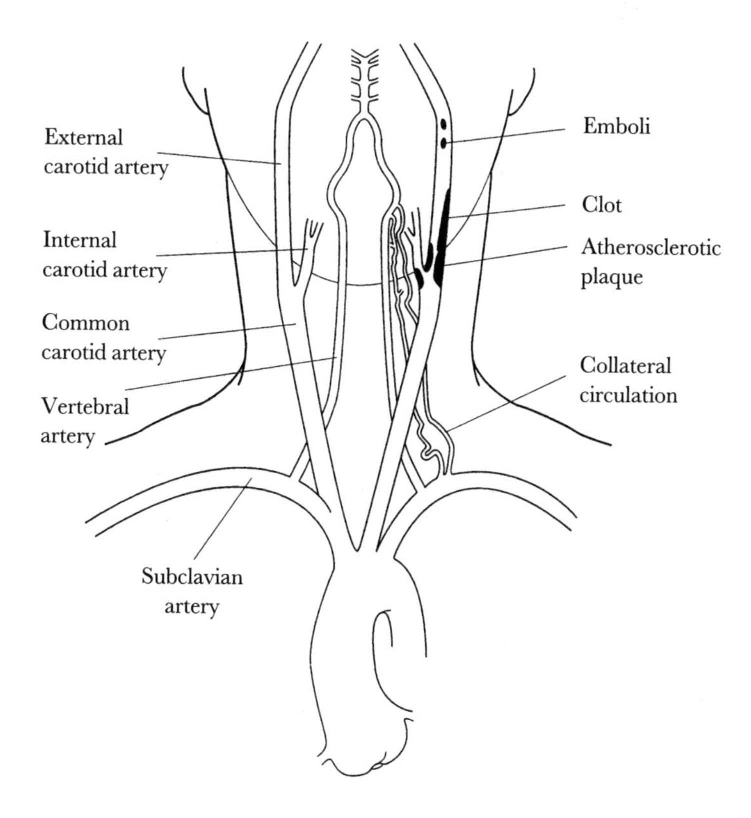

Figure 13.1 Carotid arteries with the most common sites of atherosclerotic plaque.

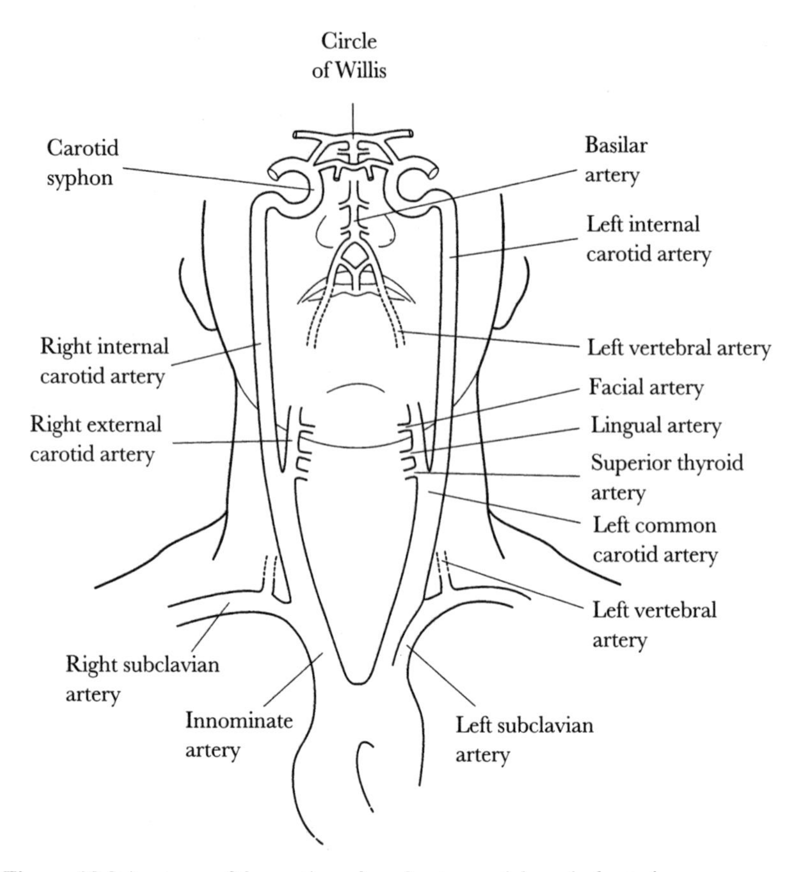

Figure 13.2 Anatomy of the aortic arch and extracranial cervical arteries.

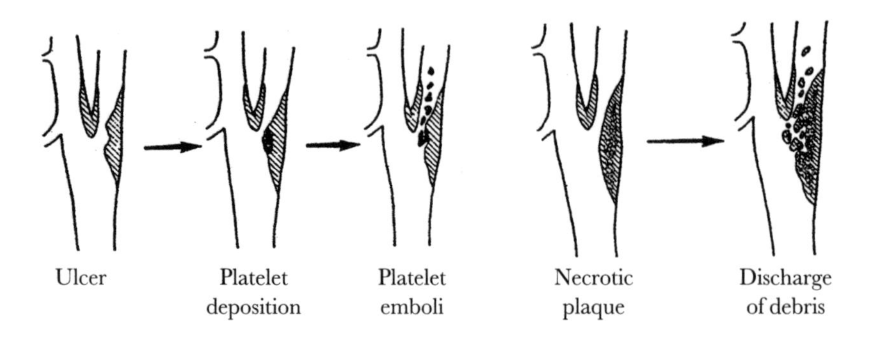

Figure 13.3 Emboli development from a carotid plaque.

Features of carotid disease

The symptoms of interrupted blood flow to the brain due to carotid disease are almost invariably sudden focal neurological deficits such as loss or difficulty with speech, weakness or numbness in one or both contralateral limbs, or transient monocular blindness. Transient monocular blindness is often described as a blind being pulled down or across one eye. The symptoms of carotid disease are rarely global, such as coma, general dizziness or unsteady gait.

Sudden onset of focal neurological deficit lasting less than 24 hours is called a *transient ischaemic attack* (TIA). The symptoms often last for only 5–10 minutes and rarely more than an hour (Table 13.2). TIAs may be multiple.

If the symptoms last more than 24 hours, but then rapidly resolve completely, the episode is called a reversible ischaemic neurological deficit (RIND).

When the symptoms do not resolve within 7 days it is called a cerebrovascular event (CVE).

The presence of a carotid bruit (audible turbulence of blood flow at the bifurcation of the carotid artery) is an unreliable guide to the presence or severity of carotid disease (Wolfe et al., 1981).

All patients suffering a TIA, RIND or CVE with good recovery should have a duplex ultrasound scan of their carotid arteries to identify and quantify carotid artery disease. The degree of stenosis is accurately measured from the increase in blood flow velocity produced by the carotid stenosis and the plaque morphology may be assessed. Carotid angiography remains the gold standard investigation, although there is an associated 1% risk of stroke/death (NASCET, 1991). Therefore in many vascular units surgery is now performed on the basis of non-invasive scanning rather than carotid angiography. For patients with critical stenosis of over 99%, duplex scanning may have limitations in defining patency of the vessel and

Table 13.2 Symptoms of a transient ischaemic attack

Symptoms
Ipsilateral transient monocular blindness (same side as carotid disease)
Contralateral hemiparesis (opposite side to carotid disease)
Contralateral hemiparaesthesia (opposite side to carotid disease)
Aphasia/dysphasia

in these situations carotid angiography may be used. Recent evidence suggests that magnetic resonance imaging (MRI) may be as sensitive with no associated morbidity but this remains unproven (Donayre et al., 1994).

Screening for asymptomatic carotid disease

The natural history of asymptomatic carotid disease is not well defined and therefore the role of screening and surgery remains controversial (Panayiotopoulos et al., 1996). Perhaps one of the strongest arguments in favour of surgery for asymptomatic patients is based on the fact that only one-third of strokes are preceded by transient ischaemic attacks (Kyriazis, 1994).

There are four large clinical trials on asymptomatic patients (Towne et al., 1990; CASANOVA, 1991; Toole et al., 1992; Halliday et al., 1995); however, the results are inconclusive. The asymptomatic carotid artery stenosis trial (ACAS, 1995) revealed a 55% relative risk reduction in patients having medical treatment. This trial continues to investigate the predictive role of plaque morphology detected by duplex scanning, which may help identify a subgroup at high risk of stroke.

The risk of stroke in a patient with asymptomatic disease and greater than 70% stenosis is much lower than with symptomatic disease. Consequently, surgery is more difficult to justify unless the perioperative stroke/death rate is very low. A conservative management approach by reducing risk factors and prescribing antiplatelet treatment such as low dose aspirin may be more beneficial for these patients. Alternatives to aspirin, such as clopidogrel, are emerging following publication of the CAPRIE study (CAPRIE, 1996).

Carotid endarterectomy (CEA)

Patients who are symptomatic (have suffered TIA, transient monocular blindness or stroke), and are found to have a greater than 70% stenosis of the appropriate carotid artery, benefit from carotid endarterectomy. This is a surgical procedure to remove the atherosclerotic plaque which has developed within the carotid artery. Clinical trials have shown that CEA in this group of patients reduces subsequent stroke risk by 17% at two years, providing that there is a surgical mortality and morbidity of less than 7% (NASCET, 1991;

ECST, 1998). Surgical risk depends on the patient's medical fitness, the technique used and the skill of the operating team.

Carotid angioplasty with or without stent is a less invasive treatment for symptomatic disease which still requires further evaluation (CAVATAS, 1998).

CEA is occasionally indicated when the stenosis is less than 70%, if the patient continues to be symptomatic despite antiplatelet or anticoagulant therapy. Patients having crescendo TIAs (TIAs which are increasingly frequent and with increasingly profound neurological symptoms), and where no cerebral infarction has incurred, may benefit from urgent CEA. In these patients a computed tomography scan (CT) of the brain should be undertaken to exclude an expanding infarct or haemorrhage. CEA should be considered following a minor ischaemic stroke with full recovery, although a patient with profound neurological deficit following a major stroke will probably not benefit from carotid surgery. The criteria for performing CEA can be seen Table 13.3.

Timing of carotid surgery after a stroke is controversial. A delay of 6 weeks is often preferable to allow cerebral autoregulation to recover and to reduce the risk of perioperative stroke (Giordano, 1998).

Table 13.3 Criteria for carotid endarterectomy

Symptomatic with >70% stenosis
Symptomatic despite medical treatment with <70% stenosis
Crescendo TIA
Unstable or ulcerated plaque

Informed consent

The relative risks and benefits of surgery should be carefully discussed with the patient and family by the surgeon in the outpatient department to help them make an informed decision about the proposed surgery. However, a second consultation by an experienced vascular nurse specialist is advisable to ensure that the patient fully understands the very real, but small, risk of perioperative stroke compared to the much greater risk of stroke if no operation is performed (Table 13.4). Having discussed the comparative risks and been given the time and opportunity for questioning and empathic listening, the nurse may even identify that the patient does not actually want to undergo surgery. Additionally, the nurse may uncover some aspect of previous medical history that has not been noted by the surgeon. This may significantly raise the perioperative stroke risk to an unacceptable level (e.g. unstable angina) or alter the decision to offer surgical treatment (e.g. carcinoma with poor prognosis). These findings should be discussed immediately with the surgeon. If the CEA is to be performed under regional block anaesthesia the vascular nurse should be present throughout the operation and perform continual neurological assessment. This consultation is the perfect opportunity to get to know the patient and allay any anxieties about having the operation performed 'awake'. On admission the vascular nurse will be a familiar face and advocate to the patient. Questions such as 'what if I want to cough or move?', 'how will I know if the anaesthetic has worked?', 'what if I feel some pain?', 'can I tell anyone if I am not comfortable?' can be answered and this in itself will reduce patient anxiety and perioperative stroke risk.

A leaflet with all appropriate advice and information, as well as a contact telephone number for further discussion, should be given to the patient to take home and read at their own leisure. This leaflet should be available to GPs and community, outpatient and ward nurses so that consistent information, health promotion advice and reassurance is offered.

Table 13.4 Risks and benefits of carotid endarterectomy

Risks of major stroke or death at 2 years without surgery – 26% (NASCET, 1991)
Risk of major stroke or death at 2 years with surgery – 9% (NASCET, 1991)
Risk of major stroke or death within 30 days of surgery under general anaesthetic – 7% (ECST, 1998)
Risk of major stroke or death within 30 days of surgery under regional block with eversion technique – 2.5% (Darling et al., 1996)

Preoperative health promotion

Patients with carotid artery disease are usually elderly with multiple medical problems such as cardiac, pulmonary and renal disease. These conditions, increasing age, and presence of severe contralateral carotid disease increase the risk of perioperative stroke and death.

To ensure the patient is as fit as possible prior to surgery associated risk factors as discussed in Chapter 3, such as smoking, obesity, hypertension, hypercholesterolaemia, diabetes and ischaemic heart disease, should be identified and if possible modified (Table 13.5).

Table 13.5 Modifiable risk factors affecting stroke incidence

Risk factor	Action/Evidence
Smoking	Strongly discourage
Hypertension	Control within safe limits (systolic <160 mmHg, diastolic <100 mmHg). Reduction by 5–6 mmHg reduces risk of stroke by 35–40% and myocardial infarction by 20–25%
Raised lipids	Lipid-lowering therapy. Total cholesterol <5.0 mmol/l reduces the incidence of symptomatic coronary heart disease
Diabetes	Recognise, treat and control. Prevention of hyperglycaemia attenuates stroke severity
Ischaemic heart disease	Treat appropriately. Angioplasty or coronary bypass may be performed before CEA or as a synchronous procedure
Alcohol	Reduce intake. May be associated with hypertension and haemorrhagic stroke

Source: Fox et al. (1996).

High-risk patients

The patient's preoperative general state of health needs to be defined and high-risk patients identified. A history of angina, myocardial infarction (MI) and untreated hypertension indicates a high-risk patient. The nurse should document and report this to ensure that medical treatment is optimised prior to surgery. Blood pressure should be monitored 4-hourly preoperatively after admission to determine the patient's normal range. Those patients who are still smoking prior to surgery may have increased risk of postoperative pulmonary complications (Warner et al., 1984). Patients should be told this and all help offered to enable them to stop smoking prior to admission. If there is a cough with green sputum, the nurse should send off a sputum specimen to the laboratory for culture, and ensure that antibiotics are prescribed if indicated.

All patients with confirmed carotid disease should have routine urinalysis, which may indicate previously undiagnosed diabetes. Optimising management of the diabetic patient pre-admission, and monitoring and controlling glucose levels preoperatively, avoids hypoglycaemic reactions and hyperglycaemic complications.

Patients on anticoagulants, such as aspirin, Persantin and warfarin have a higher risk of postoperative haematoma formation. Patients on warfarin should be fully anticoagulated with intravenous heparin before surgery and converted back after surgery. The international normalised ratio (INR) and the activated partial thromboplastin time (APTT) are checked prior to surgery. Antiplatelet therapy is stopped on the morning of surgery and subcutaneous heparin is given twice daily throughout inpatient stay to prevent deep venous thrombosis. Anti-embolism stockings are not routinely prescribed, as atherosclerosis is a systemic disease and these patients often have well-established limb disease which would be further compromised by the use of restrictive anti-embolic stockings.

Patients with contralateral carotid occlusion or who have had a recent stroke also have a high risk of perioperative stroke.

Preoperative investigations

Routine preoperative tests to ascertain patient fitness for surgery will include:

- Electrocardiogram (ECG).
- Chest X-ray.
- Full blood profile.
- Fasting blood cholesterol (preferably performed when carotid disease is first diagnosed in order to identify hypercholesterolaemia, or to optimise treatment of known hypercholesterolaemia).

A full neurological assessment is performed to identify any neurological deficit from a previous stroke, such as limb or facial weakness or altered speech. Ideally this should be performed by a neurologist. However, in centres where access to a neurology opinion is limited, the admitting surgical team should document any neurological deficit. Theatre and recovery nursing staff should be informed so that postoperative neurological changes can be identified. Most of these investigations can be performed in a pre-admission clinic one week prior to the operation. This enables the patient to be admitted the day before surgery. A repeat duplex scan is performed on admission to check that the internal carotid artery has not occluded. Occlusion eradicates risk of further TIA or stroke and negates the need for surgery.

Cross-matching of blood is usually unnecessary. Fully informed consent is obtained by a senior surgeon after discussing all aspects of the procedure, including risk of potentially fatal complications (Table 13.6).

The anaesthetist will discuss the anaesthetic procedure with the patient and may prescribe a premedication. Patients having a general anaesthetic should be fasted prior to surgery and should take all essential hypertensive and cardiac oral medication. Insulin-dependent diabetics and those on oral hypoglycaemics will need an intravenous infusion and a sliding scale of insulin prescribed. The neck should be shaved as necessary, preferably in theatre immediately before surgery.

An arterial line will be inserted in the anaesthetic room, allowing continuous monitoring of pulse and blood pressure, access for blood gas and glucose analysis, and the introduction of vasoactive drugs if there is haemodynamic instability.

Table 13.6 Postoperative complications following carotid endarterectomy

Neurological deficit
Hypotension/hypertension
Bradycardia/tachycardia
Haematoma/haemorrhage
Local nerve injury

Surgical procedure

After skin preparation the carotid bifurcation is exposed by gentle dissection, taking care not to dislodge unstable plaque or thrombus within the lumen of the vessel or to damage surrounding nerves.

Intravenous heparin is given prior to cross-clamping of the carotid arteries if a policy of selective shunting is used. A longitudinal arteriotomy is made and the vessel endarterectomised by selecting a plane between the diseased intima and the circular fibres of the media, allowing complete removal of the atheromatous plaque. Those patients who are intolerant to cross-clamping will benefit from the insertion of a temporary shunt to re-establish cerebral blood flow. These are typically patients with a stenosed or occluded contralateral carotid artery, known disease of the circle of Willis or those with a recent stroke. However, the shunt itself can cause complications, such as creating an intimal flap, which may promote thrombosis formation and plaque dislodgement resulting in cerebral emboli, air emboli, or obstruction of the surgical field.

Under general anaesthetic, cerebral ischaemia may be detected by back pressure measurement in the internal carotid artery of less than 25–50 mmHg, transcranial Doppler assessment or perioperative EEG abnormalities.

When the arteriotomy is closed, a synthetic or vein patch may be used to widen the arterial lumen if the vessel is small. After closure of the arteriotomy, adequacy of blood flow can be assessed by simple palpation, handheld Doppler or transcranial Doppler.

If there is concern about flow, thrombus formation, residual debris or kinking of the vessel, an on-table duplex scan or angiogram may be performed.

A vacuum drainage bottle is inserted prior to skin closure to reduce the risk of haematoma formation.

CEA under regional block anaesthesia

Although CEA is usually performed under general anaesthesia an increasing number of centres are using regional block anaesthesia. This facilitates continuous perioperative neurological monitoring to detect early signs of cerebral ischaemia, particularly at the time of cross-clamping of the carotid artery. These patients need only be fasted of food prior to surgery and can have free fluids until one hour prior to going to the anaesthetic room and again soon after arrival in the recovery room. Essential hypertensive, cardiac and diabetic medication should be given as normal. Insulin-dependent diabetics rarely require a sliding scale of insulin prescribed. The vascular nurse who has already met, assessed and counselled the patient in the outpatient department prior to admission escorts the patient from the ward and gives reassurance and support while the deep cervical plexus and superficial nerve block is performed. The nurse will help transfer the patient to the operating table and make sure that the head is tilted in a comfortable and appropriate position for both patient and surgeon. The surgical drapes are arranged so that the surgical field is clear, but the patient feels cool and is not claustrophobic. The nurse performs continuous neurological monitoring by verbal response command and contralateral grip power. In simple terms, this means generally chatting to the patient, asking easy mental arithmetic questions and requesting squeezing of the small bag placed in the patient's contralateral hand. This fluid-filled bag has a pressure sensor attached to the monitor so that each bag squeeze is seen as a peak on the monitor screen. Early signs of cerebral ischaemia at the time of cross-clamping, such as slurring of speech, slow or non response to verbal commands, reduction or loss in power of bag squeezing, agitation or confusion, are very easily identified in an awake patient. A definitive decision can then be made to shunt only those patients found to be intolerant of cross-clamping. Centres using a regional block claim a reduced perioperative stroke and death risk of only 1–2% (Lawrence et al., 1998). Regional anaesthesia requires a willing and cooperative patient, an anaesthetist competent in the technique, and a surgeon who is willing to operate on an awake patient.

Postoperative care and complications

Most postoperative complications occur during the first 4 hours (Table 13.6). Patients who have had surgery under general anaesthesia will usually go direct to the intensive care or high dependency unit. Those who have had a regional block anaesthesia can return straight to the ward after 4 hours in the recovery room, where they will require very close monitoring.

As soon as the patient leaves theatre, a neurological assessment using the Glasgow Coma Scale is performed to identify neurological deficit, in particular motor function and speech deficit. This deficit may be due to intraoperative hypoxia during clamping, intraoperative embolisation, or postoperative occlusion or embolisation. Urgent transcranial Doppler or duplex scan will identify whether the carotid artery is patent or occluded. If occluded, the patient should be returned to theatre immediately for re-exploration and thrombectomy. If the carotid arteries appear widely patent, supportive nursing care should be given and a CT brain scan performed in 12–24 hours to localise the cerebral infarct area and assess the amount of cerebral oedema or haemorrhage.

Hypertension may be the first sign of intracerebral haemorrhage or oedema, and hypotension may cause thrombosis of the endarterectomised vessel. It is essential that the blood pressure is checked regularly (every 15 minutes for 2 hours, half-hourly for 6 hours, hourly overnight and then 2-hourly). The systolic blood pressure should be maintained within 15% of the preoperative pressure. The doctor must be informed of any hypo/hypertension and administer Gelofusine or nifedipine as prescribed depending on the systolic blood pressure. A small rise in blood pressure may simply be a physiological response to pain, discomfort or bladder distension.

Reperfusion syndrome caused by revascularisation of a previously ischaemic area of the brain may present with severe headache.

Hypotension with tachycardia and excessive Redivac drainage indicates severe haemorrhage. Again, the patient will need to be returned to theatre immediately for exploration of the arteriotomy.

Wound haematoma may cause visible swelling of the wound site and deviation of the trachea. Stridor, low oxygen saturation level or cyanosis indicates airway obstruction. The anaesthetist should be urgently called to obtain or maintain the airway before the patient is returned to theatre for exploration and evacuation of haematoma. Small haematomas may be left alone and usually resolve within 7–10 days without complication or infection.

Local cranial nerve injury may be identified as a drooping lip, difficulty in swallowing, speech or mastication, hoarseness, or paraesthesia of the face and ear. Symptoms caused by cranial nerve injury resulting from retraction trauma will resolve in 2–6 months. This should be explained to the patient; time and reassurance is all the treatment most patients require.

Intravenous fluids and sliding scale insulin are discontinued as soon as normal diet and fluids are tolerated.

Minor discomfort is experienced and is relieved with regular oral analgesia. Full mobilisation is encouraged from the first postoperative day.

The vacuum drainage is usually minimal and the drain is removed on the first postoperative day. Aspirin is represcribed on the evening of the operation day.

Discharge arrangements

Most patients are ready for discharge on the third to fifth postoperative day. Patients who live alone or are the main carer for their elderly spouse will be able to plan their discharge, if forewarned, prior to admission, e.g. arrange for a friend or neighbour to move in for a few nights, or to stay with relatives short term.

On discharge, patients should have an information leaflet including health promotion advice and a contact phone number.

The patient should be informed that mild headaches and neck stiffness are normal and are usually due to positioning during surgery, especially if there is cervical arthritis. Driving can be resumed when neck discomfort no longer restricts range of movement.

The incision should be kept dry until the sutures/clips are removed by the community nurse on the fifth postoperative day. The patient should again be reassured about numbness around the scar and symptoms of transient nerve damage.

If the patient has had a synthetic patch inserted, they should be advised to request antibiotic cover before invasive medical or dental treatment is performed. The importance of regularly taking hypotensive, diabetic and antiplatelet medication should be stressed.

Relevant lifestyle changes should be encouraged such as low cholesterol diet, review of diabetic diet, weight reduction, smoking cessation or stress reduction.

A follow-up appointment with the consultant and check duplex scan should be arranged 6 weeks following discharge home.

Recurrent symptomatic carotid stenosis is rare and affects 1–3% of patients after CEA (Hallet et al., 1995). This generally requires repeat scanning or angiography followed by repeat endarterectomy with patch angioplasty.

Asymptomatic restenosis is detectable in 10–20% of patients following CEA, but risk of further stroke in this group is low (Hallet et al., 1995). Patients with known contralateral asymptomatic 50–70% stenosis have a significant risk of becoming symptomatic, especially if the stenosis progresses (Hallet et al., 1995). Ongoing duplex monitoring may be necessary in this latter group until criteria for CEA are reached.

Conclusion

There is an increasing role for nurses to play in the care of patients with carotid disease. People are aware of the devastating effect that a stroke can have on their life or that of their relative. Patients, their carers and relatives require much psychological support, advice and information when they are given the results of an abnormal carotid duplex scan and are informed that they have a significant risk of stroke. A well-informed nurse can provide such support as well as highlight and optimise risk factors, and offer health promotion advice. It is important to remember that many patients with carotid disease are highly likely to also have significant ischaemic heart disease and peripheral vascular disease and therefore an holistic approach to their nursing care and management is essential.

References

ACAS Study Executive Committee (1995) Endarterectomy for asymptomatic carotid artery stenosis. JAMA 273(18): 1421–1428.

American Heart Association (1991) Heart and Stroke Facts: 23.

Bamford J, Sandercock P, Dennis M., Warlow C, Jones L, McPherson K, Vessey M, Fowler G, Molyneux K, Hughes T, Burn J, Wade D (1988) A prospective study of acute cerebrovascular disease in the community: the Oxfordshire Community stroke project 1981–86. Journal of Neurology, Neurosurgery and Psychiatry 51(11): 1373–1380.

CAPRIE steering committee (1996) A randomised blinded trial of clopidogrel versus aspirin in patients at risk of ischaemic events. Lancet 348(9038): 1329–1339.

Carotid Artery Stenosis with Asymptomatic Narrowing Operation versus Aspirin (CASANOVA) study group (1991) Stroke 22(10): 1229–1235.

CAVATAS Investigators results of the Carotid and Vertebral Artery Transluminal Angioplasty Study (CAVATAS) (1998) Proceedings of the Annual Vascular Society Meeting of Great Britain and Ireland, Hull, UK, November 1998.

Darling R, Paty P, Shah D, Chang B, Leather R (1996) Eversion endarterectomy of the internal carotid artery: technique and results in 449 procedures. Surgery 120(4): 635–640.

Department of Health (1992) The Health of the Nation. A summary of the strategy for health in England. London: HMSO.

Donayre C, Wilson S, Hobson R (1994) Extracranial carotid artery occlusive disease. In: Veith F, Hobson R, Williams R, Wilson S (eds) Vascular Surgery: Principles and Practice, vol. 2, pp 649–664. New York: McGraw-Hill.

European Carotid Surgery Trialists (ECST) Collaborative Group (1998) Randomised trial of endarterectomy for recent symptomatic carotid stenosis: final results of the MRC European Carotid Surgery Trial. Lancet 351: 1379–1387.

Fox A, Budd J, Horrocks M (1996) Who needs carotid endarterectomy? The Practitioner 240(1558): 29–32.

Giordano JM (1998) The timing of carotid endarterectomy after acute stroke. Seminars in Vascular Surgery 11(1): 19–23.

Hallet J, Brewster D, Darling R (1995) Handbook of Patient Care in Vascular Surgery 11: 137–153.

Halliday A, Thomas D, Manfield A (1995) The asymptomatic carotid surgery trial(ACST). Interim Angiology 14(1): 18–20.

Kyriazis M (1994) Developments in the treatment of stroke patients. Nursing Times 20(90): 30–32.

Lawrence P, Alves J, Jicha D, Bhirangi K, Dobrin P (1998) Incidence, timing and causes of cerebral ischaemia during carotid endarterectomy with regional anaesthesia. Journal of Vascular Surgery 27(2): 329–337.
North American Symptomatic Carotid Endarterectomy Trial (NASCET) collaborators(1991) Beneficial effect of carotid endarterectomy in symptomatic patients with high grade stenosis. New England Journal of Medicine 325: 445–453.
Panayiotopoulos Y, Padayachee S, Taylor P (1996) Surgery for asymptomatic carotid artery stenosis. British Journal of Clinical Practice 50(6): 335–338.
Toole J, Hobson R, Howard V, Chambless L (1992) Nearing the finishing line? The asymptomatic carotid atherosclerosis study (ACAS). Stroke 23(8):1054–1055.
Towne J, Weiss D, Hobson R (1990) First phase report of co-operative Veterans Administration asymptomatic carotids stenosis study – operative morbidity and mortality. Journal of Vascular Surgery 11(2): 252–259.
Warner M, Divertie M, Tinker J (1984) Pre-operative cessation of smoking and pulmonary complications in coronary artery bypass patients. Anesthesiology 60(4): 380–383.
Wolfe P, Kannell W, Sorlie P, McNamara P (1981) Asymptomatic carotid bruit and risk of stroke. The Framingham Study. JAMA 245(14):1442–1445.

Further reading

Frattini W (1996) Update for nurse anaesthetists – carotid endarterectomy, anaesthetic complications. Journal of the American Association of Nurse Anaesthetists 64(2): 175–185.
Herbert L (1997) Caring for the patient undergoing carotid endarterectomy. In: Caring for the Vascular Patient, pp 221–232. London: Churchill Livingstone.
MacVittie B (1998) Carotid endarterectomy. In: Vascular Surgery. Mosby's Perioperative Nursing Series, pp 131–142. St Louis: Mosby.
Wolfe J (1996) Carotid endarterectomy. In: ABC of Vascular Diseases: pp 63–65. Coventry: Clifford Press.

CHAPTER 14

Wound Care in Vascular Disease

JANE HOLDEN

Greater understanding of wound healing processes and influencing factors has increased over the past decade. Nevertheless, the ambiguous pathogenesis of certain wounds, controversy over management techniques and lack of appropriate wound models to evaluate the numerous treatment regimes available, challenges those caring for patients with wounds. Fundamentally, these healthcare professionals can claim some reassurance from the fact that effective care is dependent on holistic assessment, individualised plans and multidisciplinary involvement. It is all too easy to focus on the wound itself and fail to identify the systemic factors which directly influence any intervention bestowed on the injured part. Never was this more true than in the patient with underlying vascular disease, as the nature of the disease process lends itself to impaired healing (Turner, 1986; Ting, 1991; Herbert, 1997).

This chapter will consider the physiology of wound healing with direct relation to clinical application, and highlight some factors thought to influence the healing process, including nutrition, infection, psychological factors and wound management. Novel approaches such as larval therapy and topical negative pressure will be explored and management recommendations for some of the wound types facing the vascular nurse will be highlighted. Finally, the role of the multidisciplinary team will be mentioned.

Physiology of wound healing

A wound can be defined as a break in skin integrity as a result of physical, mechanical, thermal or biological damage (Thomas, 1990).

Destruction of the skin jeopardises the body's first line of defence (Roitt, 1991), therefore injury demands a prompt response to ensure survival (Martin, 1997). Wound healing is a complex process of regeneration and replacement (Thomas, 1990; Doughty, 1992; Clark, 1996), with the ultimate aim of repairing the deficit and returning to normal function (Bryant, 1992; Garrett, 1997).

Descriptions of wound healing outline an initial period of *haemostasis* (Achan et al., 1996), an *inflammatory phase*, during which neutrophils and macrophages combat bacteria (Diegelmann et al., 1981), a *proliferative phase*, which re-establishes dermal integrity, cutaneous cover and neovascularisation (Clark, 1996), and finally the *maturation phase*, during which repaired and regenerated tissue is reorganised (Alison, 1992). However, this description fails to reflect the complexities of the process or to highlight the impact cellular activity, cytokines and extracellular matrix have on one another (Adzick and Longaker, 1991; Clark, 1993). Nevertheless, insight into the physiology can be useful to the nurse who needs to consider its relevance to her/his clinical practice (Table 14.1).

Table 14.1 Physiology of wound healing and clinical application

Phase	Physiology	Clinical implications
Haemostasis	Loss of blood vessel continuity results in bleeding which is followed by a complex cascade of events to achieve haemostasis (see Chapter 1). In addition to this main function of blood coagulation, other roles of this phase include providing the provisional matrix for recruitment of cells to the injured site and generating products which are fundamental in the initial stages of the healing process (Clark, 1993)	The nurse must monitor for bleeding and consider the impact of anticoagulant therapy. Should haemorrhage occur, pressure should be applied; where vascular reconstruction has been carried out this pressure should be applied above the anastomosis in an attempt to protect the graft (Herbert, 1997). Development of a haematoma may be obvious in terms of clinical signs but may also manifest slowly. Potential skin damage and infection may result from haematoma formation, which may require surgical evacuation
Inflammation	Damaged cells release histamine, prostaglandins and kinins, resulting in vasodilatation and increased	The classical signs of inflammation, redness, swelling, heat and pain, should be expected. Management should focus on allowing the process

(contd)

Table 14.1 (contd)

Phase	Physiology	Clinical implications
	permeability. The destructive element of this phase lasts 1–6 days and involves migration of neutrophils and monocytes into the damaged area drawn by a process of chemotaxis. Neutrophils destroy bacteria and monocytes develop into the key cell of the healing process, the macrophage. Both white blood cells clear the wound of bacteria and foreign material. The macrophage also stimulates the fibroblast, one of the key cells in the proliferative phase (Clark, 1993, 1996)	to continue unhalted, protecting the area from contamination and supporting the patient with adequate pain relief. Exudate will be produced and provides the medium in which healing can occur
Proliferation	This is a rebuilding period involving 4 activities: granulation, angiogenesis, epithelialisation and contraction (Clark, 1993). The fibroblast is concerned with depositing the extracellular matrix of the wound, which replaces the damaged dermis. The production of new blood vessels is known as angiogenesis. The epithelium is regenerated by the proliferation and migration of epithelial cells across the newly forming extracellular matrix, both elements of the wound interacting and dependent on each other for development (Donaldson and Mahan, 1983). Contraction of the wound reduces the surface area promoting wound closure. However this can result in altered function if over joints and can prompt aesthetic problems	The macrophage is sensitive to drops in temperature, pH and hypoxia and therefore management should consider the influence treatments may have on inactivating the macrophage and therefore delaying healing. Maintain a warm and undisturbed environment if possible. Avoid the use of antiseptics in the absence of infection. Epithelial cells require moisture and oxygen for proliferation and migration. Minimal intervention and careful handling is important, as is a well-balanced diet

Maturation	Once the epithelium has covered the wound further reorganisation of the underlying collagen occurs in order to achieve tensile strength (Clark, 1993, 1996). This process will continue from the point of epithelium closure up to 1–2 years post injury.	Epithelialisation is complete but the area is vulnerable and needs protection. It will never regain the original strength. Vascularisation reduces and the wound changes in colour. Patients need education regarding protection, cleansing, moisturising and information about the way it will continue to change over the coming year. Complications such as hypertrophic and keloid scarring may present themselves during this phase

Factors affecting wound healing

Numerous factors influence the healing process, highlighting the need for comprehensive, holistic assessment. Morison (1992), categorises these factors as intrinsic and extrinsic (Table 14.2).

Table 14.2 Intrinsic and extrinsic factors influencing healing

Intrinsic	Extrinsic
Local condition at the wound bed: • poor blood supply resulting in hypoxia • oedema • infection • foreign bodies (haematoma; slough; stitches, prosthetic graft) • age of the wound • position of the wound	Inappropriate wound management: • incorrect wound assessment • inappropriate topical products • inappropriate dressing selection • careless techniques • pressure • mechanical stress on the wound • temperature
Pathophysiology: • malnutrition, e.g. obesity • metabolic disorders, e.g. diabetes • anaemia • immunosuppressive disorders • other underlying diseases, e.g. rheumatoid arthritis	Other therapies: • drugs, e.g. steroids, anti-inflammatory, nicotine • radiation • repeated trauma to the area
Ageing process: • slower maturation phase • underlying disease processes	The patient: • lifestyle, e.g. smoking, poor diet • self-interference with wound

Inevitably the healthcare professional should aim to identify factors which may influence the healing process and if possible counteract them so that natural healing can progress (Negus, 1995). In situations where this does not occur, either because the assessment has not been comprehensive enough or because the problems cannot be counteracted, one can expect healing to be compromised. Fundamental to the healing process is the presence of an adequate blood supply so that oxygen, nutrients and key cells for healing are delivered to the injured area and all waste products are removed (Westerhof, 1993; McCollum, 1994; Cullum and Roe, 1995). Without a blood supply wounds will not heal (Negus, 1995; Paquet and Lapiere, 1993; Herbert, 1997). Individual patient assessment is essential and the multidisciplinary team needs to realistically plan goals of care with the patient. As a result of this process, the aim to heal the wound may not always be appropriate and further surgery, amputation or palliative care may become the main focus.

Nutrition

The growing body of knowledge about the impact of nutrition on wound healing suggests that good nutrition optimises the environment for healing to occur and poor nutrition increases morbidity and mortality in patients undergoing operations (Casey et al., 1983; Dickhault et al., 1984; Ruberg, 1984; McClaren, 1993; Osak, 1993). This includes problems with delayed wound healing and an increased susceptibility to infection (Doughty, 1992; Osak, 1993; Konstantinides and Lehmann, 1993; Ondrey and Hom, 1994), indicating an important consideration for the nurse caring for patients undergoing vascular reconstruction, especially with the evidence that moderate to severe protein-calorie malnutrition is not uncommon among surgical patients (Bistrian et al., 1974; Hill et al., 1977; Bobel, 1987).

Nutritional deficits may be associated with severe catabolic stress caused by surgery and nosocomial infection (Bobel, 1987). Intermittent periods of fasting necessitated by repeated visits to theatre for those patients whose vascular reconstruction is not totally successful may complicate this further. It is important to note that only one of the essential elements may be deficient but result in prolonged healing, and that the emphasis on adequate nutrition needs to focus on whole body nutrition and not individual nutrients (Schilling, 1976; Osak, 1993). The key nutrients that provide the raw materials for healing include protein, carbohydrates, fats, vitamins and minerals (Table 14.3).

Table 14.3 Examples of the influence some nutrients have in wound healing

Nutrient	Role in wound healing
Carbohydrates	Associated with increased metabolic needs of the stressed and traumatised patient (Young, 1988; McClaren, 1993; Hallett, 1995)
Protein	Protein deficiency has been associated with a prolonged inflammatory phase (Schilling, 1976; McClaren, 1993), impaired angiogenesis, fibroblast proliferation, proteoglycans and collagen synthesis and wound remodelling (Young, 1988; Lotti et al., 1998), including the rate at which a wound gains tensile strength (Ruberg, 1984). Protein will be sacrificed for gluconeogenesis when carbohydrates are not readily available, and negate healing (Bobel, 1987; Lee and Stotts, 1990; Pinchoky-Devin, 1994)
Vitamin C	Essential component for collagen formation via hydroxylation of proline (Stone and Meister, 1962; Schilling, 1976; Ruberg, 1984; Goode et al., 1992; Osak, 1993), and in increasing lymphocyte proliferative responses (Goode et al., 1992)
Vitamin A	Vitamin A may be another cofactor in collagen synthesis (Ruberg, 1984; Osak, 1993), and is thought to promote epithelialisation (Osak, 1993), because it has a role in epidermal growth and differentiation (Harper and Savage, 1980). Vitamin A has also been identified as an immunostimulant in humans specifically relating to the postoperative responses of patients to supplementary vitamin A as compared with groups of patients who did not receive the vitamin (Cohen et al., 1979)
Zinc	Zinc deficiency has been associated with reduced epithelialisation and reduced wound strength (Ruberg, 1984; Konstantinides and Lehmann, 1993). However, such effects remain a topic of controversy with some studies negating that oral zinc has any effect on the healing of leg ulcers (Greaves and Ive, 1961). The suggestion that zinc acts primarily at the wound site where it could be incorporated into the various enzyme systems (Pories et al., 1967) highlights the importance of adequate delivery of minerals, as with other nutrients, which is dependent on the arterial supply. To guarantee liberation at the appropriate site, topical application of nutrients such as zinc has become an alternative option to nutritional intake (Williams, 1996). However, further investigation is warranted to confirm this

Further research will be required to determine how dietary intake needs to be manipulated in order to optimise the supply of nutrients for the healing process (McClaren, 1993), especially in the patient whose circulatory problems complicate the mechanisms by which these factors are delivered to the wound site.

Infection

Diagnosing wound infection in clinical practice can be problematic with misdiagnosis leading to inappropriate treatment (Tonge, 1997). Nursing care involves monitoring wounds for infection, detecting and eradicating infection while systemically supporting the patient. A reduction in the efficiency of circulation to extremities, as seen in patients with vascular disease, increases the patient's susceptibility to infection (Turner, 1986), and therefore heightens the importance of considering this in aspects of nursing care, especially as advancing infection can prove fatal (Negus, 1995). The presence of resistant organisms such as methicillin-resistant *Staphylococcus aureus* (MRSA), and strains of *Acinetobacter* heightens this challenge further. This highlights the importance of detecting such organisms in existing wounds prior to arterial reconstructive procedures where the synthetic graft material provides an excellent focus of additional infection and subsequent graft failure.

Nurses need to be able to differentiate between inflammation associated with the healing process and that relating to infection. Offensive odour, copious amounts of exudate, pus, increasing pain and systemic temperature all contribute to the clinical signs of infection. In addition, lack of healing or deterioration of the wound may indicate an infective process. The use of the bacteriological swab to investigate the presence of bacteria on the wound bed is well established in wound management practice, yet its limited diagnostic potential needs to be acknowledged by those using it (Tonge, 1997). The wound biopsy has been proposed as a preferred method but this too has its disadvantages and is often impractical to perform (Lawrence and Ameen, 1998). Greater investigation into how wounds can be more effectively investigated in terms of bacterial growth is very much needed. When wound swabbing is used, close liaison with the microbiologist and clear indication of the clinical presentation of the wound will aid in the appropriate choice of therapies (Tonge, 1997).

The challenge for the nurse is that there is no consensus on how to prepare the wound prior to swabbing or how to best take the swab (Lawrence and Ameen, 1998; Gilchrist, 1996). The recommendation of taking a swab using a zigzag motion in order to cover the entire surface of the wound, while simultaneously rotating the swab between thumb and forefinger to utilise the entire surface area of the swab (Lawrence and Ameen, 1998), seems logical yet is not scientifically supported.

Parenteral antibiotics are preferable to topical preparations (Negus, 1995). However, systemic antibiotics may not adequately permeate necrotic avascular tissues and hence may not be able to eliminate an infection (Hellgren and Vincent, 1993). The importance of removing necrotic tissue from the wound is vital as it removes non-viable tissue which presents as a focal point for infection (Hellgren and Vincent, 1993).

Patients who have undergone revascularisation procedures (see Chapter 10) have the added potential of developing an infected prosthesis. If this occurs, graft removal may be required for the infection to be eradicated and the wound to heal but this is obviously at the expense of the revascularised limb.

Psychological impact

Altered body image can occur at any time due to illness, disease, trauma, treatment regimes and ageing (Cronan, 1993; Magnan, 1996). A change in the functional ability of a part that may result from vascular disease and/or physical mutilation resulting from surgery irrespective of extent or visibility can affect self-esteem, having an impact on body image (Wassner, 1982; Herman, 1986; Drench, 1994). This highlights the considerable impact such a disease process may have at various times, as patients undergoing vascular reconstruction may be challenged by the underlying disease, surgical procedure, ongoing wound problems and/or treatment regimes, and this will manifest in a variety of ways. Key issues for the vascular nurse to consider include the process experienced when the change or loss occurs, the knowledge of the healthcare team about the interrelationship between body image and its disruption, and the reintegration of the patient into society (Henker, 1979; Wassner, 1982; Piff, 1986; Partridge, 1990; Price 1990a).

Previous losses, physiological factors, prognosis of treatment, cultural attitudes and the stigma associated with the change are thought to influence a person's reaction to mutilation (Goffman, 1963; Bishop, 1963). Adaptation takes time as the person needs to reorganise the values they associate with certain images (Henker 1979; Wassner, 1982; Price, 1990b). However, if the person is unable to accommodate the change, body image problems may arise and specialist input may be required, such as counselling.

Members of the healthcare team need to consider personal beliefs and assumptions that have formulated as a result of socialisation (Price, 1990b). Routine association with patients undergoing extensive vascular surgical procedures influences this and may not reflect society's norms or mirror the expectations of the patient; hence there is a danger of neglect where the alteration is considered by the healthcare professionals to be minor (Drench, 1994). The nurse's role has been highlighted consistently as pivotal because they deal with the affective domain and provide close continuous care which focuses on holism (Fawcett and Frye, 1980; Price, 1990b; Newell, 1991; Cronan, 1993; MacGinley, 1993; Magnan, 1996; Salter, 1997). However, this highlights major assumptions that nurses know what altered body image is, the influence it has on health and more importantly that they have the skills to offer some form of intervention (Price, 1990b). It is possible that the skills used to deal with such a complex area are largely developed by trial and error and although psychological care is recognised as important, it may well be overlooked.

Emphasis has been placed on preoperative assessment and providing information and explanations (Wilson-Barnett and Osborne, 1983; Price, 1990b; Cronan, 1993). This includes the assessment of care available from, and response of, a spouse towards the impending treatment (Dyk and Sutherland, 1956). However, the initial assessment period is limited, especially when emergency vascular procedures are required, and it is important to consider that preoperative teaching does not ensure expectations will be met, nor does it prepare for the unexpected (Kelly, 1985; Magnan, 1996). This is an important consideration for patients undergoing vascular surgery that may result in unpredictable outcomes such as limb amputation or large open wounds.

Advice and strategies for nurses involved with patients with altered body image are well documented (Price, 1990a, 1990b; Carpenito, 1993; MacGinley, 1993; Drench, 1994; Magnan, 1996; Salter, 1997), but rigorous evidence supporting these suggestions is not recorded, making evaluation of techniques impossible. Nevertheless, it is evident that all members of the multidisciplinary team have a role in working through issues with the patient with the aim of planning gradual and successful reintegration into society and their home environment (Henker, 1979; MacGinley, 1993). However, in a climate where time and resources are limited the ability to follow these recommendations can be challenged.

Ongoing support following discharge from community healthcare professionals and support networks is essential (Dyk and Sutherland, 1956; Cronan, 1993; Drench, 1994). Family and friends are seen as important because they provide the mirror for the individual to gather cues about their image; through their response to the altered image the individual may be able to restore self-esteem and engage in social interaction (Dyk and Sutherland, 1956; Griffiths, 1989; Partridge, 1990). If healthcare professionals intend to rely on the family to provide emotional support as the patient adapts to the altered body image, they need to consider ways of preparing them for that role. Reactions of the relatives to the patient's wounds can vary from total commitment to revulsion (Partridge, 1990), the second of which intimates how involvement of some family members may not be appropriate.

Wound management

The dynamic process of wound healing means that wounds will have varied presentations throughout the healing process, and therefore demand ongoing reassessment, with a treatment plan being based on a holistic approach (Herbert, 1997). Certain principles such as cleansing, debridement and topical treatment are important. Nevertheless, the nurse is wise to remember that if the underlying cause of the wound is not resolved, whether it is a poor blood supply or infection, it will not heal. This equally applies before and after revascularisation procedures, e.g. angioplasty; bypass grafts.

The nurse should document the following in her/his local wound assessment:

- Wound size. Nurses in the clinical area do not usually have access to sophisticated measuring devices (Vowden, 1995), but depend on methods that are available, practical and cheap. Tools to achieve this need to be minimally invasive, safe and produce precise data (Goodson and Hunt, 1982; Melhuish et al., 1993; McTaggart 1994). Although the shape of a wound may not lend itself to measurement of any kind, some form of measurement is required to provide a baseline against which intervention can be evaluated and progress monitored (Bale, 1997). Methods may include linear measurements, perimeter tracings, surface area calculations, photographs or moulds to estimate depth. Each method has advantages and disadvantages and different wound types demand different forms of measurement.
- The type, consistency and amount of exudate.
- The condition of the surrounding skin.
- Bacterial status including the dates of recent swabs and a record of results from previous swabs.
- The appearance of the wound including the type of tissue present.

Wound tissue may be infected, as already discussed, necrotic, sloughy, granulating or epithelialising, all of which require different approaches in their management.

Necrotic/sloughy wounds

Dead tissue obstructs granulation, provides a focal point for infection and therefore needs to be removed (Hellgren and Vincent, 1993; Bale, 1997) (Figure 14.1). The most efficient method of debridement involves surgical excision down to the viable tissue. However, this is not always practical in terms of the patient's sutiability for anaesthesia, coagulation status or wound area requiring debridement (Hellgren and Vincent, 1993). Sharp debridement at the bedside may be possible with adequate pain relief (see Chapter 6). Additional approaches that may be used as an adjunct to sharp debridement include: autolysis facilitated by the application of dressings that maintain a moist environment at the wound bed, enzymatic with the application of topical enzymes (Table 14.4) and biological as in the use of larvae (Bale, 1997).

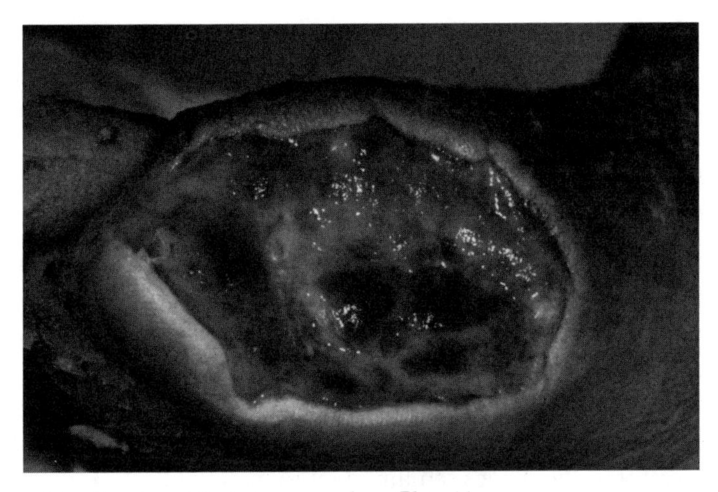

Figure 14.1 Slough and fibrin in a wound; see Plate 11.

Healthy tissue needs protection through this process and the nurse should expect the wound initially to increase in size as all the dead tissue is removed and the true size of the injured area revealed. Each patient must be assessed holistically when considering the most appropriate method, which should be evaluated for its advantages and disdvantages. Sharp debridement may not be appropriate for the confused agitated patient and nurses who have not developed competence in this should not perform it. Ischaemic areas are susceptible to infection and therefore dry necrosis should not be moistened in the patient with ischaemia, hence autolytic debridement is not appropriate. Certain enzymatic preparations may be contraindicated in certain patient groups, and hospital wound dressing formularies may be reluctant to recommend them due to lack of clinical evidence to support their efficacy (Wandsworth Community Health and St George's Healthcare NHS Trusts, 1996).

Granulating wounds

Granulation occurs in a moist, warm, slightly acidic environment and once all the slough and necrotic tissue is removed management should focus on facilitating a favourable environment. Tissue is very fragile and needs protection; therefore frequency of dressing changes can be reduced in accordance with the exudate and type of wound care product applied. Nevertheless, areas may overgranulate, requiring treatments to flatten raised granulation so that the epithelial cells can continue to migrate over the surface. Throughout this entire period strategies should be employed to prevent contamination and cross-infection.

Epithelialising wounds

This final visual phase of healing requires high oxygen tension at the wound surface and the importance of moisture is well established (Winter, 1962; Hinman and Maibach, 1963; Winter, 1965). Epithelialisation is dependent on healthy granulation tissue to migrate across but will be halted by overgranulation. These cells are fragile and trauma to the area needs to be avoided. Until this layer of the skin is restored the tissues remain open to infection.

It is possible that a variety of tissues will be present at any one time. In addition, the wound may also display bone, muscle, tendon, ligament, deep fascia and/or subcutaneous fat. All of these should be commented on in the wound assessment together with any indication of foreign bodies present such as haematoma (Figure 14.2), sutures, clips or synthetic bypass graft material.

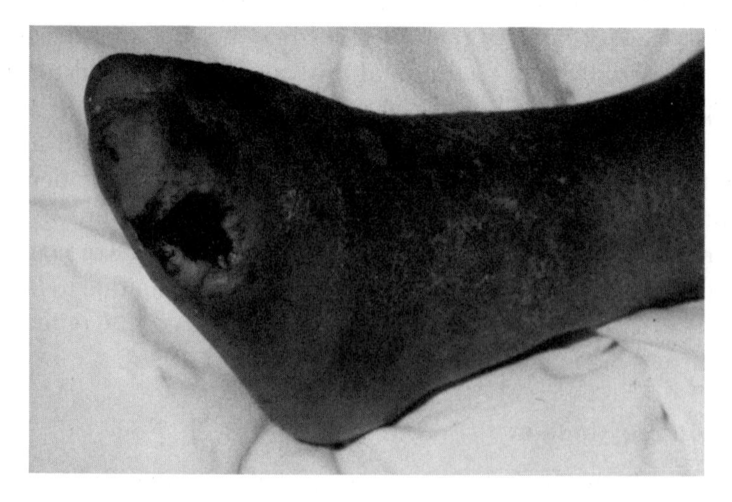

Figure 14.2 Haematoma in the base of a wound; see Plate 12.

Selecting appropriate dressings

The majority of uncomplicated wounds heal spontaneously. However, the vascular patient, as a result of the disease process and/or surgical intervention, may present with a variety of wound types ranging from the simple sutured wound to those which are much more complicated. There are numerous texts to guide the clinician in selecting appropriate dressings for the variety of wounds that may be presented by the patient with vascular disease (Thomas, 1990; Bryant 1992; Morison, 1992; Dealey, 1994; Bale and Jones, 1997). Nevertheless, nurses need to consider the overall assessment and identify aims of care rather than focusing solely on the dressing type. Dressing selection should also be guided by hospital formularies and for those patients whose transfer to the community setting is imminent it is important to choose products that will be available on prescription, once discharged from the hospital setting.

Numerous products exist, some examples of which are included in Table 14.4. However, selecting from the variety of products is complicated by the lack of scientific evidence to suggest that one is better than another, and the heavy dependence on the animal as a wound model (Ordman and Gillman, 1966; Cullum and Roe, 1995; Negus, 1995).

Recent advances in wound care

Examples of the advances in wound care over the last 10 years include numerous types of dressing products, developments in tissue engineering (Mulder, 1999), growth factors, larval therapy and negative pressure. All of these methods may be used in the patient with vascular disease, although emphasis still needs to be on treating the underlying problem (Negus, 1995). Clinical trials and case studies supporting in vogue therapies need to be scrutinised closely with respect to the patients selected and the follow-up periods. Larval therapy and negative pressure therapy are examples of such therapies adopted in the management of wounds of patients with vascular disease.

Larval therapy

The 1990s have seen the repopularisation of larval debridement, which dates back to Napoleon, the American Civil War and World War I (Edwards, 1997; Waters, 1998). Although the use of maggots has been reported as beneficial in wound management, the claims are based largely on anecdotal evidence and limited numbers of case

Table 14.4 Dressing products

Category	Examples	Uses	Advantages	Disadvantages
Alginates	Comfeel Seasorb Kaltostat Sorbsan Tegagel	For autolytic debridement in medium to heavily exuding sloughy wounds Exudate control	Absorbent Conforms to cavities Readily available	Always requires a secondary dressing Will stick in low exudate wounds May cause discomfort on application Not the dressing of choice in infected wounds
Deodorising	Actisorb Plus Clinisorb Lyofoam C	Activated charcoal dressings reduce offensive odours	Reduces odour Some types absorb excess exudate	Some must not be used directly over the wound Can be difficult to obtain in the community
Enzymes	Varidase	Debridement	Topical debriding agent	Poorly documented efficacy of current products limits use Costly
Foams	Allevyn Cavicare Flexipore Lyofoam Tielle	For autolytic debridement in heavily exuding sloughy wounds Exudate control Primary or secondary control	Conforming Absorbent Provides thermal and mechanical protection	Can be difficult to apply in awkward areas Some brands may adhere to the wound bed Some require skill in preparation (cavicare) Brands without an adhesive border require a secondary dressing
Hydrocolloids	Aquacel Combiderm Comfeel Plus Cutinova Foam	For autolytic debridement in low exuding necrotic wounds Exudate control Primary or secondary dressing	Available in a variety of forms Does not adhere to wound bed	Produces a liquid with odour at the wound bed Can ruck up Should not be used in the presence of untreated anaerobic infection

	Duoderm Granuflex Tegasorb	Maintains a moist wound environment	Maintains moist, acidic environment Can be left up to 7 days	Can cause maceration to surrounding tissue Can result in over granulation tissue
Hydrogels	Geliperm GranuGel Intrasite Nu-Gel Purilon Gel	For autolytic debridement in low exuding/necrotic wounds and dry sloughy wounds Maintains a moist environment	Maintains moisture Encourages autolysis Can be a medication carrier Can be left for several days Can be used during all stages of wound healing	Requires secondary dressing Can cause irritation and maceration Caution in the presence of anaerobic organisms Should not be left to dry out No value in heavily exuding wounds
Low adherent dressings	Mepitel NA Ultra Release Tricotex	Minimal exudate Epithelialising wounds	Caters for low exudate wounds Readily available No loose fibres	Poor absorption May result in maceration to surrounding skin May adhere to wound bed
Medicated dressings	Bactigras Chlorhexitulle Inadine Iodoflex M&M tulle Poviderm	Infected wounds Povidone iodine may have a role in infection containment in the presence of MRSA	Carries medications Some brands are relatively cheap	Ineffective unless used for appropriate organism May stick to wound May leave particles in wound bed Limited support of efficacy in some brands Sensitivities

(contd)

Table 14.4 (contd)

Category	Examples	Uses	Advantages	Disadvantages
Semi-permeable films	Bioclusive Epiview Mefilm Opsite Flexigrid Tegaderm	As a secondary dressing over alginates or hydrogels Primary dressing in low exuding, superficial wounds Skin protection	Allows monitoring of the wound Vapour permeability Adheres securely to the area/ conforms Maintains moisture	Leaks if exudate is heavy Exudate cools area Can be awkward to apply Rucks in dressing provide channels for bacteria Can cause sensitivities Can be painful to remove

Sources: Thomas (1990), Heenan (1999).
The examples have been divided into the identified categories by the author for illustration purposes; manufacturers' descriptions may differ. The examples listed are not exhaustive of the products on the market and various sizes are available.

studies; rigorous research into the mechanisms involved and resulting outcomes is noted for its absence (Sherman et al., 1996; Edwards, 1997; Thomas et al., 1998a; Waters, 1998). The basic role of larvae is debridement, but they may also have a role in pain management and odour reduction (Thomas, 1997; Thomas et al., 1998a). Numerous factors influence healing but fundamental to any of the phases is the vascular status of the wound; hence although the clinical application of larvae may be indicated in vascular wounds, there is a need for caution. The decision to use larvae must be based on holistic assessment and be part of a larger plan of wound management. It is not a definitive treatment in its own right as debridement is only one aspect of a complex course of events involved in the healing process and should not be considered in isolation. In essence, although debridement can easily be achieved using larvae (Figures 14.3 and 14.4), it must be emphasised that if the underlying vascular problem has not been treated the wound will not heal. Randomised controlled trials are now in process to compare the use of larvae with more conventional treatments, as well as investigations into their antibacterial and proteolytic activity (Thomas, 1997).

Additional information can be obtained from the Surgical Materials Testing Laboratory at Bridgend in Wales and readers are directed to the references in the paragraph above for details about mode of action, implications for use and method of application.

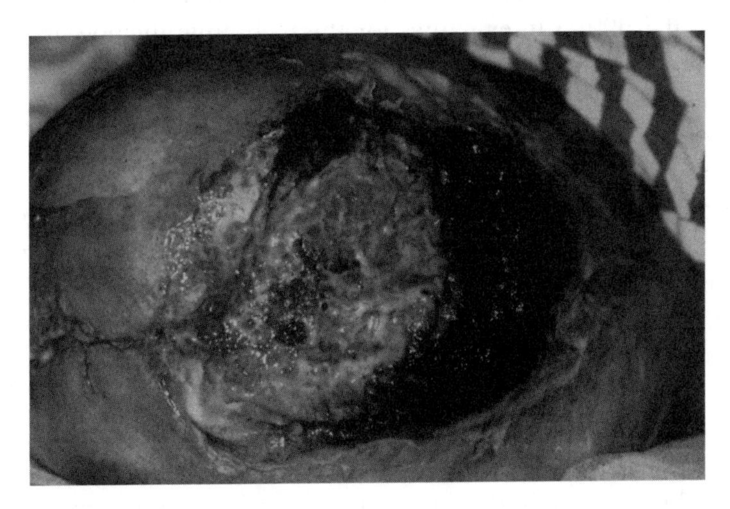

Figure 14.3 Necrotic tissue in stump wound to which larvae are to be applied; see Plate 13.

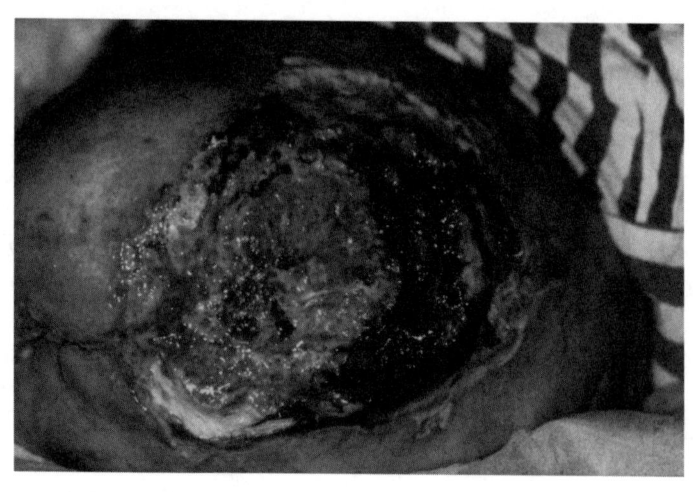

Figure 14.4 Necrotic tissue in stump wound reduced following application of larvae; see Plate 14.

Negative pressure dressings

A recently popularised development in wound management is the application of sub-atmospheric or negative pressure (Valenta, 1994; Fowler et al., 1995; Fleischmann et al., 1995; Argenta and Morykwas, 1996; Baxandall, 1997; Morykwas et al., 1997a, 1997b; Collier, 1997; Deva et al., 1997; Mullner et al., 1997; Genecov et al., 1998; Masters, 1998; Mendes-Eastman, 1998; Schneider et al., 1998; Banwell, 1999). Other names for the technique include negative pressure dressing, foam suction dressing, sub-atmospheric pressure therapy, vacuum sealing technique, vacuum-assisted closure (VAC), and topical negative pressure.

Fundamentally, these terms represent the application of sub-atmospheric pressure, measured in mmHg, from an adjustable source directly to a wound bed, via tubing inserted into or between pieces of open-cell foam dressing. A closed, controlled wound environment is then achieved by applying an adhesive polyurethane dressing over the top and sealing the edges.

The mechanism by which this dressing facilitates the healing process is ambiguous but several suggestions have been made:

- Reducing localised oedema resulting in an improved blood supply to the tissues.

- Facilitating a moist environment.
- Enhancing epithelial migration.
- Promoting angiogenesis and granulation tissue formation.
- Controlling exudate.

Clinical evidence supporting this therapy is considerable but scientific support remains limited. Nevertheless, additional work is currently underway (Banwell, 1999). Its role in the management of wounds in patients with vascular disease can be applied to the fasciotomy wound, amputation stump wound, dehisced groin wound, skin graft and slow healing wounds such as leg ulcers (Morykwas and Argenta, 1993; Argenta and Morykwas, 1995a, 1995b, 1996, 1997). Nurses are referred to the above references for more information about this method of wound management.

Management of different types of wound

The vascular nurse can consult various texts for directions on wound management, yet specific detail about the wounds facing the vascular nurse are lacking (Bryant, 1992; Morison, 1992; Dealey, 1994; Bale and Jones, 1997). Texts focus on the management of leg ulcers or drain and suture/clip removal (Herbert, 1997), which fails to highlight the diverse types of wounds the vascular nurse has to manage and the considerable problems they pose. Some general points will be considered here.

Sutured wounds

At 24 hours dry suture lines can be considered sealed. Stitches and staples can get caught if not covered so simple dressings may be used in an effort to protect the suture line from mechanical trauma and infection. Closed vacuum drains which are inserted prior to closure following bypass grafts and amputations are usually removed at 24–48 hours postoperatively. Drainage sites should be considered as a wound and a potential site for infection and therefore management should focus on minimising trauma and contamination to the area.

Diabetic foot ulcers

Wounds in the diabetic foot occur as a result of neuropathy and/or vascular disease, and these lesions can be complicated further by infection (Knowles, 1996). In both neuropathic and neuro-ischaemic lesions the original problem may be caused by minor trauma, poor hygiene or ill-fitting footwear, yet the damage can be considerable as the altered circulation and/or sensation impacts upon the patient's perception of the problem and the healing (Krone and Muller-Wieland, 1990). Care needs to focus on preventing the damage and highlights the importance of teamwork between various healthcare professionals and the patient. Prevention includes blood sugar control, health promotion (see Chapter 3), appropriate footwear, ongoing chiropody, good foot hygiene, skin care and lifetime foot inspection. The debridement of callus, trimming of toe nails and management of minor foot injuries in these patients should be directed to experienced personnel such as the chiropodist or podiatrist (Negus, 1995; Knowles, 1996).

Malodorous wounds

Offensive wound odour has been attributed to a mixture of agents produced by anaerobic bacteria together with metabolic products from other bacteria (Thomas et al., 1998b). These malodorous wounds can be very distressing to patients, with the extent of the problem varying between wounds. The nurse must consider the problem from the patient's perspective and care focuses on eliminating the bacteria so that the odour is reduced or employing means to mask the odour in situations where eliminating the bacteria is not possible.

Systemic antibiotics may be required but may have a limited effect in reducing odour as concentrations at the wound bed where the infection is may be limited, especially in the patient with altered blood supply (Thomas et al., 1998b). Topical antiseptics may reduce odour in certain circumstances but remain an issue of controversy especially in the light of the negative impact they have on the healing process (Tatnal et al., 1987). The application of metronidazole gels has been effective in certain situations, and other products such as honey, live yogurt and larvae have been reported as beneficial (Thomas et al., 1998b). Additionally, there are a number of charcoal impregnated dressings on the market, although different types may vary in their efficiency in reducing odour. A study comparing the efficacy of five different types of dressings used in malodorous wounds highlighted considerable variation between products, concluding that those that combine a physical absorbent element with a charcoal component have the better performance (Thomas et al., 1998b).

In situations where the elimination of bacteria causing the problem is not possible the nurse needs to employ a variety of other means to reduce the odour. This may include more frequent dressing changes and the use of air freshners including aromatherapy oils. Nurses may encounter malodorous wounds in patients with end-stage vascular disease where management will focus on symptom control together with other palliative care interventions (see Chapter 15).

Fasciotomy

Inflammatory oedema occurs in response to acute ischaemia, such as thrombosis or embolism, and pressure within muscle groups of upper and lower limbs will increase as the fascia which surrounds them does not expand, this can lead to compartment syndrome (Perry, 1988; Herbert, 1997). If pressure is not reduced, tissue damage will occur. This can also occur in patients who have undergone arterial reconstruction or as a result of vascular damage resulting from trauma (Perry, 1988). Hence a fasciotomy – a procedure that aims to adequately and promptly release the pressure – may be performed as a prophylactic procedure if compartment syndrome is suspected or in response to clinical presentations (Hirshberg et al., 1996). Attention has focused on methods of assessing the need for such a procedure and approaches to take, but less information is available about the management of the wounds once the fasciotomy has been performed (Mbubaegbu and Stallard, 1996). The aim of management is to keep the area moist and free from infection in the interim period before closure can be achieved. Methods of closure range from simple primary closure once the swelling has resolved to the use of techniques to bring skin edges closer together to facilitate delayed primary closure (Mbubaegbu and Stallard, 1996; Narayanan et al., 1996). Alternatively, split thickness skin grafting may be required, while small wounds may be allowed to heal by secondary intention (Perry, 1988).

Although it is desirable to close the wound promptly (Perry, 1988), in situations where the swelling is slow to resolve this may not be possible. Dressing management can be challenging as these wounds may produce large amounts of exudate and therefore require bulky dressings. In addition, there is the potential for infection for as long as the skin is not intact. If the management plan for the wound is to heal by secondary intention, the dressing products chosen will vary during the healing period, being selected according to the presentation of the wound, needs of the patient and resources available. Alginates are a popular choice for managing exudate and maintaining a moist wound environment (Thomas, 1990). However, if the management plan is to perform a split-thickness skin graft once the swelling has settled, it should be remembered that there is a risk of fibres of certain alginate dressings becoming incorporated into newly forming granulation tissue and obstructing the microcirculation that forms during skin graft take. Tulle gras is frequently the primary dressing of choice with gauze padding to absorb exudate. Although this may be simple and cheap to apply it will stick if it is not changed at least daily and is not appropriate if the wound is to heal by secondary intention. In addition, these dressings can be cumbersome and uncomfortable. Foam dressings can be useful if there is enough exudate in the wound to prevent the wound bed drying out. Alternatively negative pressure dressings have the advantage of maintaining moisture while managing excess exudate and preparing the wound bed for secondary procedures such as delayed primary closure or skin grafting.

Amputation stump wounds

A variety of amputations may be required by a patient suffering from lower limb ischaemia and this provides unique challenges for nurses caring for them (see Chapter 11). In terms of wound healing, it may be that in an attempt to preserve length of the limb the wound may be in an area where perfusion is not optimal, or repair may be challenged by the presence of advancing vascular disease (Spark et al., 1998). Problems that may arise include:

1. Wound infection.
2. Erosion of bone through the skin flap.
3. Swelling with hyperpigmentation and skin changes.
4. Ischaemic failure and further necrosis.
5. Old prosthetic graft material providing a source for infection in limb amputation stumps.

The same principles applied to other wound types should be followed when managing these wounds such as protecting the area, preventing infection, debriding if necessary and using dressing products that facilitate healing depending on the presentation of the wound. Additional challenges are the practical ways to secure dressings while caring for vulnerable surrounding skin (Figure 14.5), and pain management. Light elastic tubular bandages such as tubinette, elastic tubinette or Tubifast provide a method of securing dressings that can be adapted to the body surface while having the unique benefit of not exerting inappropriate compression (Asmussen and Sollner, 1995). In addition, they assist in reducing oedema and shaping the stump. Negative pressure dressings, although they may be awkward when applying to an amputation stump wound, have the advantage of contouring to the wound and preparing the wound bed for subsequent grafting or closure (Blackburn et al., 1998). In transmetatarsal amputations where skin opposition is possible, they will be closed primarily. Alternatively, the amputation stump wound may be left open to heal by secondary intention or skin grafted.

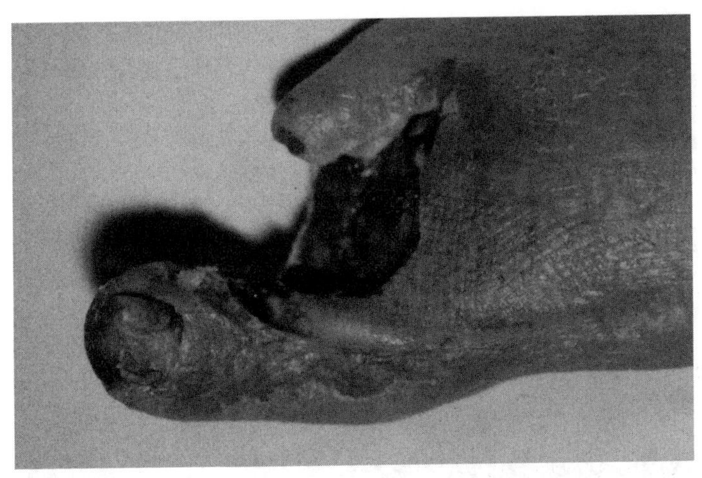

Figure 14.5 Amputation stump wound with fragile surrounding tissue; see Plate 15.

Post-bypass groin wounds

The groin is a common site for wound infection in post-vascular reconstruction patients (Herbert, 1997), especially where perspiration creates a continually damp area and in obese patients whose folds of skin provide an ongoing problem with friction and pressure. In addition, the formation of a haematoma may provide a focus for infection and necessitate a surgical evacuation. Infection in this area can be difficult to treat as there may not be an adequate blood supply to the area to ensure appropriate levels of antibiotic reach the infected tissue. The presence of synthetic graft material heightens the problem should the area become infected. Necrotic tissue or slough overlying a vascular graft needs cautious management, and a multidisciplinary approach is important in considering all the patient's options (Herbert, 1997). The potential for synthetic graft exposure highlights the importance of thorough and ongoing assessment and demands early intervention. In situations such as this, and in wounds where tissue damage is extensive, more complicated plastic surgery reconstruction may be required such as myocutaneous flaps (Figure 14.6). Alternatively, negative pressure dressings in the less severe wounds may be adequate in encouraging granulation tissue to fill the defect so that split-thickness skin grafting can be performed (Blackburn et al., 1998).

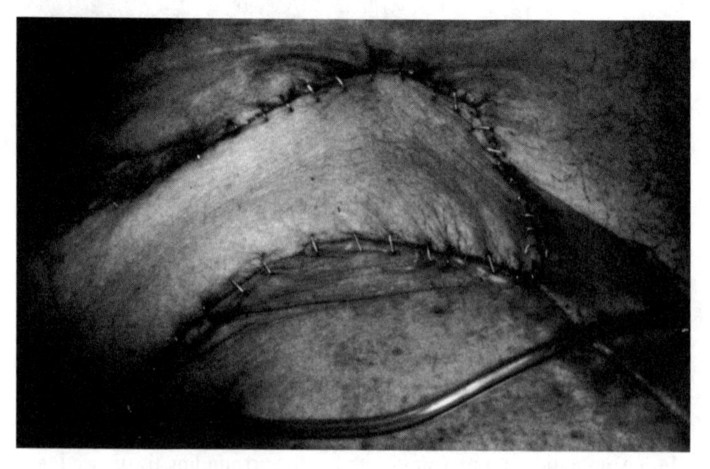

Figure 14.6 Myocutaneous flap to reconstruct a groin wound post-bypass; see Plate 16.

Skin grafts

A skin graft is a segment of dermis and epidermis that is removed in a sheet from its own blood supply, *the donor site*, and placed onto another area of the body to repair a cutaneous defect, *the recipient site*

(Grabb and Smith, 1979; McGregor and McGregor, 1995). Skin grafts are used in patients with vascular disease to repair ulcer sites following revascularisation, to provide cutaneous cover in fasciotomy wounds or amputation stump wounds and to achieve wound closure in venous ulcers with adjunctive support therapy after grafting.

Skin grafts can be full thickness, containing the entire thickness of epidermis and dermis, or split thickness containing the entire thickness of the epidermis but various degrees of the dermis (McGregor and McGregor, 1995). Split-thickness skin grafts are the type most commonly encountered by nurses working in the vascular specialty. Once removed from the donor site, the graft, irrespective of its thickness, will require a good blood supply for its survival. This has implications for the type of wound bed upon which the graft is laid, vascular status of the area and post-grafting support mechanisms to maintain adequate circulation. There are a variety of skin grafting techniques used including sheet, meshed, pinch and postage (Nanninga et al., 1993; McGregor and McGregor, 1995). The process of healing following skin graft application, otherwise know as *skin graft take*, is explained physiologically in Table 14.5.

Reasons for skin graft failure include shearing movement of the graft or fluid collection beneath it, both of which prevent the graft becoming adhered to the wound bed and therefore deter a new circulation becoming established. The most problematic aspect of the skin graft is the challenge posed by the donor site, which can be a very difficult wound to manage, especially in terms of exudate control and pain management (Negus, 1995). Fundamentally, this is an epithelialising wound but in the initial days there will be copious amounts of exudate which reflect the inflammatory phase of the healing process (Table 14.1). Initially dressings need to provide adequate absorption characteristics but should not be so heavy that they pull on the wound causing tissue damage and pain. Once exudate is more manageable, lighter dressings such as a combination of alginate and polyurethane film can be used (Table 14.4).

A multidisciplinary team approach

The multifactorial nature of wound healing demands expertise from a variety of sources and close collaboration between all the team members involved (Davey et al., 1994; Lawrence, 1994). It is important that professionals acknowledge their own limitations and utilise

Table 14.5 Physiological process of skin graft 'take'

Physiology of 'take'	Implications for clinical practice
Application of skin graft to wound bed ⇩	Thorough preparation of wound bed Non-infected wound bed Requires good blood supply Requires granulating surface
Adherence of graft through fibrin network (imbition) ⇩	Very fragile Easily dislodged Graft needs stability by immobilisation
Plasmatic circulation becomes established ⇩	Protection of graft ongoing by immobilisation and leaving it undisturbed
Capillary buds grow into the graft (inosculation 3 days) ⇩	May need early inspection at this time if the surgeon is concerned about the viability of the wound bed Can be inspected at this time if care is taken
Vascular link up (capillary ingrowth 5 days) ⇩	Routine first inspection at 5 days is traditional rather than scientific Careful removal of dressing is important Sutures around edges of graft can be removed at this stage Subsequent dressings need to provide a firm splint to the graft Mobilisation may be permitted at this time depending on the position and condition of the graft and the ability to support it Dressing frequency will depend on the assessment of the wound at this stage
Fibroblast activity and increasing strength as graft matures ⇩	Graft will become more stable and any raw areas need to be assessed as any wound would be
Lymphatic and nerve link up 'Graft take' ⇩	Needs moisturising and ongoing skin care The wound will never obtain its original strength An improvement in the appearance can be expected over the following 12 months

Sources: Kemble and Lamb (1984), McGregor and McGregor (1995).

their colleagues, as wounds demand different approaches from members of the healthcare team who have varied perspectives and approaches to management. This includes doctors, who may be drawn from a variety of specialties such as vascular, dermatology and plastic surgery, nurses, podiatrists, chiropodists, dieticians, physiotherapists, occupational therapists, social workers, mental health professionals, infection control specialists and/or other clinical nurse specialists.

Multidisciplinary leg ulcer clinics have become well established in dealing with the multiple problems of this patient group (see Chapter 8). In addition, there are claims that the key to reducing the incidence of diabetic foot ulceration is the establishment of multidisciplinary foot care teams with the key person in that team being the patient (Apelquist et al., 1993; Boulton, 1994). This perhaps is a key issue for consideration in that the patient has a prominent role to play in the process of wound management. Hence the nurse needs to incorporate health promotion into patient care (see Chapter 3), and consider her role as the coordinator of all members of the team, for in situations where joint collaboration is not well established, there may be confusion, conflict and a limited patient-focused approach.

References

Achan V, Jurd KM, Hunt BJ (1996) Haemostasis and the systemic inflammatory response syndrome. British Journal of Intensive Care July/August: 223–230.

Adzick NS, Longaker MT (1991) Scarless fetal healing. Annals of Surgery 215(1): 3–7.

Alison MR (1992) Repair and regeneration. In: McGee J O'D, Isaacson PG, Wright NA (eds) Oxford Textbook of Pathology, Volume 1: Principles of Pathology, chapter 5.3, pp 365–388. Oxford: University Press.

Apelquist J, Larson J, Agardh C (1993) Long-term prognosis for diabetic patients with foot ulcers. 2nd Conference on Advancement in Wound Management Proceedings. London: Macmillan Magazines.

Argenta L, Morykwas M (1995a) Vacuum assisted closure (VAC therapy) for secondary closure of dehisced and infected wounds. Presented: 5th Annual Meeting European Tissue Repair Society, Padua, Italy, August.

Argenta L, Morykwas M (1995b) Vacuum assisted closure (VAC therapy) for treatment of leg ulcers. Presented: 5th Annual Meeting European Tissue Repair Society, Padua, Italy, August.

Argenta LC, Morykwas MJ (1996) New concepts in wound healing In: Jackson IT, Sommerlad BC (eds) Recent Advances in Plastic Surgery, chapter 2, pp 13–26. Edinburgh: Churchill Livingstone.

Argenta LC, Morykwas MJ (1997) Vacuum-assisted closure: a new method for wound control treatment: clinical experience. Annals of Plastic Surgery 38: 563–577.

Asmussen PD, Sollner B (1995) Wound Care, Wound Management: Principles and Practice. Hamburg: Biersdorf.

Bale S (1997) A guide to wound debridement. Journal of Wound Care 6(4): 179–182.
Bale S, Jones V (1997) Wound Care Nursing A Patient Centre Approach. London: Baillière Tindall.
Banwell PE (1999) Topical negative pressure therapy in wound care. Journal of Wound Care 8(2): 79–84.
Baxandall T (1997) Healing cavity wounds with negative pressure. Elderly Care 9(1): 20–22.
Bishop E (1963) The Guinea Pig Club. Holburn: Macmillan.
Bistrian BR, Blackburn GL, Hallowell E, Heddle R (1974) Protein status of general surgical patients. Journal of the American Medical Association 230: 858–860.
Blackburn JH, Boemi L, Hall WW, Jeffords K, Hauck RM, Banducci DR, Graham WP (1998) Negative pressure dressings as a bolster for skin grafts. Annals of Plastic Surgery 40: 453–457.
Bobel LM (1987) Nutritional implications in patients with pressure sores. Nursing Clinics of North America 22(2): 379–390.
Boulton AJM (1994) The diabetic foot. In: Harding K, Dealey C, Cherry G, Gottrup F (eds) Proceedings of the 3rd European Conference on Advances in Wound Management, pp 102. London: Macmillan Magazines.
Bryant RA (ed.) (1992) Acute and Chronic Wounds. St Louis: Mosby Year Book.
Carpenito LJ (1993) Nursing Diagnosis Application to Clinical Practice, 5th edn. Philadelphia: JB Lippincott.
Casey J, Flinn WR, Yao JST, Fahey V, Pawlowski J, Bergan JJ (1983) Correction of immune and nutritional status with wounds and complications with patients undergoing vascular operations. Surgery 93: 822–827.
Clark RAF (1993) Mechanisms of cutaneous wound repair. In: Fitzpatrick TB, Eisen AZ, Freedberg IM, Frank K (eds) Haematology in General Medicine, chapter 38, pp 473–486). New York: McGraw-Hill.
Clark RAF (ed.) (1996) The Molecular and Cellular Biology of Wound Repair, 2nd edn. New York: Plenum Press.
Cohen BE, Gill G, Cullen PR, Morris PJ (1979) Reversal of post-operative immunosuppression in man by vitamin A. Surgery, Gynecology and Obstetrics 149: 658–662.
Collier M (1997) Know how: vacuum-assisted closure (VAC). Nursing Times 93(5): 32–33.
Cronan L (1993) Management of the patient with altered body image. British Journal of Nursing 2(5): 257–261.
Cullum N, Roe BH (1995) Leg Ulcers Nursing Management A Research-based Guide. London: Scutari Press.
Davey L, Soloman J, Freeborn SA (1994) A multidisciplinary approach to wound care. Journal of Wound Care 3(5): 249–252.
Dealey C (1994) The Care of Wounds. Oxford: Blackwell Science.
Deva AK, Siu C, Nettle WJS (1997) Vacuum-assisted closure of a sacral pressure sore. Journal of Wound Care 6(7): 311–312.
Dickhault SC, Delee JC, Page CP (1984) Nutritional status: importance in predicting wound healing after amputation. Journal of Bone and Joint Surgery 66A: 71–75.
Diegelmann RF, Kelman Cohen I, Kaplan A (1981) The role of macrophages in wound repair. Journal of Plastic and Reconstructive Surgery 6: 107–113.
Donaldson D, Mahan JT (1983) Fibrinogen and fibronectin as substrates for epidermal cell migration during wound closure. Journal of Cell Science 62: 117–127.

Doughty DB (1992) Principles of wound healing and wound management. In: Bryant RA (ed) Acute and Chronic Wounds, chapter 2, pp 31–68. St Louis: Mosby Year Book.

Drench ME (1994) Changes in body image secondary to disease and injury. Rehabilitation Nursing 19(1): 31–36.

Dyk RB, Sutherland AM (1956) Adaptation of the spouse and other family members to the colostomy patient. Cancer 9: 123–138.

Edwards J (1997) Larval therapy. The British Association of Plastic Surgery Nurses. Magazine, Winter: 7–8.

Fawcett J, Frye S (1980) An exploratory study of body image dimensionality. Nursing Research 29(5) 324–327.

Fleischmann W, Becker V, Bischoff M, Hoekstra H (1995) Vacuum sealing: indication, technique and results. European Journal of Orthopaedic Surgery and Traumatology 5: 37–40.

Fowler J, Mchone J, Morykwas M, Argenta L (1995) Acute/traumatic wounds with massive soft tissue loss: enhanced outcomes with negative pressure therapy. Presented: 25th Annual Conference Wound, Ostomy and Continence Nurses, San Antonio: July 10–15.

Garrett B (1997) The proliferation and movement of cells during re-epithelialisation. Journal of Wound Care 6(4): 174–177.

Genecov DG, Schneider AM, Morykwas MJ, Parker D, White WL, Argenta LC (1998) A controlled subatmospheric pressure dressing increases the rate of skin graft donor site reepithelialization. Annals of Plastic Surgery 40: 219–225.

Gilchrist B (1996) Sampling bacterial flora: a review of the literature. Journal of Wound Care 5(6): 386–388.

Goffman E (1963) Stigma Notes On The Management Of Spoiled Identity. Harmondsworth, Middlesex: Penguin Books.

Goode HF, Burns E, Walker BE (1992) Vitamin C depletion and pressure sores in elderly patients with fractured neck of femur. British Medical Journal 305: 925–927.

Goodson WH, Hunt TK (1982) Development of a new miniature method for the study of wound healing in human subjects. Journal of Surgical Research 33: 394–401.

Grabb WC, Smith JW (eds) (1979) Plastic Surgery, 3rd edn. Boston: Little, Brown and Company.

Greaves MW, Ive FA (1961) Serum zinc and the healing of venous ulcers. Lancet ii: 1261.

Griffiths E (1989) More than skin deep. Nursing Times 85(40): 34–36.

Hallett A (1995) Vital ingredients. Nursing Times 91(5): 76, 78.

Harper RA, Savage CR (1980) Vitamin A potentiates the mitogenic effect of epidermal growth factor in cultures of normal adult human skin fibroblasts. Endocrinology 107(6): 2113–2114.

Heenan A (1999) Wound dressings and the drug tariff. Journal of Wound Care 8(2): 69–72.

Hellgren L, Vincent J (1993) Debridement: an essential step in wound healing. In: Westerhof W (ed.) Leg Ulcers: Diagnosis and Treatment. Amsterdam: Elsevier Science.

Henker FO (1979) Body-image conflict following trauma and surgery. Psychosomatics 20(12): 812–820.

Herbert LM (1997) Caring for the Vascular Patient. New York: Churchill Livingstone.
Herman JA (1986) Nursing assessment and nursing diagnosis in patients with peripheral vascular disease. Nursing Clinics of North America 21(2): 219–231.
Hill GL, Pickford I, Young GA, Schorah CJ, Blackett RL, Burkinshaw L, Warren JV, Morgan DB (1977) Malnutrition in surgical patients. Lancet i: 689–692.
Hinman C, Maibach H (1963) Effects of air exposure and occlusion on experimental human skin wounds. Nature 200: 377–378.
Hirshberg A, Sherr-Lurie N, Adar R (1996) Compartment haematoma complicating closed fasciotomy. British Journal of Surgery 83: 951–952.
Kelly MP (1985) Loss and grief reactions as responses to surgery. Journal of Advanced Nursing 10: 517–525.
Kemble JVH, Lamb BE (1984) Plastic Surgical and Burns Nursing. Current Nursing Practice. Eastbourne: Baillière Tindall.
Knowles A (1996) Special foot clinics for patients with diabetes Critique II. Journal of Wound Care 5(5): 241–242.
Konstantinides NN, Lehmann S (1993) The impact of nutrition on wound healing. Critical Care Nurse 13(5): 25–33.
Krone W, Muller-Wieland D (1990) Special problems of the diabetic patient. In: Dormandy J, Stock G (eds) Critical Leg Ischaemia, its Pathophysiology and Management, chapter 10, pp 145–157. Berlin: Springer-Verlag.
Lawrence J (1994) Dressing and wound infection. American Journal of Surgery 6(2): 12–13.
Lawrence JC, Ameen H (1998) Swabs and other sampling techniques. Journal of Wound Care 7(5): 232–233.
Lee KA, Stotts NA (1990) Support of the growth hormone–somatomedin system to facilitate healing. Heart and Lung 19(2): 157–163.
Lotti T, Rodofili C, Benci M, Menchin G (1998) Wound-healing problems associated with cancers. Journal of Wound Care 7(2): 81–84.
MacGinley KJ (1993) Nursing care of the patient with altered body image. British Journal of Nursing 2(22): 1098–1102.
Magnan MA (1996) Psychological considerations for patients with acute wounds. Critical Care Nursing Clinics of North America 8(2): 183–193.
Martin P (1997) Wound healing – aiming for perfect skin generation. Science 276: 75–81.
Masters J (1998) Reliable, inexpensive and simple suction dressings. British Journal of Plastic Surgery 51(3): 267.
Mbubaegbu CE, Stallard MC (1996) A method of fasciotomy wound closure. Injury 27(9): 613–615.
McClaren S (1993) Nutritional factors in wound healing. Wound Management 3(1): 8–10.
McCollum C (1994) Ischaemia and wound healing. In: Harding K, Dealey C, Cherry G, Gottrup F (eds) Proceedings of the 3rd European Conference on Advances in Wound Management, pp 7–8. London: Macmillan Magazines.
McGregor IA, McGregor AD (1995) Fundamental Techniques of Plastic Surgery, 9th edn. Edinburgh: Churchill Livingstone.
McTaggart JH (1994) An area of clinical neglect: Evaluation of healing status in wound care. Professional Nurse 9: 600, 602, 604, 606.

Melhuish JM, Plassmann P, Harding KG (1993) Volume and circumference of the healing of wounds. In: 3rd European Conference on Advances in Wound Management Proceedings, pp 41–43. London: Macmillan Magazines.

Mendes-Eastman S (1998) Negative pressure wound therapy. Plastic Surgical Nursing 18(1): 27–29, 33–37.

Morison MJ (1992) Patient assessment. In: A Colour Guide to the Nursing Management of Wounds. Chapter 2, pp 22–30. London: Mosby Year Book.

Morykwas MJ, Argenta LC (1993) Use of negative pressure to promote healing of pressure sores and chronic wounds. Presented: 25th Annual Conference, Wound, Ostomy and Continence Nurses Association, San Antonio, July 10–15.

Morykwas MJ, Argenta LC, Salem W (1997a) Non surgical modalities to enhance healing and care of soft tissue wounds. Journal of Southern Orthopaedic Association 6(4): 279–288.

Morykwas MJ, Argenta LC, Shelton-Brown EI, McGuirt W (1997b) Vacuum assisted closure: A new method for wound control and treatment: Animal Studies and Basic Foundation. Annals of Plastic Surgery 38(6): 353–362.

Mulder GT (1999) The role of tissue engineering in wound care. Journal of Wound Care 8(1): 21–24.

Mullner T, Mrkonjic L, Kwasny O, Vecsei V (1997) The use of negative pressure to promote the healing of tissue defects: a clinical trial using vacuum sealing technique. British Journal of Plastic Surgery 50: 194–199.

Nanninga PB, Mekkes JR, De Vries HJC, Westerhof W, Teepe RGC, Barradon Y (1993) Grafting techniques. In: Westerhof W (ed.) Leg Ulcers: Diagnosis and Treatment, chapter 21, pp 335–348. Amsterdam: Elsevier Science.

Narayanan K, Latenser BA, Jones LM, Stofman G (1996) Simultaneous primary closure of 4 fasciotomy wounds in a single setting using the sure-closure device. Injury 27(6): 449–451.

Negus D (1995) Leg Ulcers A Practical Approach to Management, 2nd edn. Oxford: Butterworth Heinemann.

Newell R (1991) Body-image disturbance: cognitive behavioural formulation and intervention. Journal of Advanced Nursing 16: 1400–1405.

Ondrey FG, Hom DB (1994) Effects of nutrition on wound healing. Neck Surgery 110(6): 557–559.

Ordman LJ, Gillman T (1966) Studies in the healing of wounds. Archives of Surgery 93(6): 857–882.

Osak MP (1993) Nutrition and wound healing. Plastic Surgery Nursing 13(1): 29–36.

Paquet P, Lapiere CM (1993) Causes of delayed wound healing. In: Westerhof W (ed.) Leg Ulcers: Diagnosis and Treatment, chapter 16, pp 281–290. Amsterdam: Elsevier Science.

Partridge J (1990) Changing Faces. The Challenge of Facial Disfigurement. London: Penguin Books.

Perry MO (1988) Compartment syndrome and reperfusion injury. Surgical Clinics of North America 68(4): 653–864.

Piff C (1986) Let's Face It. London: Sphere Books.

Pinchoky-Devin G (1994) Nutrition and wound healing. Journal of Wound Care 3(5): 231–234.

Pories WJ, Henzel JH, Rob CG, Strain WH (1967) Acceleration of wound healing in man with zinc sulphate given by mouth. Lancet i: 121–124.
Price B (1990a) Body Image Nursing. Concepts and Care. New York: Prentice Hall.
Price B (1990b) A model for body-image care. Journal of Advanced Nursing 15: 585–593.
Roitt I (1991) Essential Immunology, 7th edn. Oxford: Blackwell Scientific Publications.
Ruberg RL (1984) Role of nutrition in wound healing. Surgical Clinics of North America 64(4): 705–714.
Salter M (1997) (ed) Altered Body Image: The Nurse's Role, 2nd edn. London: Baillière Tindall.
Schilling JA (1976) Wound healing. Surgical Clinics of North America 56(4): 859–874.
Schneider AM, Morykwas MJ, Argenta LC (1998) A new and reliable method of securing skin grafts to the difficult recipient bed. Journal of Plastic and Reconstructive Surgery 102(4): 1195–1198.
Sherman R, My-Tien T, Sullivan R (1996) Maggot therapy for venous stasis ulcers. Archives of Dermatology 132: 254–256.
Spark I, Vowden K, Vowden P (1998) Lower-limb amputation: wound care and rehabilitation. Journal of Wound Care 7(3): 137–140.
Stone N, Meister A (1962) Function of ascorbic acid in the conversion of proline to collagen hydroxyproline. Nature 194: 555–557.
Tatnal FM, Leigh IM, Gibson JR (1987) Comparative toxicity of anti microbial agents on transformed human keratinocytes. Journal of Investigative Dermatology 89: 316–317.
Thomas S (1990) Wound Management and Dressings. London: The Pharmaceutical Press.
Thomas S (1997) The use of fly larvae in the treatment of wounds. Nursing Standard 12(12): 54–59.
Thomas S, Andrews A, Jones M (1998a) The use of larval therapy in wound management. Journal of Wound Care 7(10): 521–524.
Thomas S, Fisher B, Fram PJ, Waring MJ (1998b) Odour-absorbing dressings. Journal of Wound Care 7(5): 246–250.
Ting M (1991) Wound healing and peripheral vascular disease. Critical Care Nursing Clinics of North America 3(3): 515–523.
Tonge H (1997) The management of infected wounds. Nursing Standard 12(12): 49–53.
Turner JA (1986) Nursing intervention with patients with peripheral vascular disease. Nursing Clinics of North America 21(2): 233–240.
Valenta AL (1994) Using the vacuum dressing alternative for difficult wounds. American Journal of Nursing April: 44–48.
Vowden K (1995) Common problems in wound care: wound and ulcer measurement. British Journal of Nursing 4(13): 775–779.
Wandsworth Community Health and St George's Healthcare NHS Trusts (1996) Pressure Sore Prevention and Wound Management. Hull: Smith and Nephew.
Wassner A (1982) The impact of mutilating surgery or trauma on body image. International Nursing Review 29(3): 86–90.
Waters J (1998) The benefits of larval therapy. Nursing Times 94(2): 62–63.
Westerhof W (1993) Introduction. In Westerhof W (ed.) Leg Ulcers: Diagnosis and Treatment, chapter 1, pp 1–4. Amsterdam: Elsevier Science.

Williams DR (1996) Trace element starvation and wound healing problems. Journal of Wound Care 5(4): 183–189.
Wilson-Barnett J, Osborne J (1983) Studies evaluating patient teaching: implications for practice. International Journal of Nursing Studies 20(1): 33–43.
Winter GD (1962) Formation of the scab and the rate of epithelialization of superficial wounds in the skin of the young domestic pig. Nature 193: 293–294.
Winter GD (1965) A note on wound healing under dressings with special reference to perforated-film dressings. Journal of Investigative Dermatology 45(4): 299–302.
Young ME (1988) Malnutrition and wound healing. Heart and Lung 17(1): 60–67.

Chapter 15

Palliative Care Provision for Vascular Patients

LOUISE M. WILSON

Introduction

There have been huge technological advances in the field of vascular surgery in the last 15 years, although little attention has been paid to the chronic aspects of vascular disease. Management of people with vascular disease is usually by surgical teams with the emphasis on cure. In the acute setting, it is easy to overlook the chronic nature of the disease. The breadth of skills and facilities needed to manage the critically ill postoperative patient alongside those with end-stage vascular disease (ESVD) are seldom available.

Palliative care is an issue rarely discussed in relation to people with peripheral vascular disease. Some might argue that much of the treatment received by those with severe symptoms of this chronic condition is palliative. However, this is not the main focus of this chapter. Instead the difficulty in providing a palliative care approach to those individual patients with end-stage vascular disease is highlighted together with a brief overview of their palliative care requirements. Although a relatively small number of people with peripheral vascular disease die as a direct result of this, the majority dying from other causes such as myocardial infarct or stroke, the demographic changes resulting in increased death from degenerative disease may see this situation change. In addition, because of a lack of focus on palliative care provision the size of the problem is difficult to quantify and may be larger than realised. Little is understood of the specific needs of this group of patients and as a result palliative care provision has not been addressed. For those that die from peripheral vascular disease, whether in an acute unit or at home, service provision is at best patchy, at worst non-existent.

To date, development in care for the dying and specialist palliative care services have focused almost entirely on patients with cancer and those with HIV. This has overshadowed the needs of the greater number of patients dying from other diseases.

Although an expert report (Standing Medical Advisory Committee and Standing Nursing and Midwifery Advisory Committee, 1992) argued that palliative care services should be developed for patients other than those with cancer, little progress has been made.

A search of the literature has produced no information on the needs and experiences of people with ESVD.

The World Health Organisation defines palliative care as 'the active total care of patients and their families by a multi-professional team, when the patient's disease is no longer responsive to curative treatments' (World Health Organisation, 1990).

Principles of palliative care

The principles of palliative care for patients with non-malignant diseases have been further elucidated by the National Council for Hospice and Specialist Palliative Care Services (1998) as:

- A focus on quality of life, including good symptom control.
- A whole person approach taking into account a person's past life experiences and current situation.
- Care which encompasses both the dying person and those who matter to that person.
- Respect for patient autonomy and choice.
- An emphasis on open and sensitive communication.

Some might argue that these principles should be threaded into all health care. However, the reality may be somewhat different. For instance, when palliative care provisions are stretched to maximum capacity meeting the needs of those with malignant disease, those dying from non-malignant disorders may have difficulty accessing appropriate support. Nurses working in an acute vascular care setting may have encountered specific difficulties in trying to apply palliative care principles to those with ESVD, which is demonstrated in the case study (Box 15.1).

Box 15.1 Case study

John, a man in his sixties, underwent a series of arterial bypass procedures over a number of years. He reached the end stages of the disease when his infected aorto-bifemoral graft had to be removed and his lower limbs became non-viable. During the course of his final illness, John made it clear that he wished to die at home. John's family was supportive, and wanted to do their best to respond to his wishes.

John had very poor perfusion from the waist down and therefore needed to be nursed on a special bed. Provision of this bed was straightforward in the hospital setting, but obtaining funding for transfer to the community was a logistical nightmare and the referring health authority would not fund the bed. Although the district nurses were supportive of John's return home, their managers were not sure that this was practical due to the nursing input required. Many hours were spent trying to arrange John's transfer, with support and advice from the hospital's Macmillan nurses. After contacting many charities, funding was obtained for the bed hire for 10 days only. Sending John home with this limitation was a difficult decision to make but the nurses sensed that once home, John would be at peace and able to slip away comfortably.

Considerable effort was made to ensure John and his family had sufficient support to make discharge arrangements workable, and that contingency plans were in place in case all did not go smoothly. John's local hospice were unable to guarantee a bed for him if arrangements did not work out and any consequent failure in the discharge plans would have meant transfer back into an acute care setting. John died at home, as was his wish, within 10 days; therefore the need to apply for further funding for the bed fortunately did not arise.

Reflecting on the difficulties of meeting John's request to return home, it was clear that had the same situation arisen for a patient with an illness with a major supporting charity, e.g. heart disease, stroke or cancer, the discharge planning and support services would have been easier.

The issues raised by this case study highlight many of the difficulties encountered when trying to provide a first class service to a patient whose disease is poorly understood, both within healthcare circles and by the general public. At the time, the difficulties encountered in accessing appropriate levels of support to ensure that palliative care principles were met were a great burden to those caring for John. Nurses involved in his care felt disillusioned with a system that could provide easy access to relevant support to some but only if they had specific diseases. As suggested by Field (1994, p 61), 'Perhaps the "five star" care for the select few provided by hospice organizations should be replaced by "three star" for all.'

Which vascular patients may need palliative care?

As can be seen from the definitions of palliative care already given, any vascular patient in whom the emphasis has moved from curative treatments to symptom control and care, may benefit from a palliative care approach (Table 15.1).

Table 15.1 Vascular patients needing palliative care

- Those with critical limb ischaemia who refuse or are unfit for major bypass surgery or limb amputation
- Those in whom high level limb amputation fails to heal and is associated with repeated sepsis and ischaemia
- Those where major bypass surgery has failed, resulting in critical limb ischaemia with or without sepsis, where no other treatment options remain
- Those with slowly leaking aneurysms, who refuse or are unfit for surgery
- Those where aortic aneurysm surgery has failed or graft material has become infected and further surgery is impossible

What are the palliative care needs of vascular patients?

In common with other patients needing palliative care, physical, social and psychological care needs should all be considered.

Physical

Pain is perhaps the most commonly experienced problem of patients with ESVD, and may be difficult to manage. Symptom relief is a cornerstone of palliative care, and effective pain control is essential. Old prejudices and concerns about the use of opioid analgesics still linger; these are best overcome by education, and the involvement of specialists in pain management at an early stage.

Referral patterns and available expertise vary between centres although the following may be useful sources of advice:

- palliative care teams
- acute pain teams
- anaesthetists
- pharmacists

- hospices (including Marie Curie cancer care centres and Macmillan cancer relief).

Discussion of the pain management techniques is beyond the scope of this chapter and the reader should refer to Chapter 6 for further discussion, and to the further reading section at the end of this chapter.

Constipation is often a problem resulting from immobility, and as a side effect of opioid analgesia. Laxatives may be needed and should be prescribed regularly for patients having opiate analgesia. Nausea and vomiting may also arise with opioid administration and will require an anti-emetic to reduce symptoms.

Recognition that the terminal phase of the disease has been reached may be hard to accept, but failure to do so represents a significant barrier to appropriate patient management. Nursing staff have an advocacy role in representing the wishes of patients and their carers to medical staff, who may often focus only on curative strategies.

The majority of patients with ESVD will have extensive, disfiguring wounds due to tissue ischaemia. Some patients will have sepsis and will also be at risk of pressure sore development. In the presence of terminal ischaemia, wound healing is an inappropriate target and management should focus on achieving patient comfort (see Chapter 14). Frequency of dressing change will be an important consideration, since frequent changes are likely to be very painful for the patient. Additional short-acting analgesia prior to dressing changes will often be needed (see Chapter 6). Staff involved in caring for these wounds, which may be the most demanding that a nurse will ever encounter, need to be experienced, confident and competent.

Malodorous wounds need to be managed carefully both for the benefit of the patient, and for their visitors. Appropriate specialist beds and pressure-relieving mattresses can be used to prevent further tissue breakdown, and to maintain overall patient comfort. Expert advice from tissue viability and wound care nurses can be valuable (see Chapters 5 and 14), as can contact with a specialist vascular unit.

Psychosocial

Psychological aspects of terminal disease include anxiety and distress, uncertainty, loss of independence, fear of the unknown, spiritual concerns and body image problems.

The psychosocial needs of those facing end-stage vascular disease are often complex and poorly addressed within the acute ward environment. Actual recognition that a patient has reached the terminal phase of their illness can in itself be a hurdle that many professionals in the acute environment, where the emphasis is on cure, find difficult to cross. These factors on their own stand as a huge potential barrier to effective symptom management and psychosocial support. Some critics of the medicalisation of death argue that increasing medicalisation of life has diminished people's ability to manage their own health or to cope with their pain and suffering (Illich, 1990). Illich argues that death is often seen less as an inevitable part of life and more as a failure of treatment. It is certainly true that the past century has seen a sharp decline in home deaths even though the preferred place of death for many is their own home. If acute hospital wards are to be the place of death for those with end-stage vascular disease, health professionals must endeavour to ensure that the psychosocial needs of patients are met. Mills et al. (1994) reported that two-thirds of dying patients in the hospital studied did not receive adequate nursing care, with 22 of 23 patients being alone for at least 75% of the observation period. In contrast, pulse and temperature were monitored until death in 84% of patients. Thus it is important that we achieve the right focus for individual patient needs and make good use of that valued commodity – time. The pioneering work of Kubler-Ross (1970) gives us insight into the psychological distress experienced by the dying.

Communication skills are the key to enable carers to provide patient-centred care, and to meet the psychological needs of the dying. If care is not taken it is all to easy for the patient with end-stage vascular disease to become isolated from those who are close to them and indeed their nurses and doctors. Carers may feel inadequately trained to meet the complex needs of the patient. They may use distancing techniques to avoid confronting the emotional needs of the patient. Wound management and pain management may be difficult to manage without specialist input, thus potentially reinforcing the carers' need to withdraw in what may be seen as a hopeless situation. Malodorous wounds may also exacerbate a patient's sense of social isolation. Giving patients the opportunity to discuss their fears and uncertainty is imperative. A nurse may also question how often are patients with end-stage vascular disease actually aware they are dying. The disease trajectory often is difficult to predict and the sense of helplessness sometimes experienced among surgical teams when all has not gone as planned can affect the level of open discussion with the patient.

When planning care, the needs of the family as a whole must not be forgotten. It is imperative that communication channels are established to enable discussion of concerns, and that support systems are available to provide practical help. As poignantly suggested by Monroe (1996), professionals need to help families create good enough memories for the future, and they will need to feel that whilst the patient was still alive they did what they could to help. It is imperative that a multidisciplinary approach to care is applied when meeting the needs of those dying from end-stage vascular disease. Occupational therapists, doctors, nurses, social workers, link psychiatrists, counsellors and specialist vascular nurses, amongst others, should be involved in care provision, whether the patient is in an acute or community setting.

Conclusion

A nurse faced with John's situation today would hopefully not face so many barriers, though this is still not universally true. Support for patients needing non-malignant palliative care is more readily available in some areas of the country than in others, with more palliative care teams available to provide both short-term interventions for special problems, and on-going support. Broader access to care is developing through groups such as Macmillan Support, although where resources are limited, a higher priority will be given to those with cancer.

Vascular nurses as a group must set the tone by ensuring service development for this group of patients. A clearer understanding of both the physical and psychosocial needs of those facing end-stage disease is needed. Service development must be guided by evidence of need; therefore research is needed to provide this body of knowledge. At an individual level, careful attention to verbal and non-verbal patient communication is vital in order to elicit the real needs of patients.

Nurses must be aware of the service provision within their area and must actively seek to promote development in the interests of their client group. Vascular nurses are starting to raise the profile of this sphere of care within the profession and must also continue to raise public awareness, and that of other healthcare providers.

Palliative care principles can be used as a guiding model for much of the care provided to this group of patients, even from early in the disease process, as long as we do not believe that palliative care means terminal care. Much of the force behind cancer service development came from private/charitable organisations. Obtaining a similar level of provision for vascular patients will require clarity of vision, leadership and the development of a wide-ranging coalition of interest and support.

References

Field D (1994) Palliative medicine and the medicalization of death. European Journal of Cancer Care 3: 58–62.

Illich I (1990) Limits to Medicine: Medical Nemesis: The Expropriation of Health. London: Penguin.

Kubler-Ross E (1970) On Death and Dying. London: Tavistock.

Mills M, Davies HTO, Macrae WA (1994) Care of dying patients in hospital. British Medical Journal 309: 583–586.

National Council for Hospice and Specialist Palliative Care Services (1998) Reaching Out: Specialist Palliative Care for Adults with Non-Malignant Disease. Occasional Paper 14. London: National Council for Hospice and Specialist Palliative Care Services and Scottish Partnership Agency for Palliative and Cancer Care.

Monroe B (1996) Terminal illness and the family. In: Ford G, Lewin I (eds) Managing Terminal Illness. London: Royal College of Physicians of London.

Standing Medical Advisory Committee and Standing Nursing and Midwifery Advisory Committee (1992) The Principles and Provision of Palliative Care. London: HMSO.

World Health Organisation (1990) Cancer Relief and Palliative Care. Technical Report Series 804. Geneva: World Health Organisation.

Further reading

Bircumshaw D (1993) Palliative care in the acute hospital setting. Journal of Advanced Nursing 18: 1665–1666.

Clark D (ed.) (1993) The Future for Palliative Care. Buckingham: Open University Press.

Dunlop R, Hockley J (1990) Terminal Care Support Team: The Hospital–Hospice Interface. Oxford: Oxford Medical Publications.

Ford G, Lewin I (eds) (1996) Managing Terminal Illness. London: Royal College of Physicians of London.

Lendrum S, Syme G (1992) Gift of Tears: A Practical Approach to Loss and Bereavement Counselling. Tavistock: Routledge Publications.

Levitt M (1990) Family recovery after vascular surgery. Heart and Lung Journal of Critical Care 19: 486–490.

Murray-Parkes C (1993) Bereavement: Studies of Grief in Adult Life, 2nd edn. London: Routledge Publications.

Nash A (1993) Reasons for referral to a palliative nursing team. Journal of Advanced Nursing 18: 707–713.

Report of a working party (1995) Specialist palliative care: A statement of definitions. Occasional Paper 8. London. National Council for Hospice and Specialist Palliative Care Services.

Ronayne R (1989) Uncertainty in peripheral vascular disease. Canadian Journal of Cardiovascular Nursing 1: 26–30.

Saunders C (1990) (ed.) Hospice and Palliative Care: An Interdisciplinary Approach. London: Edward Arnold.

Seers K, Friedli K (1996) The patients' experiences of their chronic non-malignant pain. Journal of Advanced Nursing 24: 1160–1168.

Index